EMERGENCY NEURORADIOLOGY

T. SCARABINO · U. SALVOLINI · J.R. JINKINS

(Editors)

EMERGENCY NEURORADIOLOGY

With 294 Figures in 793 Parts and 10 Tables

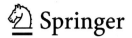 Springer

EDITORS

Tommaso Scarabino

Department of Neuroradiology, Scientific Institute "Casa Sollievo della Sofferenza", San Giovanni Rotondo (FG), ITALY
Department of Radiology, ASL BA/1, Hospital of Andria (BA), ITALY

Ugo Salvolini

Neuroradiology and Department of Radiology, University of Ancona, ITALY

J. Randy Jinkins

Department of Radiology, Downstate Medical Center, State University of New York, Brooklyn, NY, USA

This edition of **Emergency Neuroradiology** by **Scarabino – Salvolini – Jinkins** is published
by arrangement with Casa Editrice Idelson-Gnocchi srl, Naples, Italy

ISBN-10 3-540-29626-3 Springer Berlin Heidelberg New York
ISBN-13 978-3-540-29626-3 Springer Berlin Heidelberg New York

Library of Congress Control Number: 2005934099

Springer is a part of Springer Science+Business Media
http://www.springeronline.com

© Springer Berlin Heidelberg 2006

Printed in Germany

Editor: Dr. Ute Heilmann
Desk Editor: Meike Stoeck
Production Editor: Joachim W. Schmidt
Cover Design: eStudio Calamar, Spain

Typesetting: FotoSatz Pfeifer GmbH, 82166 Gräfelfing, Germany
Printed on acid-free paper – 24/3151 – 5 4 3 2 1 0

CONTRIBUTORS

R. Agati, M. Armillotta, S. Balzano, A. Bertolino, M.G. Bonetti, M. Cammisa, A. Carella, A. Carriero, A. Casillo, M. Caulo, A. Ceddia, G. Cerone, S. Cirillo, P. Ciritella, C. Colosimo, V. D'Angelo, P. D'Aprile, R. De Amicis, G.M. Di Lella, F. Florio, A. Fresina, M. Gallucci, T. Garribba, S. Ghirlanda, G.M. Giannatempo, M. Impagliatelli, A. Lorusso, S. Lorusso, P. Maggi, A. Maggialetti, N. Maggialetti, M. Maiorano, M. Mariano, C. Masciocchi, F. Menichelli, M. Nardella, F. Nemore, M. Pacilli, T. Parracino, U. Pasquini, L. Pazienza, C. Piana, F. Perfetto, S. Perugini, G. Polonara, T. Popolizio, M. Rollo, B. Rossi, R. Rossi, M. Schiavariello, C. Settecasi, A. Simeone, L. Simonetti, A. Splendiani, A. Stranieri, V. Strizzi, A. Tarantino, T. Tartaglione, G. Valle, N. Zamponi, N. Zarrelli

FOREWORD

Encouraged by the success of the Italian editions, the Authors have decided to publish an English version taking into account the latest technical and methodological advances and the consequent new acquisitions in clinical practice. The contribution of Professor R. Jinkins has been essential to carry out both these tasks.

The resulting work is an up-to-date technical tool that preserves its original aim of contributing to the training of those radiologists who work in emergency departments.

We hope that this revised and extended English version will have the same success as the previous Italian editions, thereby confirming the validity of our initiative.

The work of all the friends and colleagues who have contributed to the making of this book is gratefully acknowledged.

Tommaso Scarabino
Ugo Salvolini

CONTENTS

I

CEREBROVASCULAR EMERGENCIES

1.1

CLINICAL AND DIAGNOSTIC SUMMARY

T. Scarabino, G.M. Giannatempo, A. Maggialetti

Stroke, a clinical diagnosis of acute, sudden-onset neurological deficit, is one of the main causes of death and permanent disability in the industrialized world. Pathologically the process may be an ischaemic or a haemorrhagic event, or both. About 85% of cerebrovascular accidents result from ischaemia, predominantly secondary to carotid thromboembolism.

The stroke patient may clinically present with typical symptoms of focal neurological deficit, a combination of deficit with coma, a meningeal irritation syndrome in the form of headache, vomiting and neck stiffness, or less frequently with the gradual appearance of an extrapyramidal or pseudo-bulbar syndrome often associated with progressive mental deterioration.

The clinical picture in stroke patients can be classified according to how long the neurological deficit lasts, or alternatively whether or not the deficit is permanent. Four different such clinical categories can be distinguished. The *transient ischaemic attack* (TIA) is represented by a sudden, focal non-convulsive onset of a neurological deficit that usually subsides in a few minutes and always resolves within 24 hours; the *reversible ischaemic neurological deficit* (RIND) lasts at most for a period of 48 hours followed by a return to complete normality within 3 weeks; *progressive ictus* is a tem-

porally worsening clinical condition during the first 24 to 48 hours following acute onset associated with persistent functional deficit; *complete ictus* is a clinically stable condition, with the deficit being present from the outset, though some improvement may be observed in the long term.

NEURORADIOLOGICAL PROTOCOL

The role of the neuroradiologist in stroke cases is to provide the clinician with the maximum morphological and functional information concerning the condition of the cerebral parenchyma as is possible, as well as the condition of the intra- and extracranial brachiocephalic blood vessels. One should particularly assess whether or not there is a direct causal relationship between the craniocervical vascular pattern and the stroke, whether the lesion is ischaemic or haemorrhagic, if there are signs of other vasculopathic changes, and if the aetiologic factors responsible for the stroke are intra- or extracranial.

The recent development of specific fibrinolytic treatments that can potentially reverse ischaemic injury in the early stages has changed the role of imaging in this area (5). It is no longer sufficient to simply distinguish ischaemic alteration from primary haemorrhage. It is now necessary to identify cerebral ischaemia within the first few hours when treatment can be most effective. It is also important to quickly distinguish normal cerebral tissue from that which is "at risk", and that parenchyma which is irreversibly damaged. Thus, the medical imaging investigation is now a fundamental part of planning effective emergency treatment potentially capable of preventing irreversible cerebral damage and long-term patient disability. The neuroradiologist must therefore find the optimal means of supplying the required information through both invasive and non-invasive investigative methods.

Angiography has to date been the most commonly used of the available tools to analyse the brachiocephalic vascular system directly. Less invasive methods include computed tomography (CT), ultrasound and magnetic resonance imaging (MRI), both conventional (basic morphological imaging and angiography) and functional (spectroscopy, diffusion and perfusion). Single photon emission computed tomography (SPECT) and positron emission tomography (PET) are able to show local changes in blood flow and metabolism, respectively, both markers for cerebral damage. However, these latter methods are not commonly available, and require the injection of radioactive tracers.

In emergency situations, the cerebral investigation of choice is CT due to its non-invasiveness, the fact that it is widely available, its ease and speed of use and its relatively low cost (7). CT distinguishes between haemorrhagic and ischaemic stroke at an early stage, a factor that may be of vital importance in prognosis and treatment. If the CT is negative or incongruous in some way with the clinical picture, MRI makes possible a more detailed brain investigation to be carried out non-invasively.

HAEMORRHAGIC STROKE

CT has always been considered useful in analysing cerebral haemorrhage, whether subarachnoid or intraparenchymal in location. Intracranial haemorrhage is apparent on CT im-

mediately after the bleeding episode due to its high density relative to brain tissue. However, haemorrhage has a more complex appearance and explanation on MRI. An acute cerebral haemorrhage is primarily oxyhaemoglobin, a substance with no paramagnetic properties that behaves much like an aqueous solution, almost indistinguishable from an area of parenchymal ischaemia. In subacute haemorrhage, the parenchymal blood that was originally oxyhaemoglobin first turns into deoxyhaemoglobin, and then into intracellular and next into extracellular metahaemoglobin. These substances are paramagnetic and/or magnetically susceptible and therefore are able to influence relaxation times and change the MR signal in a somewhat predictable manner.

Recently released high field strength, high speed MR equipment and imaging sequences are particularly sensitive to magnetic susceptibility differences (e.g., echo planar imaging: EPI) has demonstrated that it is possible to clearly reveal even small areas of cerebral haemorrhage on MRI (15). Because of this ability of MRI to distinguish between non-haemorrhagic ischaemia and haematoma, MRI may replace CT at some time in the future where this is practicable. However, the fact that high field strength, high speed gradient performance MRI is presently less widely available and more costly than CT determines that CT will still be the first diagnostic imaging examination carried out in such situations for the foreseeable future. On the other hand, emergency angiography should be reserved for cases of subarachnoid haemorrhage in order to search for causative pathology of stroke (i.e., haemorrhage) such as aneurysms or vascular malformations (3).

ISCHAEMIC STROKE

CT has been shown to be unable to document the presence of non-haemorrhagic ischaemic alteration in the first few hours following the clinical onset of stroke. Over a period of hours and with proper experience, it is in practice possible to identify the subtle initial signs of ischaemic tissue damage as relatively lower attenuation brain tissue resulting from cytotoxic oedema, and major cerebral arterial hyperdensity (e.g., middle cerebral artery stem, basilar artery) due to vascular embolus/thrombosis (12, 14, 16).

Although *conventional* T2-weighted MRI (e.g., spin echo, fast spin echo) is particularly sensitive to changes in the water content of tissue and therefore to oedema, it is still frequently negative in cases of hyperacute stroke (i.e., first 1-6 hours). This is due to the fact that only 3% of the water in the cellular cytoplasm consists of free water, which is the principal type of water molecule capable of altering MRI signal intensity in instances of cytotoxic oedema.

MR *diffusion* weighted imaging (DWI), however, can visualize hyperacute cerebral ischaemia with some degree of certainty. Nevertheless, DWI does not indicate whether the involved tissue is irreversibly damaged or is still vital, and therefore amenable to benefiting from interventional recanalization treatment (9, 10, 11). For this purpose MR *perfusion* imaging can be used to evaluate the presence or absence of discrepancy between the diffusion and perfusion of affected tissue. If such discrepancies exist, for example in a case of a circumscribed area having abnormal diffusion but showing greater relative perfusion, then it is apparent that the "shadow" tissue area or ischaemic penumbra may benefit from recanalization; conversely, where there is no such ischaemic penumbra, it is unlikely that fibrinolytic therapy will be successful (2, 4). MR *spectroscopy* may provide yet further information on the viable status of ischaemic brain tissue, even if at the present time this is limited to some extent by the long examination times involved (13).

In a similar manner to what has been shown with functional MRI, recent studies have shown that it may also be possible to obtain functional data with CT (8). Therefore, it may be that emerging technologies will have an impact on the diagnosis and treatment of patients with cerebral stroke.

In order to identify suitable candidates for thrombolytic therapy, it is necessary to know clearly whether there has actually been a vascular occlusion. If this is indeed the case, an MR (or CT) angiographic study acquired during the acute clinical stage is imperative (1). With MR *angiography* it is possible to evaluate the arterial anatomy of the major vessels at the base of the brain. Good anatomical imaging shows either the normal vessels composing the circle of Willis, or their absence in the ischaemic cerebral area. This may at times be the key to the diagnosis of major vascular occlusion, in which case it is useful to extend the MR angiographic examination to the vessels in the neck and even the aortic arch, the latter requiring intravascular gadolinium injection and timed imaging of the aortic arch and cervical region. These techniques can also be useful as a treatment-monitoring tool, serially imaging the vascular stenoses and occlusions non-invasively in patients on specific therapy. However, there are some limitations associated with the MR angiographic technique, such as less temporal and spatial resolution as compared to digital angiography. It is partly for this reason that conventional invasive angiography remains the investigative method of choice when the imaging diagnosis of vasculitis, vascular dissection or embolism is in doubt, and also for purposes of unequivocal vascular examination in suspected cases of cerebral cortical venous and cranial venous sinus thrombosis (3, 6).

Some authors have advocated the use of CT angiography, in part because of its ability to show associated dystrophic atherosclerotic calcification of arterial walls in addition to the vascular luminal characteristics. However, the need to introduce contrast media as a part of the CT angiographic technique, involving in most cases high dosages of 100 to 200 cc, is a relative contraindication in cases of suspected ischaemia with blood-brain barrier disruption. In such cases the possible further adverse effects of extravasated contrast material upon the underlying cerebral parenchyma must be considered, as the tissue is already ischaemically injured. For this reason MR angiography is preferred because of the small quantities of intravascular gadolinium contrast agent required and the essentially harmless nature of the paramagnetic contrast medium used. MR angiography has the additional advantage of showing not so much the flow itself, but instead the "cast" of the arterial lumen, with the imaging findings being very similar to those of digital angiography.

CONCLUSIONS

In conclusion, the neuroradiologist today has many means available to him for the investigation of the lesions associated with clinical stroke and their underlying pathophysiology. Ideally, all of the neuroradiological investigations outlined in this discussion should be carried out in within the first few hours of onset of the stroke. In such cases the imaging protocol must include: 1) a CT examination and, when possible, 2) a basic MRI to confirm the clinical diagnosis and to exclude other acute onset non-ischaemic pathological process potentially responsible for the neurological deficit; 3) MR diffusion weighted imaging to evaluate the extent of the ischaemic injury; 4) MR perfusion imaging to show the extent of the remaining vital tissue; and 5) MR angiography to establish the presence or absence of a vascular luminal defect with certainty so that fibrinolytic therapy can be initiated when appropriate. In this way it is possible within 45-60 minutes to have a morphological and pathophysiological assessment of the ischaemic injury, an assessment that may also be useful for prognostic purposes.

However, for this to be possible, much depends on environmental factors such as equipment availability, compliance with the constraining time elements requiring that the patient be ready for imaging analysis within a very few minutes or hours after the onset of the stroke syndrome, adequate patient cooperation and specific physician skills, competence and experience. In any case, an accurately performed and interpreted CT examination is required, and in the case of a negative CT, a baseline MR examination and MR angiogram.

REFERENCES

1. Atlas SW: MR angiography in neurologic disease. Radiology 193:1-16, 1994.
2. Barber PA, Darby DG, Desmond PM et al: Prediction of stroke outcome with echoplanar perfusion and diffusion weighted MRI. Neurology 51:418-426, 1998.
3. Brant-Zawadzki M, Gould R: Digital subtraction cerebral angiography. AJR 140:347-353, 1983.
4. De Boer JA, Folkers PJM: MR perfusion and diffusion imaging in ischaemic brain disease. Medica Mundi 41:20, 1997.
5. Hacke W, Kaste M, Fieschi C et al: Intravenous thrombolysis with recombinant tissue plasminogen activator for acute hemisferic stroke. The European Cooperative Acute Stroke Study (ECASS). JAMA 274:1017-1025, 1995.
6. Hankey GJ, Warlow CP, Molyneux AJ: Complications of cerebral angiography for patients with mild carotid territory ischaemia being considered for carotid endarterectomy. J Neurol Neurosurg Psychiatry 53:542-548, 1990.
7. John C, Elsner E, Muller A et al: Computed tomographic diagnosis of acute cerebral ischemia. Radiologe 37(11): 853-858, 1997.
8. Koening M, Klotz E, Luka B et al: Perfusion CT of the brain: diagnostic approach for early detection of ischemic stroke. Radiology 209(1):85-93, 1998.
9. Li TQ, Chen ZG, Hindmarsh T: Diffusion-weighted MR imaging of acute cerebral ischemia. Acta Radiologica 39:460-473, 1998.
10. Lovblad KO, Laubach HJ, Baird AE et al: Clinical experience with diffusion-weighted MR in patients with acute stroke. AJNR 19:1061-1066, 1998.
11. Lutsep HL, Albers GW, DeCrespigny A et al: Clinical utility of diffusion-weighted magnetic resonance imaging in the assessment of ischemic stroke. Ann Neurol 41:574-580, 1997.
12. Marks MP, Homgren EB, Fox A et al: Evaluation of early computed tomography findings in acute ischemic stroke 30(2):389-392, 1999.
13. Mattews VP, Barker PB, Blackband SJ et al: Cerebral metabolites in patients with acute and subacute strokes: a serial MR and proton MR spectroscopy study. AJR 165:633-638, 1995.
14. Pressman BD, Tourse EJ, Thompson JR et al: An early CT sign of ischemic infarction: increased density in a cerebral artery. AJR 149:583-586, 1987.
15. Schellinger PD, Jansen O, Frebach JB et al: A standardized MRI stroke protocol: comparison with CT in hyperacute intracerebral hemorrhage. Stroke 30(4):765-768, 1999.
16. Von Kummer R, Allen KL, Holle R et al: Acute stroke: usefulness of early CT findings before thrombolytic therapy. Radiology 205:327-333, 1997.

1.2

CT IN ISCHAEMIA

T. Scarabino, N. Zarrelli, M.G. Bonetti, F. Florio, N. Maggialetti,
A. Lorusso, A. Maggialetti, A. Carriero

INTRODUCTION

Cerebral ischaemia is the pathological condition that affects the cerebral parenchyma when blood flow drops to levels that are insufficient to permit normal function, metabolism and structural integrity. The ischaemic state can be incomplete or complete, according to whether blood supply is insufficient or totally interrupted, respectively; and whether the problem is global or regional, depending on the parenchymal territory involved. By far the most frequent cause of cerebral ischaemia is arteriosclerosis of the arteries that supply blood to the brain, when an embolus or a thrombus occludes such a vessel. Other causes include emboligenic cardiopathies, sudden global drops in cerebral perfusion pressure, non-atheromatous arteritis (e.g., inflammatory, traumatic causes, etc.), haematological disorders such as polyglobulia or drepanocytosis and oestroprogestinic treatment. At the current time, CT represents the most suitable method for diagnosic imaging of cerebral ischaemic conditions, especially in cases of a complete neurological injury/deficit. It is, however, less suitable for diagnosing transient ischaemic attacks (TIA) and reversible ischaemic neurological deficits (RIND), which are temporary and subside rapidly, and in which case it is more important to assess the status of the larger intra- and extracranial vessels (for which purpose echo-Doppler and MR angiography investigations may be more appropriate).

SEMEIOTICS

The resulting CT picture obtained depends on a number of factors including the type, completeness and location of the vascular occlusion, the time required for the ischaemic process to become established and the presence or absence of anastomotic pathways. Unlike complete neurological deficits, in transitory forms of ischaemia a negative CT can be expected, and in only 14% of all cases does the site detected coincide with that region suggested by the patient's syndrome. In certain cases, however, it can reveal signs linked to the underlying vasculopathy such as the dilation, tortuosity and parietal calcification of vessel walls in the vessels comprising the circle of Willis. Although somewhat rare, in certain cases, TIA's can be accompanied by vascular malformation, a small haematoma or a neoplastic process. On the other hand, infarctions can be completely asymptomatic, especially when small and when located in mute parenchymal areas. The importance of an ischaemic lesion, as diagnosed by CT, in causing neurological signs and symptoms depends on both its age and site and can therefore only be held responsible for symptoms in progress that are in keeping; if this is not the case it must merely be considered as an incidental finding, expression of the same stroke-causing cerebrovascular pathology (18). Regardless of clinical criteria, there are a number of semeiotic CT findings to be considered in order to identify the nature of a given ischaemic lesion, namely: 1) site and morphology, 2) evolution of lesion density, 3) presence of mass effect, and, 4) enhancement following endovascular injection of contrast agents (i.e., pattern of contrast enhancement, CE) (Fig. 1.1).

Site and morphology

The site of the lesion has considerable importance in diagnosis as it reflects a vascular blood supply territory (Fig. 1.2). One or more large arterial vessel territories can be partially or totally affected (depending in part on the efficiency of any collateral circulation present) (Figs. 1.3, 1.4, 1.5, 1.6, 1.7); alternatively a reduction of cardiac output can affect the border zones between the various vascular territories or between the deep and superficial districts of the same territory (the so-called "watershed" areas), or the end point of a vascular territory (the so-called "last mea-

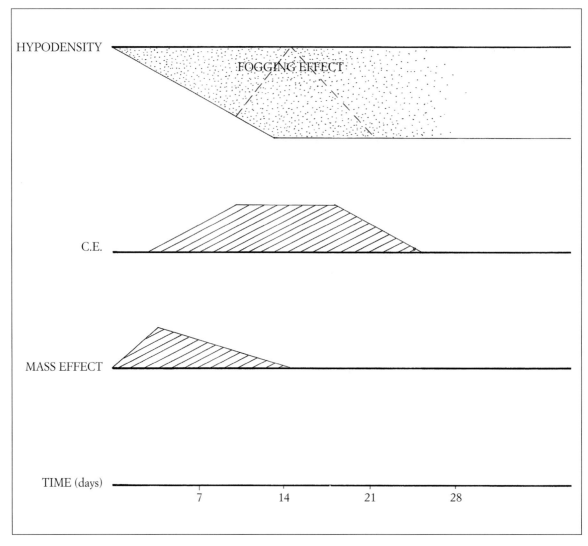

Fig. 1.1 - Evolution over time of certain aspects of CT semeiotics: density, CE and mass effect of the ischaemic lesion.

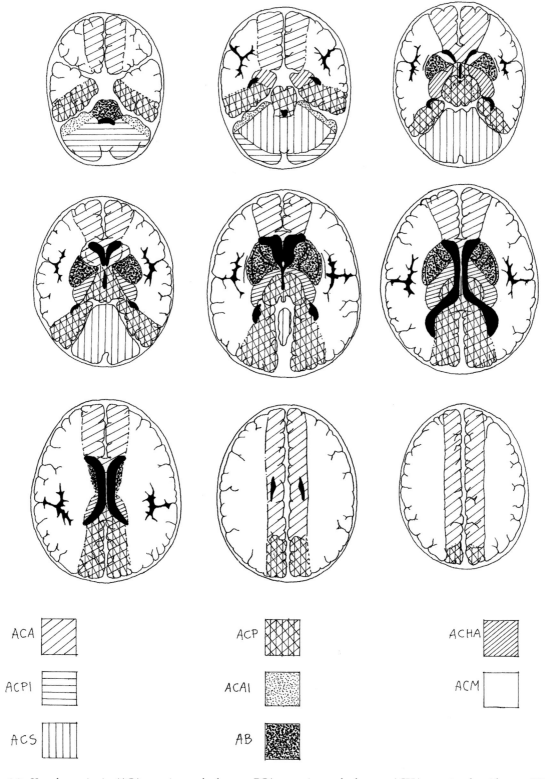

Fig. 1.2 - Vascular territories (ACA: anterior cerebral artery; PCA: posterior cerebral artery; ACHA: anterior choroid artery; PICA: posterior inferior cerebellar artery; AICA: anterior inferior cerebellar artery; MCA: middle cerebral artery; SCA: superior cerebellar artery; BA: basilar artery).

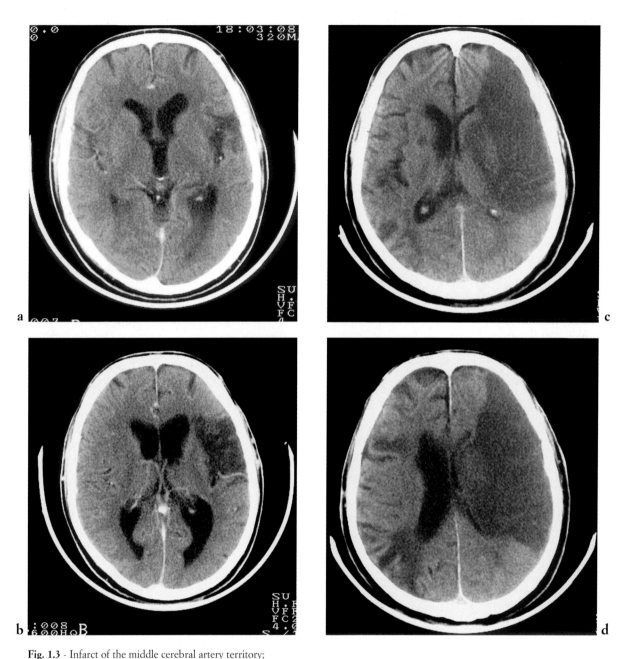

Fig. 1.3 - Infarct of the middle cerebral artery territory;
a-b) partial infarct with involvement of the superficial left district only;
c-d) complete infarct on the left with mass effect on the adjacent lateral ventricle, which appears compressed; on the right, other smaller ischaemic hypodensities can be seen.

dows"). Typical watershed infarcts are situated at the frontal-parietal border (between the anterior cerebral artery territory and that of the middle cerebral artery), at the gyrus angularis (between the territories of the anterior, middle and posterior cerebral arteries), between the putamen and the insula (on the border of the deep and super-ficial branches of the middle cerebral artery) (Fig. 1.8). "Last meadow" infarcts affect Heubner's artery (Fig. 1.9), lenticulostriate arteries or perforating arteries (31).

The most frequently affected vascular territory is that of the middle cerebral artery, followed by that of the posterior cerebral artery, the

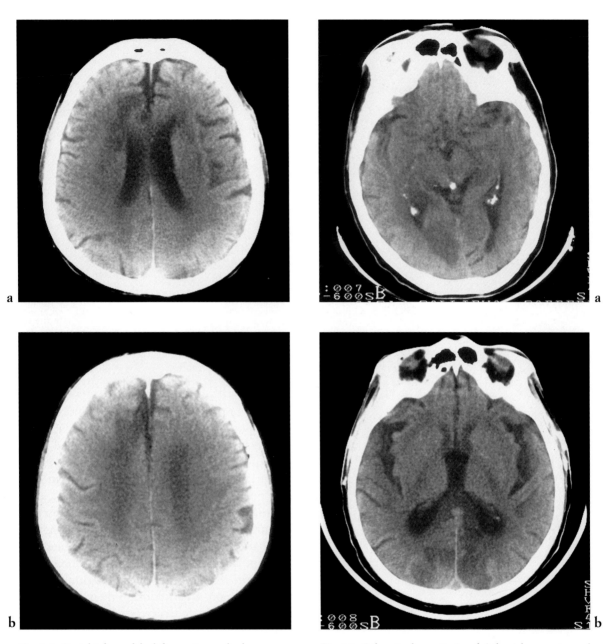

Fig. 1.4 - Partial infarct of the left anterior cerebral artery territory.

Fig. 1.5 - Infarct in the territories of **a**) the right posterior and **b**) bilateral cerebral arteries.

anterior cerebral artery and the basilar artery (Fig. 1.10). Infarcts less commonly occur in certain territories such as the brainstem (Fig. 1.11) and the thalamus (Fig. 1.12). It is also possible to observe pathologically multiple small infarcts (0.5 - 1 cm), which are somewhat problematic to detect on imaging studies, especially when situated in the posterior fossa (due to the bony arte-

facts at the base of the skull) (Fig. 1.11). As mentioned previously, the morphology of the ischaemic area is also important. The occlusion of the internal carotid artery produces an infarct throughout the ipsilateral hemisphere (Fig. 1.7) and may or may not spare the thalamus. These larger lesions may demonstrate severe mass effect and the prognosis in such cases can in

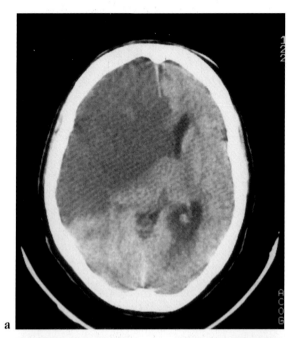

a

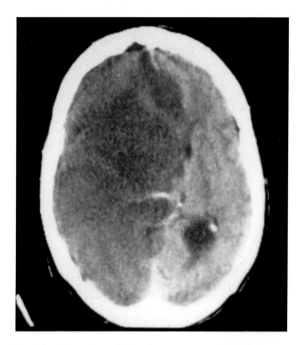

Fig. 1.7 - Vast infarct of the right anterior, middle and posterior cerebral artery territories.

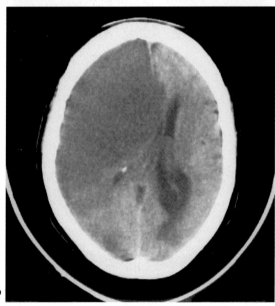

b

Fig. 1.6 - Infarct of the right anterior and middle cerebral artery territory, with clear mass effect on the shifted midline structures contralaterally.

part be dependent upon the presence of collaterals of the circle of Willis and leptomeninges.

Infarcts affecting the branches of the middle cerebral artery are wedge-shaped, with their base at the convexity and tip at the 3rd ventricle, whereas a curved trapezoid shape is typical of a distal occlusion at the beginning of the lenticu-

lostriate branches (Fig. 1.3 c-d). The occlusion of the posterior cerebral artery, which appears as a rectangular shape, affects the medial territory of the lateral ventricle junction and therefore the occipital, temporal posteromedial and posteroparietal areas and, in some cases, the thalamus (Fig. 1.5). Infarcts of the anterior cerebral artery affect the frontal parasagittal and parietal areas (Fig. 1.4); they are triangular in shape at the base of the frontal lobe but linear in the remainder of the parasagittal frontoparietal region. In addition to their site, watershed infarcts are characterized by their shape and usually have a linear appearance.

Despite the fact that they affect both white and grey matter, ischaemic alterations are more clearly visible in the former with axial CT sections. If they are of medium dimensions, they appear irregular, round or elliptical rather than triangular. Those lesions that affect the central grey matter nuclei tend to reflect the shape of these structures; those of the grey matter cortex are somewhat triangular with their base at the convexity if only one branch is occluded, and trapezoid-shaped when more than one branch is occluded.

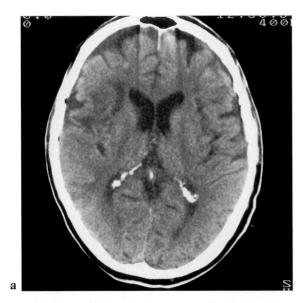

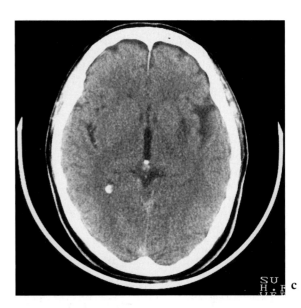

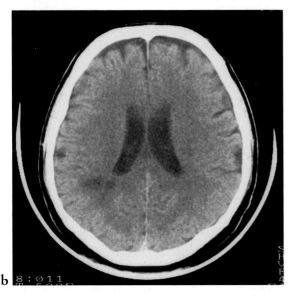

Fig. 1.8 - "Watershed" infarcts.
a) between the right anterior and middle cerebral artery territories;
b) between the right middle and posterior cerebral artery territories;
c) between the left deep and superficial middle cerebral artery territories.

Evolution with time

Four distinct temporal phases can be identified, including: 1) hyperacute, 2) acute, 3) subacute, and 4) chronic (3, 8, 10, 15, 17, 27). The hyperacute phase occurs within 6 hours from onset. From a neuropathological point of view, the main alteration is best described as cytotoxic oedema represented by the shift of water in neurons. Because this is a relatively modest change, the CT in this stage is usually negative. In this phase, the clinical and CT findings may not agree. In this early stage, despite the fact that the patient may present with complete hemiplegia and unconsciousness, the CT scan often remains normal (Fig. 1.13a). However, with the passage of time, the CT becomes positive.

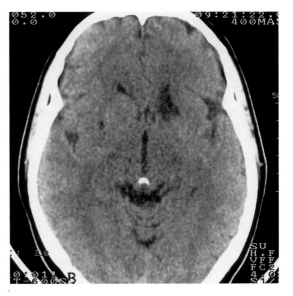

Fig. 1.9 - Ischaemic lesion at the head of the left caudate nucleus; there is also a lacunar infarct of the contralateral external capsule.

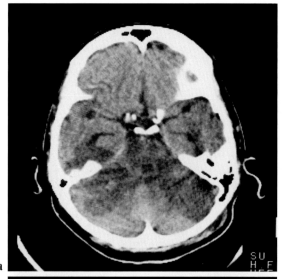

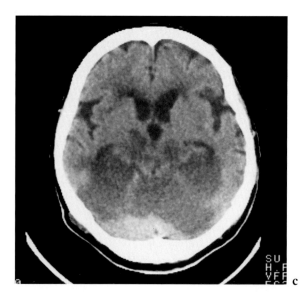

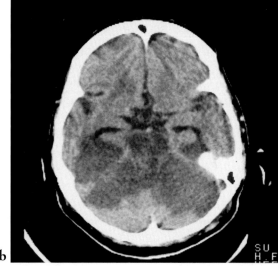

Fig. 1.10 - Infarct in the vertebrobasilar territory.
Large, non-homogeneous hypodense area involving the brainstem, the anterior and external faces of the brain hemispheres as well as the medial and posterior faces of the temporal lobes. The hyperdensity is associated as with thrombosis of the basilar stem (**b**) and the ectasia of the supratentorial ventricles (**c**).

Obviously, the clinical deficit caused by the ischaemia takes place before oedema is apparent on CT. However, negative CT scans acquired in the early stages of ischaemia are valuable in ruling out other types of pathology, and especially associated abnormalities including haemorrhage. It is therefore essential that when clinical suspicion points to hyperacute acute' ischaemia and the initial CT is negative, a subsequent scan should be performed during the upcoming hours to evaluate for evolution of the abnormality (5). On occasion, a CT scan obtained in the hyperacute phase can give direct signs (e.g., vessel hyperdensity, subtle parenchymal hypodensity) or indirect signals (e.g., sulcal effacement, gyral swelling, ventricular compression, fading of the white matter/grey matter interface) of hyperacute ischaemia. Such findings have a negative prognostic value and are directly associated with the degree of neurological disability (23). Vessel hyperdensity in major cerebral arteries or one of their branches (the middle cerebral artery is the most commonly affected) can be observed within the first minutes following the onset of neurological signs and symptoms and takes place before the appearance of CT findings of the parenchymal infarct in the corresponding territory (Fig. 1.14). This increase in intravascular density, which is visible on CT without the use of contrast agents, appears to be caused by the formation of an endoluminal clot, either by arterial thrombosis or embolism (19, 30). For this reason, when clinical signs point to cerebral infarction, a CT scan through the cerebral arteries traversing the basal subarachnoid cisterns must be performed immediately (14), acquired with multiple thin slices (e.g., 1.5 - 4 mm). In 40-60% of cases, selective angiography reveals a thromboembolic occlusion, a finding that disappears subsequently as the endoluminal clot lyses (2). Subtle pa-

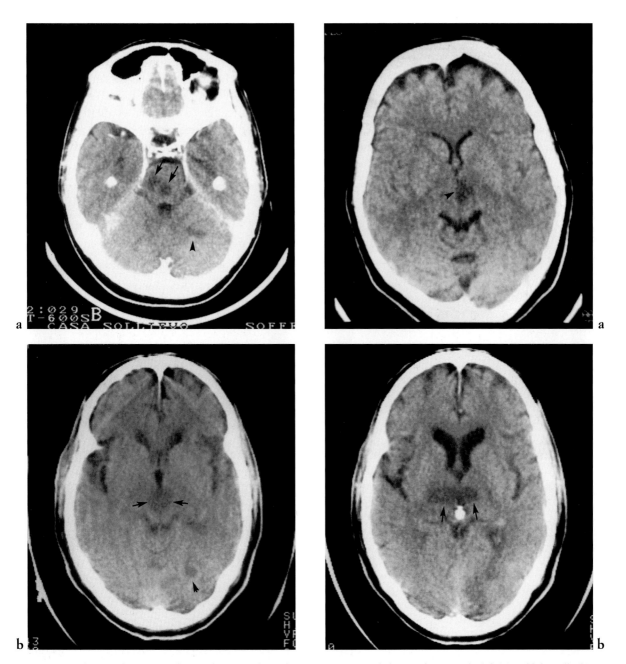

Fig. 1.11 - Infarcts in the posterior fossa and in particular in the pons (**a**), midbrain (**b**) and left cerebral hemisphere (**a-b**).

Fig. 1.12 - Thalamic infarcts: on the left (**a**) and bilaterally (**b**).

renchymal hypodensities can sometimes be observed in these early stages, as even the slightest increase in water content alters the CT attenuation coefficients, and therefore the relative tissue contrast (in particular, a 1% increase in brain water content yields an attenuation of 2.5 Hounsfield units).

– The acute phase of ischaemia occurs within the first 24 hours of the event, but typically begins within 6 hours after the stroke onset. From a neuropathological point of view, vasogenic oedema is present as supported by the filling of the extracellular spaces of the brain due to a blood-brain barrier breakdown. Because of such tissue alterations, the ischaemic area appears on CT as a poorly marginated, hypodense lesion. Retrospective analyses of CT investigations have shown that the involvement of more than 50% of the middle cerebral artery territory is associated to an 85% mortality rate (28). Moreover, data provided by the European Co-operative for Acute Stroke Study shows that the response to thrombolytic treatment can vary greatly depending in part upon the volume of the ischaemic oedematous area as shown on the initial CT (9). In fact, it has been observed that rt-PA (recombinant tissue plasminogen activator) treatment increases the risk of death in cases where the hypodense area(s) exceed 1/3 of the perfused territory of the occluded artery. In su-

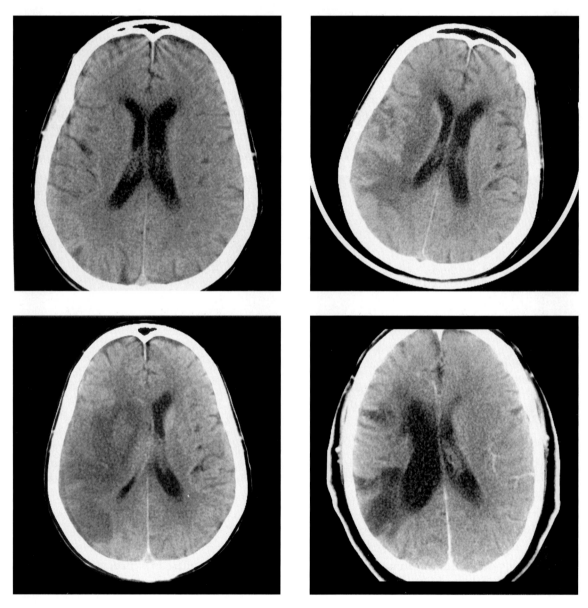

Fig. 1.13 - Typical evolution of an infarct in the right middle cerebral artery territory.
a) acute phase
b) early subacute phase (2 days from clinical onset)
c) late subacute phase (2 weeks later)
d) chronic phase (1 year later).

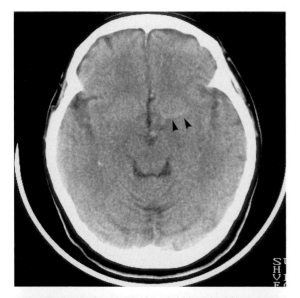

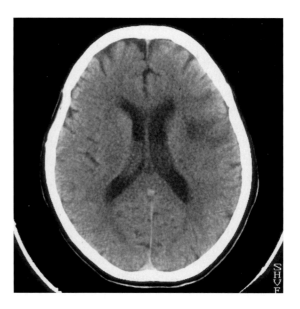

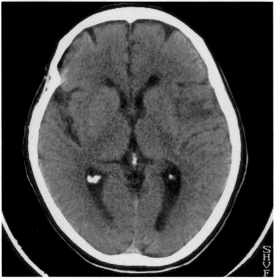

Fig. 1.14 - **a)** Thrombosis of the left middle cerebral artery (arrow head). **b-c)** CT check shortly after onset: ischaemic lesion in the corresponding vascular territory.

ch cases, therefore, patients do not benefit from fibrinolytic treatment because they are more susceptible to brain haemorrhages if such treatment is undertaken, as opposed to if they are treated conservatively.

– The subacute phase of ischaemia commences 24 hours after the event and continues until six weeks from the onset. From a neuropathological point of view, beginning in the start of the second week there is an increase in the vasogenic oedema as shown in CT by an area with increasingly low attenuation coefficients, better defined margins and mass effect (internal cerebral herniations are possible, especially in cases of massive ischaemia) (Fig. 1.13b); the ischaemic area appears most clearly two to three days after clinical onset of stroke. From the second week after the event, the oedema and mass effect gradually subside and the area of hypodensity becomes less clear (Fig. 1.13c); in some cases it disappears altogether and the ischaemic area becomes difficult or impossible to distinguish from the normal brain surrounding it. This is the so-called "fogging effect", which is supported neuropathologically by an increase in cellularity due to the invasion of microphages and the proliferation of capillaries (i.e., neoangiogenesis) (24). In massive infarctions, this process is usually partial and particularly affects the grey matter of the cortical mantle, where the cellular reaction is more marked than in the white matter. This must therefore be taken into account when evaluating the dimensions of an infarction, as scans performed one to two weeks after the stroke could result in the underestimation of its size or even failure of recognition. In this phase, CT can provide important information in terms of prognosis, such as when intraparenchymal haemorrhage (i.e., haematoma or haemorrhagic infarction) and extraparenchymal bleeding (i.e., intraventricular or subarachnoid) accompany the otherwise bland infarct. A recent study on this matter conducted by the Multicenter Acute Stroke Trial (Italy) demonstrated that in this phase, haemorrhagic transformation is frequent, and that patients who develop intraparenchymal haemorrhage, extraparenchymal bleeding or even continued cerebral oedema have an unfavourable outcome (83%, 100% and 80%, respectively) (16).

The onset of the chronic stage of ischaemia coincides with the start of the sixth week from the onset of the clinical stroke and is characterized by repair processes. Parenchymal hypodensity with well-defined margins appears with attenuation values in the CSF range (Fig. 1.13d). In the larger ischaemic foci, the necrotic areas evolve towards porencephalic cavitation with CSF density on CT. This is accompanied by the dilation of the ipsilateral ventricle and adjacent subarachnoid cisterns and, in some cases, by an ipsilateral displacement of midline structures. However, it is also possible that complete recovery takes place.

Mass effect

During the initial phases of ischaemic infarction, oedema and mass effect affect both the white and the grey matter; these alterations are present in the ischaemic area alone (Figs. 1.3 c-d, 1.6, 1.7) and they never persist beyond the third week after the event (Fig. 1.13c). Prolonged presence after week three suggests a different type of pathology such as neoplasia; in such cases an angiographic evaluation is required to distinguish between different pathological types unless prior CT scans showed haemorrhage (in fact, some neoplasms do hemorrhage, so that further caution must be exercised in such instances). If haemorrhage is present, the combination of the volume of the haemorrhage with the volume of the ischaemia may produce sufficient mass effect to worsen the prognosis. For example, in the case of large cerebellar infarctions, com-

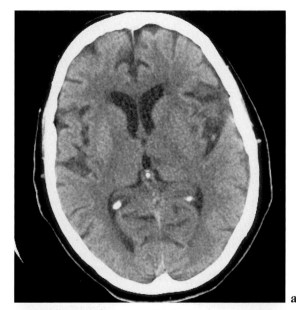

a

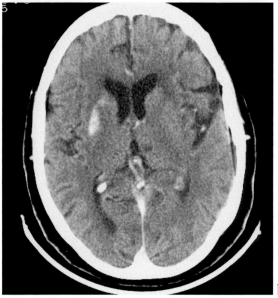

b

Fig. 1.15 - Ischaemic lesion of the lenticular nucleus (15 days from clinical onset) with nodular and homogeneous CE.
a) direct examination: small hypodense lacunar area in left thalamic location;
b) examination after contrast medium administration: marked CE in the right putamen.

pression of the lower brainstem may occur, resulting in occlusion of the fourth ventricle outlets and consequent acute triventricular hydrocephalus; in this case, suboccipital surgical decompression can be a "lifesaving" procedure (Fig. 1.10).

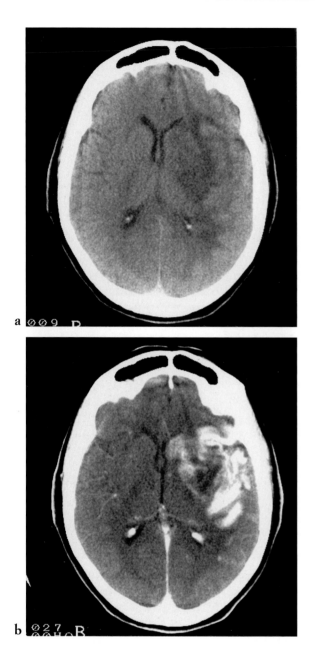

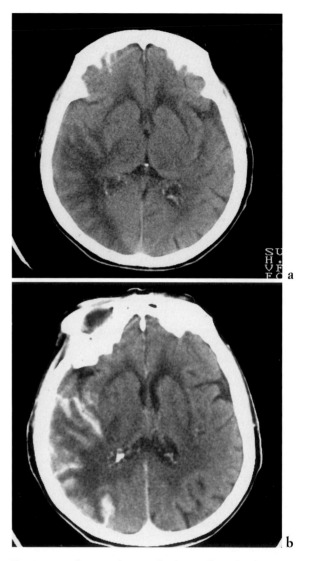

Fig. 1.17 - Right parietal-occipital infarct with gyral enhancement: **a**) direct examination; **b**) examination after contrast medium administration.

Fig. 1.16 - Widespread infarct lesion in the left middle cerebral artery territory, with non-homogeneous CE: **a**) direct examination; **b**) examination after contrast medium administration.

Contrast enhancement (CE)

Enhancement on CT following the intravenous injection of contrast agents may vary during the different stages of ischaemia. There are three types of enhancement: intravascular, meningeal and intraparenchymal. Intravascular enhancement is the first to occur, due in part to the re-duction in flow caused by stenosis or frank occlusion of the visualized vessel, an effect that is worsened by the cytotoxic oedema. Abnormal vascular enhancement can in fact be documented within two hours of the onset of signs and symptoms. This type of enhancement is present mainly in a superficial cortical location, whereas it is poorly visualized in the deep grey matter and white matter. Intravascular enhancement provides valuable information on prognosis, as it is inversely proportional to the clinical seriousness of the lesion. In the cases of both total occlusion (with retrograde collateral flow) and partial oc-

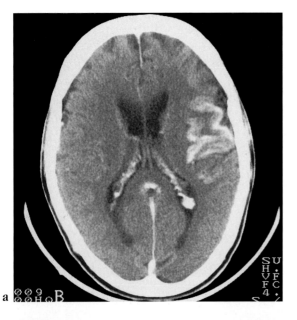

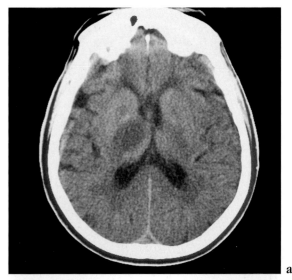

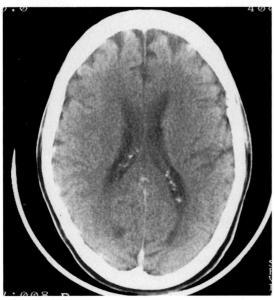

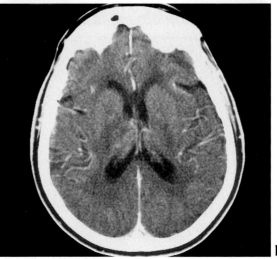

Fig. 1.19 - Ischaemic lesion of the right capsulothalamic area on direct examination (**a**); lesion visibility is reduced after contrast medium administration (**b**).

Fig. 1.18 - Fogging effect of an ischaemic lesion in the left frontal region (12 days from clinical onset); **a**) the direct examination is negative; **b**) CE of the lesion.

clusion (with direct antegrade flow), the area of the enhancing vessel's watershed is perfused, and therefore there is a possibility of recovery. Due to meningeal inflammation accompanying pial congestion, abnormal leptomeningeal enhancement is somewhat delayed when there is simultaneous parenchymal hypodensity on CT.

Both abnormal intravascular and meningeal enhancement are more clearly observed on enhanced MRI scans, having greater contrast resolution as compared to CT. Moreover, the relative degree of enhancement using paramagnetic contrast media with MRI is more conspicuous than that observed using a water-soluble iodine contrast agent with CT.

Parenchymal enhancement is usually even more delayed in appearing (in some cases, temporary hyperacute contrast enhancement may be seen on MRI). In particular, in the first 5-6 days after onset of the clinical stroke, the contrast medium does not alter or only slightly alters the attenuation values in the area of the infarction, and therefore, the presence of dense enhancement in this phase suggests an alternative pathological entity such as neoplasia. However, after the first week, some degree of parenchymal enhancement can be observed in the vast majority of cases of infarction. It is particularly evident two to three weeks after the ictus and can last up to a month or more. After this time the parenchymal enhancement gradually subsides.

Parenchymal enhancement primarily affects the grey matter of both the superficial cortical mantle and the deep basal nuclei, but the pattern of enhancement may have different appearances. For example, a nodular and homogeneous form may be seen in deep nuclei (Fig. 1.15); alternatively, a non-homogeneous pattern may be observed, especially in the white matter along the border between the superficial and deep vascular territories (Fig. 1.16); and a gyral pattern of enhancement is typical of the form encountered within the superficial cerebral cortex (Fig. 1.17). While enhancement patterns such as these are typical of cerebral infarction, they can occasionally be confused with enhancement accompanying arteriovenous malformations, cases of active meningitis, instances of recent subarachnoid haemorrhage, meningeal carcinomatosis and lymphoma.

Pathological parenchymal enhancement in the chronic phase can be attributed to the vascular proliferation of neocapillaries having abnormally permeable endothelium. This mechanism of enhancement is observed in the second and third weeks after the stroke, when this vascular proliferative process is at its most active.

In the typical case, CE is transitory and generally follows the same pattern as the fogging effect, and therefore may not be observed if only a single CT is performed, or if that study is obtained in a phase during which it is usually absent (4, 29). Scans performed at shorter time intervals will enable the visualization of CE during the evolution of the infarction as described above. This protocol of enhanced imaging can be particularly useful during the second stage, especially if the fogging effect is

present, as it tends to improve recognition of the infarction (Fig. 1.18). However, in the initial phase, the typical increase in attenuation values accompanying the administration of contrast media occurring within a hypodense ischaemic area can render it invisible (i.e., isodense enhancement as compared to the surrounding normal parenchyma); this mandates the performance of a pre-enhancement image in all cases so as not to miss the infarction altogether (Fig. 1.19). However, contrast media should only be administered in certain cases (e.g., unusual clinical presentation, atypical imaging presentation forcing a broader differential diagnosis), because the extravasation of hyperosmolar substances into the extracellular space, especially in the early stages, can hypothetically increase the cellular and vascular insult over and above that caused by the ischaemia, thereby slowing the repair processes and possibly even contributing to the final irreversible degree of injury (11). In cases where contrast agent use is mandatory upon clinical grounds, the use of a non-ionic contrast agent with less potential for harmful effects is preferable.

PARTICULAR FORMS OF INFARCTION

Lacunar infarction

Common in patients with high blood pressure, lacunar infarction usually occurs in small penetrating branches of the middle and posterior cerebral arteries, the anterior choroidal and the basilar arteries. This may be due to lipohyalinosis, fibrinoid necrosis, microatheromatous plaques or even cardiac embolism (6). These lacunar infarcts give rise to a large number of typical clinical disorders. Their recognition is proportionate to their size, and visualization largely depends upon the imaging technique used. Lacunar lesions of just a few millimetres in diameter can easily go unnoticed, whereas larger ones (from 0.5 to 1.5 cm) are more easily recognized, especially when thin imaging slices are used (Fig. 1.20).

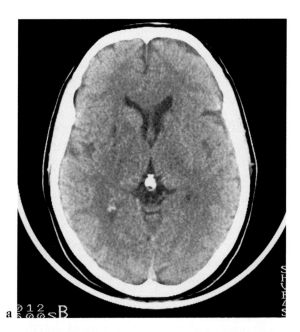

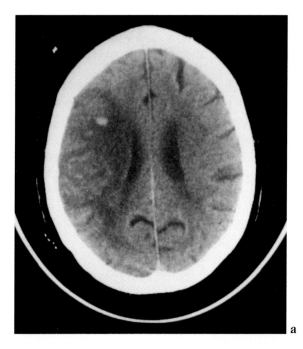

hyperdense areas in the parenchymal watershed of the involved vessel (Fig. 1.21a) (26); in certain cases, massive confluent haemorrhages can give rise to a homogeneously hyperdense lesion that can be impossible to distinguish

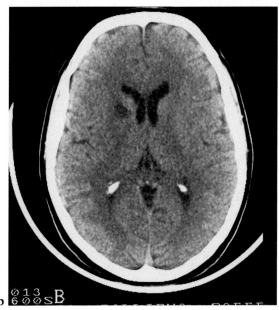

Fig. 1.20 - Multiple infarcts in the right basal ganglia region.

Haemorrhagic arterial infarcts

Ischaemic infarcts usually become haemorrhagic when blood returns to the capillary bed after a period of absence, by means of collateral circulation or due to the lysis and fragmentation of the original embolus. CT scans will usually show a mixture of hypodense and

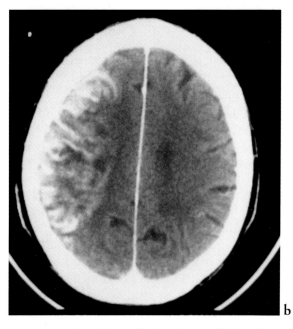

Fig. 1.21 - Infarct of the right hemisphere with hyperdense haemorrhagic component (**a**); in **b**) massive and non-homogeneous impregnation of the ischaemic-haemorrhagic region.

from a non-ischaemic haemorrhage unless its shape reflects the territorial distribution of a cerebral artery. CE can either be barely visible or massive in such cases (Fig. 1.21b).

In haemorrhage of arterial origin, the bleeding primarily takes place in the grey matter (cortical and deep grey matter) and is almost always present, on condition that the ischaemia lasted long enough to damage the capillary walls and the systemic blood pressure remained higher than 60 mm of Hg. Although in widespread infarctions the infarcted grey matter can become entirely haemorrhagic, it may only be affected peripherally.

Small, irregularly dispersed petechial haemorrhages are a very frequent microscopic finding in all infarcts; however, a diapedesis of red blood cells capable of causing a haemorrhagic infarction is observed in 20% of cases. In actual fact, it is somewhat rare to view minor haemorrhagic infarctions using CT for two reasons: 1) small petechial haemorrhages often go unnoticed due to their size, and 2) the petechial phenomenon lasts for such a short period that it can be missed unless sequential scans are performed at very short intervals.

Minor parenchymal hypodensity in the hyperacute phase, accompanied by cytotoxic oedema and detected at an early stage by CT scans, is considered a useful element for forecasting the development of a haemorrhagic infarction. This unfavourable event can be further precipitated by anticoagulation (e.g., fibrinolytic) treatment.

Venous haemorrhagic infarctions

Haemorrhagic infarctions can be caused by thromboses within the dural venous sinuses, a complication that arises in association with many pathological conditions (e.g., infections, head injuries, hypercoagulability, dehydration in newborns and infants, leukaemia) (26). The clinical presentation is often similar to that of strokes, although the picture can often be accompanied by epileptic convulsions, lethargy and signs of increased intracranial pressure (20). CT makes it possible to identify both direct and indirect signs of dural venous sinus occlusion. The former appear as small hyperdensities within the intravenous space (Fig. 1.22a). Following bolus contrast medium infusion, dural venous sinus thromboses generally appear as non-contrasted areas: the so-called

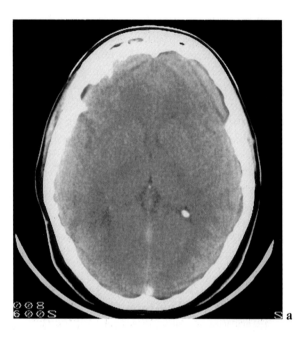

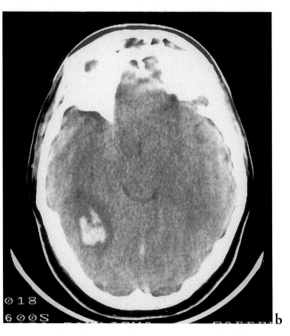

Fig. 1.22 - Hyperdensity of the upper sagittal sinus due to thrombosis (**a**) with adjacent ischaemic-haemorrhagic focus (**b**).

"empty delta sign", a finding which can be sometimes better documented by imaging with high window widths and levels. "Gyral enhancement" can also be observed, although it is uncommon (7, 20). Indirect signs, a consequence of venous obstruction, are represented by ischaemic-haemorrhagic parenchymal foci affecting the subcortical white matter (Fig. 1.22b). Venous events can sometimes be distinguished from arterial ones by the size of the haemorrhage(s) (e.g., single or multiple, unilateral or bilateral), the widespread topography that does not point to an arterial event, and by theire triangular shape with the base lying at the overlying cerebral cortex and the apex that points towards the ventricular system.

A definitive diagnosis of this condition is not always easy because bone artefacts can simulate an apparent venous filling defect at the skull base and division or duplication of the venous sinus can also result in a smaller delta sign.

DIFFERENTIAL DIAGNOSIS

Infarctions should not be confused with:

– *non-ischaemic primary haemorrhages*
Given the hyperdensity of the hemorrhagic component, this problem cannot arise during the acute and subacute phases; and a peripheral "ring enhancement" pattern following intravenous contrast administration is typical, although it is neither constant nor specific, during the subacute phase. In the late stage, a well-defined, hypodense area is observed, and therefore differentiation of a simple haemorrhage from one of ischaemic origin is only possible on the basis of whether or not the lesion conforms to a vascular territory.

– *neoplasia*
The differential diagnosis is difficult in the case of low degree, iso- or hypodense astrocytomas devoid of CE following contrast agent administration (Fig. 1.23). In such cases, it is important to determine whether or not there is a failure to respect a vascular territory, the pat-

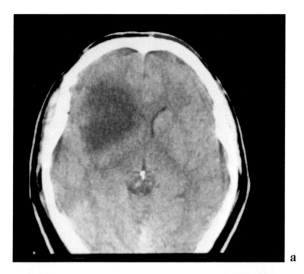

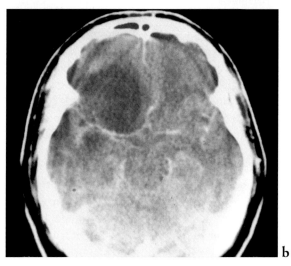

Fig. 1.23 - Low-grade astrocytoma in a right frontal position (**a**), insensitive to contrast medium (**b**).

tern of evolution over time and the clinical findings. With infarcts, the mass effect can be modest and subsides within 3 weeks; a late appearance of ipsilateral ventricular enlargement and cortical atrophic alterations can also be frequently observed in cases of ischaemia. In the case of neoplastic pathology, on the other hand, vasogenic oedema is confined to the white matter only and gradually spreads over time. Moreover, in tumours that show some degree of contrast enhancement, non-homogeneous peripheral enhancement or a "ring enhancement" can be observed, which is often not continuous but is markedly irregular. At equal lesion volumes, the neurological deficit is much less in neoplasia as compared to ischaemia.

– arteriovenous malformations

Only slightly hyperdense when imaged without contrast agents, after CE arteriovenous malformations (AVM's) show a serpentine pattern of enhancement that can spread within a vascular territory, affecting not only the superficial cortex, but also the deep grey and white matter structures. Although smaller vascular malformations do not cause visible shift of regional structures, the larger AVM's can cause a considerable degree of mass effect.

– bacterial or viral encephalitis

The encephalitides appear in the form of hypodense areas that may also be associated with mass effect; they may or may not enhance in a very irregular pattern, and they do not respect vascular territories.

– cystic formations

Leptomeningeal cysts are lesions having CSF density and are often associated with mass effect with overlying cranial deformation and thinning of the internal table of the skull. By contrast, in complete ischaemic vascular lesions, mass effect is not present, similarly to the larger porencephalic cysts or cerebral cavitations with or without communication with the ventricular system, secondary to various non-specific destructive processes as observed in the chronic stages (e.g., infectious, vascular or traumatic).

CONCLUSIONS

The ease at which machines can be accessed, the rapidity and ease of scanning (even in comatose patients), the relatively low cost, the inherent ability to frequently be able to differentiate between acute ischaemic and primary haemorrhagic events (accurately assessing their size, site, relationship to adjacent structures and presence of mass effect and haemorrhage), all contribute to making CT the imaging technique of choice in the diagnosis of stroke. Despi-

te its restrictions, CT is fundamental to following the evolution and effects of treatment in acute stroke patients.

The advent of helical CT has not brought about any significant advantages or alterations in stroke diagnosis, and the evaluation of pathological and normal cerebral structures is in fact very similar (1). However, the spiral technique is fundamental to angiographic and perfusion imaging.

Angio-CT of the basal cerebral structures enables the clinician to view the circle of Willis and therefore determine whether or not the vessel pertaining to the ischaemic cerebral area is occluded. In addition, it gives more detailed information concerning the condition of the vascular wall than is possible with MR angiography.

Perfusion CT is a rapid acquisition functional imaging technique that is capable of showing cerebral ischaemia at a very early stage (prior to the appearance of significant morphological and density variations as observed in static CT), of following sequential evolution, and above all, of providing important information concerning the best choice of treatment. In fact, by evaluating alterations in cerebral perfusion, and in particular cerebral blood flow (CBF) values, it is often possible to distinguish clearly between reversible and irreversible ischaemia areas (12, 13, 21, 25).

Thanks to this recent technological advancement, CT has become of yet greater value in stroke diagnosis than MR. However, MRI does have certain advantages, such as direct multiplanar acquisition possibilities, an absence of bone artefacts in the middle and posterior fossae, better contrast resolution and greater sensitivity in detecting abnormal variations in the water content and water diffusion characteristics during the earliest stages of ischaemia (22).

REFERENCES

1. Bahner ML, Reith W, Zuna I et al: Spiral CT vs incremental CT: is spiral CT superior in imaging of the brain ? Eur Radiol 8(3):416-420, 1998.
2. Bozzao L, Angeloni V, Bastianello S et al: Early angiographic and CT findings in patients with haemorrhagic in-

farction in the distribution of the middle cerebral artery. AJNR 2:1115-1121, 1991.

3. Bozzao L, Bastianello S, Ternullo S: Imaging anatomo-funzionale dell'ischemia encefalica. In: Pistolesi GF, Beltramello A: "L'imaging endocranico", Gnocchi Editore, Napoli, 1997:211-304.

4. Caillè JM, Guibert F, Bidabè AM et al: Enhancement of cerebral infarcts with CT. Comput Tomogr 4:73, 1980.

5. Constant P, Renou AM, Caillè JM et al: Cerebral ischemia with CT. Comput Tomogr 1:235, 1977.

6. Fisher CM: Lacunar strokes and infarcts: a review. Neurology 32:871, 1982.

7. Ford K, Sarwar M: Computed tomography of dural sinus thrombosis. AJR 2:539, 1981.

8. Gaskill-Shipley MF: Routine evaluation of acute stroke. Neuroimaging Clin N Am 9(3):411-422, 1999.

9. Hacke W, Kaste M, Fieschi C et al: Intravenous thrombolysis with recombinant tissue plasminogen activator for acute hemisferic stroke. The European Cooperative Acute Stroke Study (ECASS). JAMA 274:1017-1025, 1995.

10. John C, Elsner E, Muller A et al: Computed tomographic diagnosis of acute cerebral ischemia. Radiologe 37(11):853-858, 1997.

11. Kendall BE, Pullicini P: Intravascular contrast injection in ischaemic lesions. II. Effect on prognosis. Neuroradiology 19:241, 1980.

12. Klozt E, Konig M: Perfusion measurements of the brain: using dynamic CT for the quantitative assessment of cerebral ischemia in acute stroke. Eur J Radiol 30(3),170-184, 1999.

13. Koenig M, Klotz E, Luka B et al: Perfusion CT of the brain: diagnostic approach for early detection of ischemic stroke. Radiology 209(1):85-93, 1998.

14. Lutman M: Diagnosi precoce dell'infarto cerebrale: l'iperdensità dell'arteria cerebrale media come primo segno TC di lesione ischemica. Radiol Med 77:171-173, 1989.

15. Marks MP, Homgren EB, Fox A et al: Evaluation of early computed tomographic findings in acute ischemic stroke. Stroke 30(2):389-392, 1999.

16. Motto C, Ciccone A, Aritzu E et al: Haemorrhage after an acute ischemic stroke. MAST-I Collaborative Group. Stroke 30(4):761-764, 1999.

17. Moulin T, Tatu L, Vuillier F et al: Brain CT scan for acute cerebral infarction: early signs of ischemia. Rev Neurol 1555(9):649-655, 1999.

18. Perrone P, Landelise L, Scotti G et al: CT evaluation in patients with transient ischemic attack. Correlation between clinical and angiographic findings. Eur Neurol 18:217, 1979.

19. Pressman BD, Tourje EJ, Thompson JR: An early CT sign of ischemic infarction: increased density in a cerebral artery. AJR 149:583-586, 1987.

20. Rao KCVG, Knipp HC, Wagner EJ: Computed tomographic findings in cerebral sinus and venous thrombosis. Radiology 140:391, 1981.

21. Reichenbach JR, Rother J, Jonetz-Mentzel L et al: Acute stroke evaluated by time-to-peak mapping during initial and early follow-up perfusion CT studies. AJNR 20(10):1842-1850, 1999.

22. Schellinger PD, Jansen O, Fiebach JB et al: A standardized MRI stroke protocol: comparison with CT in hyperacute intracerebral haemorrhage. Stroke 30(4):765-768, 1999.

23. Scott JN, Buchan AM, Sevich RJ: Correlation of neurologic dysfunction with CT findings in early acute stroke. Can J Neurol Sci 26(3):182-189, 1999.

24. Skriver ED, Esbach O: Transient disappearance of cerebral infarct on CT scan, the so-called fogging effect. Neuroradiology 22:61, 1981.

25. Ueda T, Yuh WT, Taoka T: Clinical application of perfusion and diffusion MR imaging in acute ischemic stroke. J Magn Reson Imaging 10(3):305-309, 1999.

26. Vonofakos D, Artmann H: CT findings in haemorragic cerebral infarct. Comput Radiol 7:75, 1983.

27. von Kummer R, Allen KL, Holle R et al: Acute stroke: usefulness of early CT findings before thrombolytic therapy. Radiology 205:327-333, 1997.

28. von Kummer R, Meyding-Lamadè U, Forsting M et al: Sensitivity and prognostic value of early CT in occlusion of the middle cerebral artery trunk. AJN 15:9-18, 1994.

29. Wing SD, Normann D, Pollack JA et al: Contrast enhancement of cerebral infarcts in computed tomography. Radiology 121:89,1976.

30. Yock DH: CT demonstration of cerebral emboli. J Comput Assist Tomogr 5:190-196, 1981.

31. Zulck KJ, Esbach O: The interhemisferic steal syndromes. Neuroradiology 4:179-185, 1972.

1.3

CT IN INTRAPARENCHYMAL HAEMORRHAGE

N. Zarrelli, F. Perfetto, T. Parracino, T. Garribba, P. Maggi, N. Maggialetti, T. Scarabino

INTRODUCTION

The term intraparenchymal haemorrhage (IPH) refers to non-traumatic bleeding within the cerebral parenchyma. IPH accounts for 15% of all cerebrovascular disease, and statistics on this common pathological condition determine that from 10-20 new cases per annum occur for every 100,000 inhabitants in the population. This variation can be accounted for by two factors, the first being a drop in the more severe forms due to the recent progress made in treating hypertension, and the second being the improvement in diagnostic accuracy as a result of the advent of computed tomography (CT). CT now makes it possible to establish the haemorrhagic nature of certain relatively "minor" events that were previously supposed wholly ischaemic.

In 88% of cases, the haemorrage occurs within the cerebral hemispheres, in 8% in the cerebellum and in 4% in the brainstem (Fig. 1.24). IPH's located in the cerebral hemispheres can be further subdivided into two subcategories: those in typical (75%) and those is atypical (13%) positions. The former are found in the basal ganglia and are almost invariably associated with high blood pressure. The latter, also known as lobar or subcortical haemorrhages, can sometimes be attributed to hypertension,

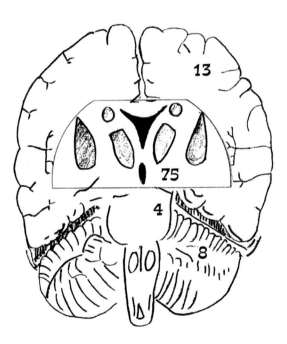

Fig. 1.24 - Modified from (12).
This diagram shows the different percentages of intraparenchymal haemorrhage distribution: 88% affect the cerebral hemispheres (75% the paranuclear structures and 13% the white matter); 8% the cerebellum and 4% the brainstem. Deep-seated haemorrhages are included inside the sector of the circle (delimited by the corpus callosum above, the external capsule to the side and the brainstem below). Superficial intraparenchymal haemorrhages develop outside this boundary. So-called "advanced" haemorrhages originate from the basal ganglia and spread through the adjacent white matter, crossing this peripheral border.

but are more commonly caused by aneurysm rupture, arteriovascular malformation rupture or by other pathology characterized by abnormal vascularization (including neoplasia). In cases of IPH, CT scanning is important as it permits the differentiation of primary haemorrhages from ischaemic forms (Fig. 1.48), which the clinical data alone is often unable to establish. In addition, the CT examination provides accurate information regarding the site, appearance, dimensions and evolution of the haemorrhagic focus.

THE ROLE OF CT

The introduction of CT immediately revealed that IPH is far more common than previously supposed on the basis of clinical data alone. Prior to the advent of this technique, only those clinical strokes in which the sudden onset and severity of symptoms were accompanied by the presence of blood in the CSF (determined by lumbar spinal tap), and in which an avascular mass was detected by selective angiography (22) were considered haemorrhagic.

Today, both of these examinations are only rarely considered due to their invasiveness and relative inaccuracy. In 50% of IPH's documented using CT, the CSF is not found to contain blood; angiography is only used very occasionally for haemorrhages in typical locations, but can be useful in confirming clinical suspicion of such underlying pathology as vascular malformations, aneurysms, angiitis and neoplasia (24).

CT is useful for documenting both larger haemorrhages, which may include ventricular rupture, as well as smaller ones with minor neurological symptoms. CT is so sensitive that it is able to document all acute, clinically symptomatic haematomas correctly (21). The clinical diagnosis is somewhat inaccurate even when sophisticated score systems are used (11), thus underscoring CT's fundamental role in evaluating neurological emergencies (2).

In the hyperacute phase that follows a clinical stroke, when the differentiation of primary haemorrhage from other pathological entities is most important, MR is only rarely used, be-

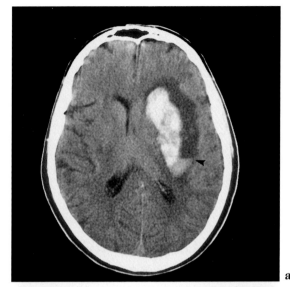

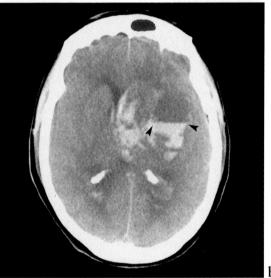

Fig. 1.25 - The presence of fluid levels is not rare (blood levels stratify in the sloping part). In (**a**) a large putaminal haematoma presents with a deep, more recent and compact component and another, superficial one characterized by a clear fluid-fluid level (arrowhead). A level can also be observed in the irregular and widespread multifocal intraparenchymal haemorrhage of a patient treated with anticoagulants for a heart attack (**b**).

cause of its relatively long scanning times. These extended examination times often make it inappropriate for use in emergency situations, as these patients are not always able to remain immobile, and continuous clinical checks are required is such cases. Moreover, on the few occasions in which it is used, the MRI signal of the haemorrhagic focus is not usually sufficient to distinguish it from other types of pathology that may bleed (3).

However, MRI can prove to be very useful in defining the anatomical-topographical nature of the IPH and, above all, in monitoring its evolution during the subacute and chronic phases (Fig. 1.26). Persistent documentation of haemoglobin derivatives makes it possible to establish the haemorrhagic nature of a vascular accident even some time after onset, a distinction that is not always possible using CT. In some cases, MRI can also contribute to identifying the pathology underlying the bleeding (Fig. 1.27), evaluate hemorrhages within the posterior fossa (where it is not hindered by artefacts such as those that occur with CT, Fig. 1.26) and thanks to its greater relative contrast resolution, it is also possible to identify smaller foci that are not visualized using CT.

Angiography is only used in cases of non-spontaneous haemorrhage, whose causes cannot be demonstrated by MR or CT (with/without contrast media) in the acute phase. It is also routinely performed in the evaluation of patients under 45 years of age, especially when the IPH has a lobar location and the patient has no past history of high blood pressure (24).

CAUSES

IPH can be attributed to a great number of causes, although by far the most common is the so-called "spontaneous" form, which is almost invariably associated with systemic high blood pressure. Haemorrhagic extravasation occurs most commonly in the basal ganglia (usually between the insula and the lenticular nucleus); it also typically affects the claustrum, the lateral portion of the putamen, and the external capsule and causes extensive injury of the surrounding cerebral parenchyma as the haematoma dissects its way through the cerebral tissue.

The haemorrhage occurs due to a rupture of an artery (usually one of the lenticulostriate arteries, which are particularly sensitive to changes in pressure), whose walls have been damaged by the chronic effects of arterial hy-

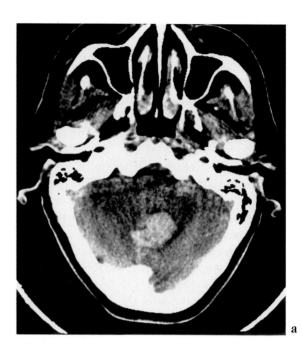

a

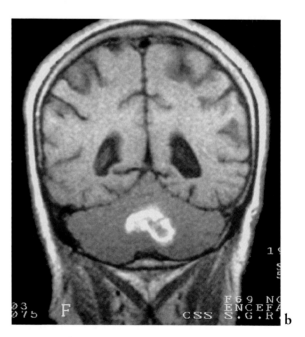

b

Fig. 1.26 - Relations between CT and MR.
A recent haematoma affects the left paramidline portion of the cerebellum (**a**). It is not subject to surgical removal (because it does not cause a «narrow» posterior fossa). It is checked one week later using MR (**b**), here represented in a coronal T1 weighted spin-echo sequence. MR is superior during the subacute phase as it better documents haemoglobin breakdown products; in particular around the posterior fossa, due to the absence of artefacts from the cranial theca that are inevitable with CT; in each phase and position due to its superior (three dimensional) spatial localization (7).

pertension. The blood flows outwardly quite violently, and due to its kinetic energy, it forms a vortex at the outlet point. Under direct observation, haemorrhagic foci are therefore masses of more or less clotted blood, with poorly defined margins (due to peripheral mingling with necrotic strands of brain tissue). The adjacent parenchyma is infiltrated with frank blood, and is more or less destroyed. The clinical presentation (most patients are in their 7th decade of life) is characterized by an abrupt onset and a rapid evolution of signs and symptoms. In 1/3 of all cases, the neurological deficit reaches a peak at onset, and in the remaining 2/3 of patients the clinical picture worsens gradually over the course of minutes or hours in proportion to the dimensions of the arteries involved and the speed at which bleeding occurs. In certain rare cases, the clinical evolution can last a number of days, thus mimicking the clinical picture typically manifested by neoplasias (19).

Prodromic symptoms such as headaches, paleness and nausea only occur somewhat rarely. In 2/3 of cases, the severe form of onset, or cerebral apoplexy, strikes patients during full activity and only rarely occurs during rest. The systemic blood pressure is high in 75-80% of cases, and therefore plays a prominent role in categorizing the likely aetiology of the haemorrhage. Unlike aneurysm ruptures (which may have multiple episodes), in most cases only one haemorrhagic event occurs, and active/progressive bleeding or late recurrence in the same site is rare.

A gradual worsening of clinical symptoms is therefore more frequently caused by a perilesional increase in oedema (with a consequential mass effect) or by the intraventricular or subarachnoid spread of the bleed rather than an increase in haematoma volume. In certain circumstances, CT images may not undergo any major change, therefore indicating metabolic factors or medical complications (22). In massive forms of IPH (Fig. 1.33), the patient is comatose and usually has severe alterations of the vegetative functions (e.g., considerable breathing difficulties, cardiovascular alterations, incontinence and hyperthermia). In this phase, neurological lateralizing signs can prove difficult to evaluate given the massive hypotonia.

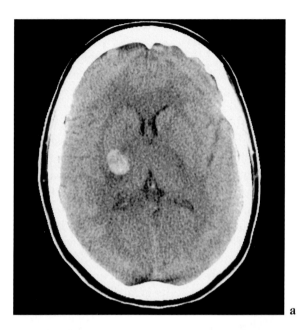

a

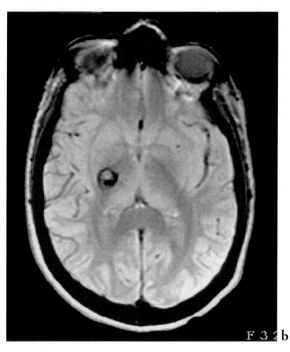

b

Fig. 1.27 - IPH caused by the rupture of a cavernous angioma. In this 22 year-old female, a localized haemorrhagic lesion affects the rear arm of the internal capsula (**a**). With its various sequences (in **b** it is represented by a PD-weighted SE sequence), MR demonstrates that it is consequential to the rupture of a cavernous angioma.

When onset is more gradual, taking a number of hours, even sluggish patients are aware of the occurrence of the neurological deficit. In

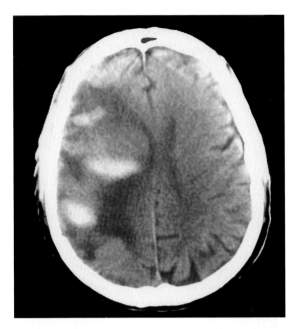

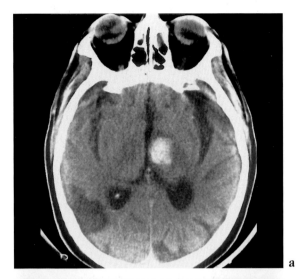

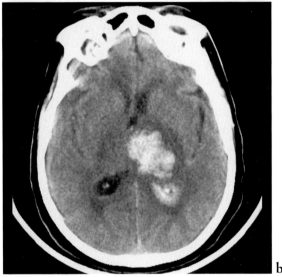

Fig. 1.28 - Large parenchymal bleed in a chronic alcoholic, with more recent, irregular hyperdense foci, alternated with areas of widespread colliquation in the white matter. The concomitance of cerebral atrophy and the somewhat limited «mass effect» caused by the lesion should also be noted.

Fig. 1.29 - Thalamic haematomas.
In (**a**) thalamic haematoma with limited extent, resolved by conservative treatment alone (note the hypodense wedge-shaped lesion in contralateral parietal location, outcome of a previous ischaemic accident). In (**b**) a coarser haematoma with marked mass effect (deformation of the 3rd ventricle) and intraventricular inundation with fatal outcome.

2/3 of cases, neurological or neurovegetative alterations tend to worsen during the first 24-48 hours, with a rapid evolution towards death, which is sometimes ultimately caused by acute pulmonary oedema.

In the so-called regressive forms, which account for the remaining 1/3 of patients, the evolution is less aggressive, and following the initial phase, which does not differ greatly from that described, within 7-10 days the patient's consciousness and neurovegetative state may stabilize or even improve.

In addition to high blood pressure, which accounts for some 80% of cases, there are many other causes of IPH. The most common are aneurysm ruptures and arteriovenous malformation (AVM) and cryptic angioma ruptures, all of which usually occur in lobar positions and are often accompanied by subarachnoid haemorrhage (Fig. 1.35).

2-10% of IPH's are caused by an underlying neoplasm, the most common metastatic forms being melanomas, kidney and lung tumours and choriocarcinomas. Primitive forms of tumours that may lead to IPH include gliocarcinomas, mesogliomas, angioblastic meningiomas and hypophyseal adenomas.

Haemorrhagic mechanisms within the tumour may be due to a number of factors, including: the rupture of pathological neovessels associated with the tumour, such as those observed in a gliocarcinoma; the rapid growth of the neoplasia outstripping its blood supply, typical of neoplastic metastases and the associated systemic

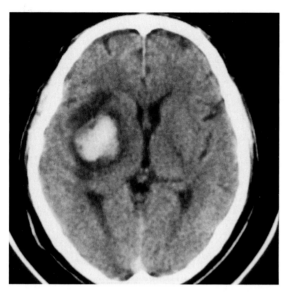

Fig. 1.30 - A «globous-midline» IPH (2), with dimensions (2.5 cm) larger than those usually observed for such formations, which completely obliterates the putamen (compare delineation with that of the healthy contralateral). The peripheral crown-shaped hypodensity is also larger than normal.

complications, such as coagulation disorders (22). In approximately one-half of these patients, the clinical onset takes the form of a haemorrhagic ictus, whereas in others the symptoms are subtler and the CT detection of peritumoral bleeding can be an unexpected finding (22).

IPH is also often caused by clotting disorders (e.g., complications of anticoagulation treatment, haemophilia, thrombocytopenic purpura, leukaemia and aplastic anaemia), where bleeding often occurs either spontaneously or secondary to minor trauma. The CT picture can be typical or can very often reveal a fluid/blood interface combined with fluid stratification as an effect of blood sedimentation below the overlying plasma (Fig. 1.25b).

IPH is also commonly observed in chronic alcoholics, being caused by a number of different pathogenic factors, especially the frequent falls to which such subjects are prone due to impaired coordination; clotting disorders, most commonly that of reduced platelet function; and cerebral atrophy that exposes brain surface vessels and bridging vessels (i.e., from brain surface to parietal dura mater) to greater risk of traumatic injury. Bleeding can be quite widespread, and usually originates in the subcortical white

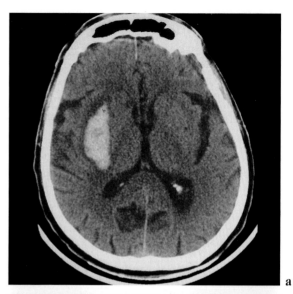

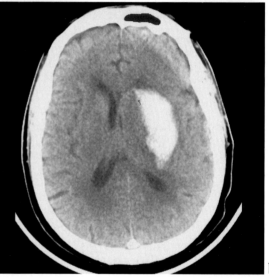

Fig. 1.31 - Two examples of putaminal haematomas spread to the external capsule, with the classic elongated shape in an anterior-posterior direction. That on the right (**a**) is smaller and surrounded by a clearer hypodense border. These forms account for 11% of all putaminal IPH's and usually have a good prognosis.

matter. For this reason the haemorrhage can thereby be differentiated from more serious post-traumatic contusive haemorrhage, which tend to be smaller and often multiple, and occupy a more superficial position (Fig. 1.28). Due to the accompanying atrophy, even when extremely widespread, the haemorrhaging gives less significant mass effect than might be expected in other forms of haemorrhage with similar dimen-

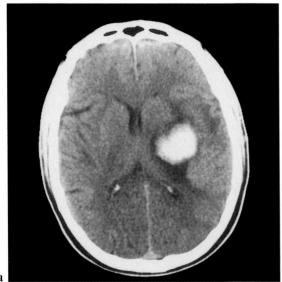

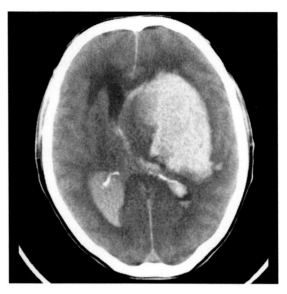

Fig. 1.33 - «Great cerebral haemorrhage».
Recent occurrence of widespread bleed massively involving the left thalamic and putaminal basal ganglia. Concomitance of: a marked mass effect (with conspicuous contralateral shift of the midline structures) and a blocking of the ventricular cavities (the homolateral ventricle is completely obliterated, the right one only in the occipital horn). However, the amount of perifocal oedema is, as usual, restricted to a peripheral border only. The patient died a few hours later.

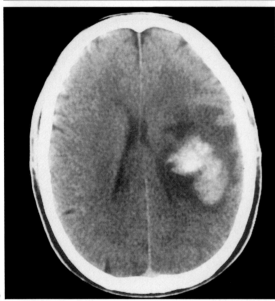

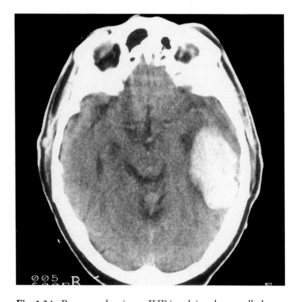

Fig. 1.32 - Typical example of putaminal haematoma that spreads to the internal capsule (**a**) and to the semioval centre (**b**). These forms account for 32% of all putaminal locations.

Fig. 1.34 - Recent, voluminous IHP involving the so-called temporal-parietal-occipital junction.

sions. Following surgical evacuation of the haematoma, the brain parenchyma often returns to its previously occupied space (22).

IPH's may also be caused by cerebral amyloid angiopathy or CAA, most commonly encountered in elderly patients (13), and in cases of sympathomimetic drug abuse, more commonly observed in the young (9).

In addition, cases of IPH are not infrequently observed secondary to arterial or venous inflammation (thrombosis/rupture of arteries and of cortical veins or the dural venous sinuses) and the forms of vascular inflammatory change occurring in systemic or infectious illnesses.

SEMEIOTICS

In comparison to the surrounding parenchyma, acute phase IPH appears on CT scans as clearly defined hyperdense, non-calcified lesions having mass (volume). The hyperdensity is linked primarily (90%) to haemoglobin and only partly (8%) to the concentration of iron (6). For this reason it is less hyperdense in patients suffering from severe anaemia, where in some unusual cases it can be difficult to perceive (14). Clot formation and its subsequent retraction cause a considerable increase in the packed cell volume and thus a further increase in density of up to 90-100 H.U. (6). IPH's usually present as round or oval in shape, but in certain haemorrhages, especially in the larger ones, the haemorrhagic mass can be irregular (Figs. 1.25b, 1.32b, 1.39a, 1.42a, 1.48a, 1.49a). The profile of the haemorrhagic mass is usually well defined, however blurred margin, tree-shaped, jagged borders or map-shaped profiles can also be observed. These shapes are a result mainly of the quantity of the extravasated blood (i.e., the greater the quantity, the greater the dissecting effect upon the surrounding neural parenchyma), although in IPH forms associated with blood dyscrasias, irregular borders are more common due to irregular clot formation (6) (Fig. 1.25b).

The appearance of the internal aspect of the haematoma can either be homogeneous or can be characterized by hyper- and hypodensities of varying degree, size and configuration (Figs. 1.28a, 1.48a). Horizontal fluid-fluid levels may also be seen (Figs. 1.25, 1.42). Occasionally, shortly after onset of the haemorrhagic event, a radiodense core surrounded by a less dense, thin circumferential border area can be observed. Over several days' time, the peripheral hypodensity is seen to enlarge and vary in width (Figs. 1.26, 1.29a, 1.30, 1.31a, 1.32a, 1.33, 1.34, 1.36, 1.41a, 1.42, 1.47, 1.49a). This peripheral oedematous layer yet later becomes visible as more extensive digitations of oedema that penetrate the white matter extending away from the haemorrhagic focus (Figs. 1.32b, 1.44, 1.45). The origin of this peripheral oedema is partly due to a serous exudation from the regional

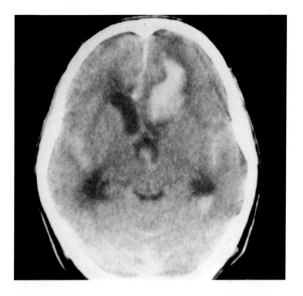

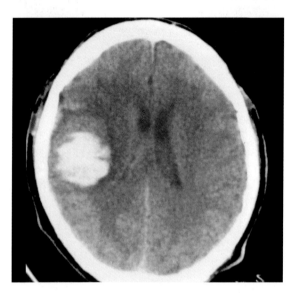

Fig. 1.35 and 1.36 - Lobar and white matter haematomas. The left frontal haematoma (Fig. 1.35) is secondary to the rupture of an aneurysm of the anterior communicating artery and is accompanied by subarachnoid bleeding, intraventricular inundation and hydrocephalus. The right parietal haematoma (Fig. 1.36) is of the «spontaneous» kind in a hypertensive patient.

blood vessels, and partly to the oedematous reaction of the surrounding neural tissue to the blood clot.

Larger hemispheric IPH's (Figs. 1.25b, 1.33) generally cause mass effect with midline shift, and eventually a transfalx internal herniation of the cingulate gyrus and downward transtentor-

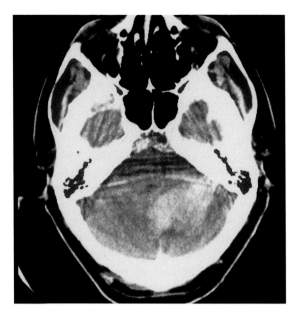

Fig. 1.37 - Voluminous IPH of the left hemisphere causes a deformation and deviation of the 4th ventricle and a closed posterior fossa condition.

ial internal herniation of the hippocampal uncus. The latter event may ultimately result in a series of secondary parenchymal softenings or haemorrhages, especially within the midbrain and pons (1).

During the first five days from IPH onset, contrast enhancement on CT is never observed, unless the haemorrhage is due to a discrete underlying pathological entity (e.g., neoplasm) (Fig. 1.42).

Some IPH's, especially those in deeper positions (and not necessarily the largest ones), rupture into the cerebral ventricles (Figs. 1.25b, 1.29b, 1.33, 1.47a, 1.49). Subarachnoid bleeding is not uncommonly encountered, but such cases usually suggest a ruptured vascular malformation or cerebral aneurysm as the underlying cause (Fig. 1.35).

Evolution

In non-fatal, conservatively treated haemorrhagic stroke cases, and especially in those in which the clinical picture progressively worsens, IPH evolution is often monitored sequen-

tially with CT. In other cases, the first scan is performed some time after bleeding commences, for example perhaps because the patient presented with a gradual progression of signs and symptoms and a less abrupt onset. For these and other reasons, it is therefore useful to know how the blood collection evolves as well as its collateral effects upon the overlying tissues in order to monitor the situation during follow-up, and be alerted to if and when further intervention may become necessary.

Diagram 1.40 shows the changes that the various IPH parameters undergo over time as judged by CT. Density tends to decrease, passing from a hyper- to an iso- and finally to an area of hypodensity (Fig. 1.41), as a result of a series of phenomena including the phagocytosis of blood pigments, the persistence of necrotic brain tissue and a mingling the whole with xanthochromic fluid (e.g., expressed serum). This

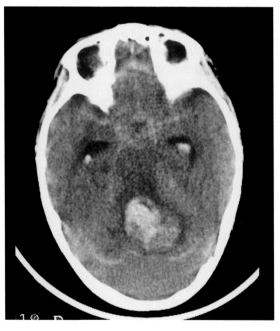

Fig. 1.38 - An eight year-old girl falls into a sudden coma. The CT picture shows a coarse IPH of the vermis with a subarachnoid haemorrhagic shift, obviously a non-spontaneous form. All the conditions (age, site and concomitant SAH) point to secondary forms. CT documents two further findings: the widespread ischaemic hypodensity of the brainstem and hydrocephalus (signalled by the ectasia of the temporal horns). There is no time to perform an angiographic check or other neuroradiological investigations. The vermis is one of the most common sites for «cryptic» angiomas (18).

progressive reduction in density that commences during the first week, continues for several months, and can usually be associated with a parallel reduction in the overall size of the IPH (19). The subacute phase, which starts 3-5 days after the haemorrhagic event, is characterized by clot lysis; the blood clot focus is surrounded by a mainly mononuclear cellular infiltrate, which causes fibrinolytic resolution, erythrocyte phagocytosis, enzymatic digestion of the molecular components and the accumulation of haemoglobin breakdown products. The CT picture shows a gradual centripetally directed reduction in density (i.e., loss of hyperdensity from the outermost layers of the blood clot, and progressing temporally inward). The IPH assumes a characteristic rosette type appearance (Fig. 1.43a), having a central hyperdense portion (represented by the centre of the clot), an intermediate hypodense area (composed of cellular debris, clot breakdown products and low haemoglobin concentration serum), and finally an even more hypodense outer portion caused by the oedema (6). In larger haemorrhages, this model can be replaced by a global, progressive reduction in clot density (4). The appearance of the IPH may also be altered by mixing with CSF or, less frequently, by rebleeding. Towards the third week, it tends to become isodense as compared to normal brain parenchyma, before subsequently becoming relatively hypodense. Two to three months after the event, the centre of the haemorrhagic focus has a density similar or near to that of CSF, transforming itself into a porencephalic cystic cavity (i.e., communicating with the cerbral ventricular system) or alternatively an area of cystic encephalomalacia (i.e., not communicating with the ventricles). The dimensions of intraparenchymal haemorrhages at this late stage are notably smaller than at onset, and an ex-vacuo dilation of the adjacent ventricularcisternal system always occurs (Fig. 1.41c).

Smaller IPH's may not leave macroscopic remains, passing from hyper- to isodensity without the subsequent evolution towards porencephaly (in such cases, the focus of the haematoma is replaced by a glial-type reaction). In the chronic phase (after 3 months), the density values can be variable, with isodensity in the case of a complete *restituto ad integrum*, hypodensity (the most frequent case) when the porencephalic/encephalomalacic cavity forms, and more infrequently, hyperdensity when calcium deposits occur. As a general rule, larger haematomas require more time to transit these phases than do smaller ones.

White matter oedema, which is visualized as hypodensity around the haemorrhage on CT, develops towards the end of the first week and subsequently diminishes in degree, although in certain cases it can persist for some time (Figs. 1.32 b, 1.41b, 1.44, 1.45). The mass effect, and in particular the compression of the cerebral ventricular system, is usually directly proportionate to the amount of oedema entity; the oedema eventually disappears after 20-30 days (Figs. 1.25a, 1.32, 1.33, 1.41b, 1.42, 1.43, 1.44, 1.45, 1.47a, 1.49a).

Evolution of the haemorrhage principally takes place in two stages: a) during the initial few days the size is related to the growth of the haematoma, and b) in the subsequent 2-3 weeks the overall mass effect is determined by the increase in the perihaemorrhagic oedema (the clinical significance of late appearing oedema is as yet unclear) (23). The progressive reduction of this mass effect is typically more rapid in the smaller initial haemorrhages and the haemorrhages associated to less perilesional oedema (4-16).

Site

Pinpointing the location of the bleed, which is usually easy with CT, is of fundamental importance as it largely determines: a) clinical symptomatology, which is closely linked to the neural structures affected by the bleed; b) aetiology and pathogenesis, because the spontaneous forms linked to hypertension develop in the basal ganglia (the typical site), whereas those due to ruptured aneurysms, AVM's or neoplasia are usually located in variable sites, (lobar, posterior fossa, etc.); c) prognosis, which correlates with haemorrhage location and extent; and d) treatment, which can differ from one form to another, as some types may benefit

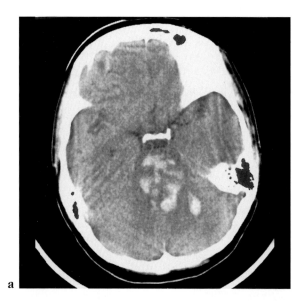

a

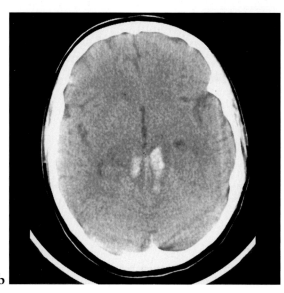

b

Fig. 1.39 - A large haematoma with a fragmented appearance massively occupies the brainstem (**a**) and spreads upwards towards the thalamic nuclei.

by surgery while others (although opinions may vary) are usually treated conservatively. Any cerebral location can be involved, albeit with varying frequency (Fig. 1.24).

The most typical hypertensive forms, which account for some three-quarters of all IPH's, can be subdivided into medial (thalamic) or lateral (putaminal) events. The former are less frequent (15-25%) and tend to be smaller due to both the smaller dimensions of the thalamic nu-

clei as well as their containing fibres that form a barrier to blood diffusion (Fig. 1.29). However, because of their deeper-seated location, these haemorrhages are more likely to rupture into the ventricular system (60% of all cases). In the larger haemorrhages, the process may reach the white matter (above) and the midbrain (below).

Putaminal haemorrhages are considerably more frequent than the thalamic and tend to have greater extension outwardly and frontally. When they are confined to the putamen (17%), they present as a rounded mass with a typical diameter of 10-18 mm. They may manifest potentially reversible symptoms as they primarily cause compression of the fibres of the internal capsule. In one-third of all cases, these haemorrhages are observed in IV drug abusers (Fig. 1.30).

However, with the exception of these more limited forms, putaminal haemorrhages tend to extend towards the surrounding neural structures, with imaging studies that depend mainly on their dimensions and expansion vectors. Lateral haematomas that extend to the external capsule (11%) commonly have an oval or comma-like shape (Fig. 1.31), a thickness that can vary between 1.5 and 2 cm, and a length of 3-5 cm. They originate in the lateral part of the putamen and principally spread in an anteroposterior direction across the external capsule; they typically do not extend either to the hemispheric white matter or deep into the internal capsule. Due to the relative lack of mass effect and absence of ventricular rupture, they commonly have a favourable prognosis and can usually be removed surgically.

Forms of haemorrhage that spread more easily to the structures noted above are included in a third group (32% of the total) and are characterized by a rounded core (2-3 cm) with linear bands that extend medially towards the internal capsule and are therefore known as capsulo-putaminal haematomas; these haemorrhages also extend rostrally towards the centrum semiovale (Fig. 1.32).

These first three groups are only rarely fatal, although in a variable percentage of cases (1/3 - 2/3) they do result in some residual neurological deficit.

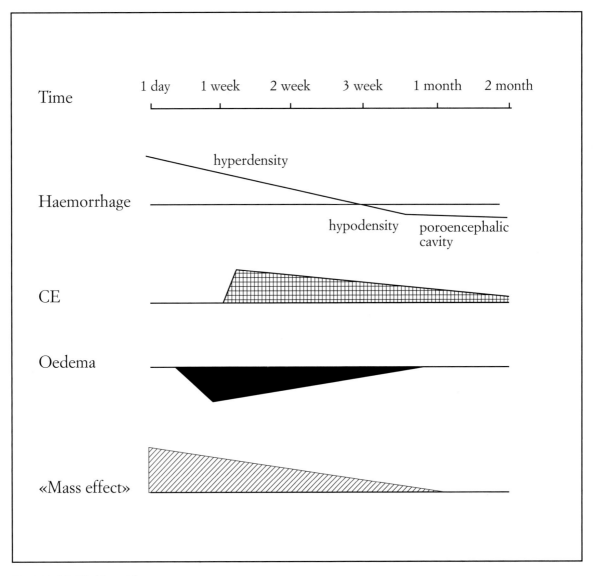

Fig. 1.40 - Modified from (4).
This chart shows the variations that the density of blood collections and other collateral parameters undergo during the phases subsequent to acute haemorrhagic accidents.

A fourth group (19%) of larger IPH's (3-5 cm) tend to expand concentrically from the putamen towards the corona radiata and the cortex of the cerebral hemispheres (frontal, temporal and parietal lobes), with either a jagged or a rounded appearance (Fig. 1.49). Unlike the forms of haemorrhage associated with middle cerebral artery aneurysm ruptures, their spread towards the Sylvian fissure is not usually accompanied by subarachnoid bleeding.

A last group (19%), with the exception of the rare bilateral haemorrhages that account for only approximately 2%, is composed of massive mixed putaminal-thalamic forms that entail complex haemorrhagic involvement of all the deep nuclear structures (22-24), (Fig. 1.33).

These latter IPH's are large (up to 7 - 8 cm), involve considerable midline shift and, in most cases, ventricular rupture. They have poor prognosis and often a rapidly fatal evolution in three-quarters of cases. Principally this is due

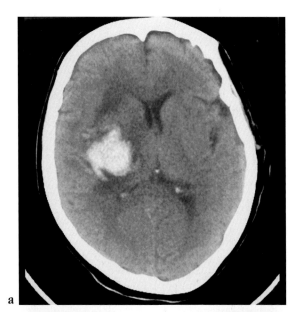

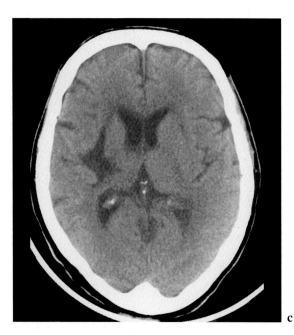

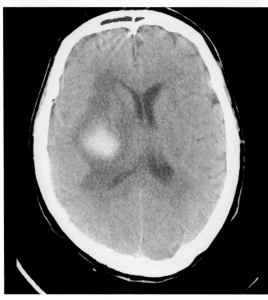

Fig. 1.41 - Evolution of IPH over time.
CT is commonly used in IPH follow-up. In (**a**) the haematoma is documented a few hours from the stroke (note the deep position, the jagged edges and the presence of small satellite foci). On a check carried out 14 days later (**b**), the haematoma presents modest reductions in volume and density; it is however, surrounded by a vaster hypodense area (with a prevalence of the oedematous component developing in the white matter). Three months later (**c**), the haematic hyperdensity is replaced by an irregular porencephalic cavity with a star shape, which produces discreet ectasia of the homolateral ventricle.

unchecked eventually results in a severe neurovegetative state (1).

It is therefore possible to formulate a progressive grading of thalamic and putaminal haemorrhages. Together with clinical grading (e.g., patient awake; drowsy with or without neurological deficit; sluggish with slight to severe neurological deficit; semi-comatose with severe neurological deficit or early signs of herniation; deep coma with decerebration), it enables an immediate prognostic assessment, which is useful in deciding upon subsequent possible courses of treatment (16). The debate between the supporters of conservative medical treatment on the one hand, and surgery on the other is still open. Whereas it seems universally accepted that surgical evacuation is the preferable treatment for lobar haemorrhages (especially when they are larger than 35-44 cm^3 and therefore have a greater probability of causing brainstem compression and herniation), the management of haemorrhages occurring in more common locations is still somewhat controversial.

It should also be pointed out that surgery is not necessarily considered as an alternative to medical treatment, but rather as a complement to it, especially when conservative management proves inadequate alone (5, 8). For example, surgery may be employed when medical therapy is unable to adequately control intracranial

to associated brainstem injury, be it direct or a consequence of transtentorial herniation, either of which worsens the degree of coma, and if

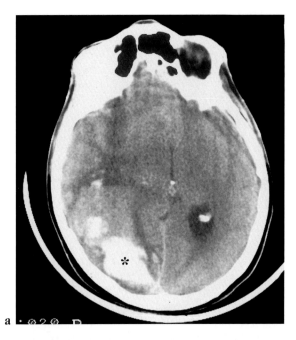

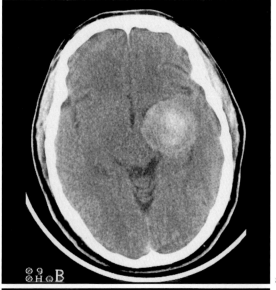

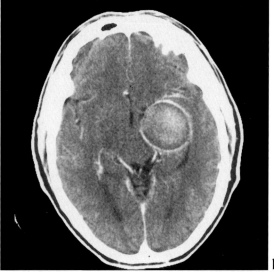

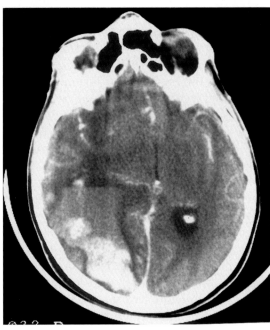

Fig. 1.42 - The use of contrast medium in atypically positioned acute haematomas. A voluminous lobar haematoma with a primarily occipital expansion (**a**) is constituted by a more hyperdense component (*), an expression of recent bleeding, and by another subacute, more widespread, and partially levelled component. The site and the lack of association with hypertension suggested a secondary haemorrhage and therefore an examination was performed after intravenous administration of contrast medium (**b**). There was no documentation of pathologically significant impregnations adjacent to the haematomas, nor alterations in density. The spontaneous haemorrhagic picture, with clots in various phases of evolution, was confirmed during surgery.

Fig. 1.43 - The use of contrast media in the subacute phase. Twenty-five days from the stroke, this haematoma presents with (**a**) a target-shaped form and a blurred central hyperdensity. The contrast medium (**b**) impregnates a thin and uniform peripheral rim. This ring is clearly distinguishable, despite the fact that the patient had received long-term steroid treatment, therefore in this «late» phase it is essentially supported by the hypervascularization of granulation tissue.

hypertension. However, generally speaking, haemorrhages in thalamic positions are not subject to surgery, because surgery at this location is associated with higher mortality rates (80%); nevertheless, these patients often require ventriculostomy, due to the frequency of associated hydrocephalus (9).

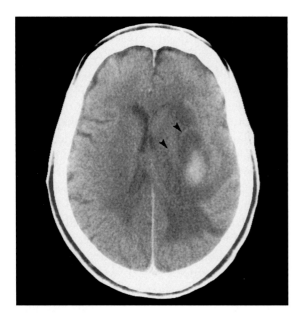

Fig. 1.44 - The influence of steroids on the outer ring. 17 days after the ictus, this IPH presents a reduction in its central density, an ample quantity of perifocal oedema and discreet mass effect. After CE it is demarcated by a ring, which because of cortisone treatment is incomplete and blurred (arrowhead).

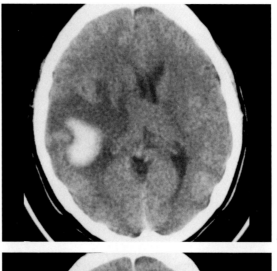

a

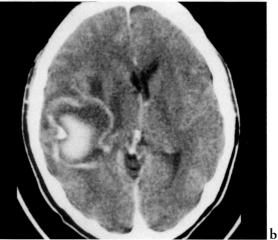

b

Fig. 1.45 - Contrast medium use in the diagnosis of forms encountered in the subacute phase only.

For approximately two weeks the patient has been suffering from worsening symptoms of intracranial hypertension, with progressive hemiplegia of the left side. Clinical suspicion points to a neoplastic pathology. The lesion documented by CT (**a**) is hyperdense as with IPH, but with atypical site (and symptomatology); it is accompanied by abundant oedema of the white matter and exerts a marked mass effect. The subsequent examination after CE, with the demonstration of the «ring» enhancement, would therefore strongly suggest a haemorrhagic nature (as confirmed by subsequent checks). It should be noted that, despite its circumvolute appearance, also in this phase the ring is thin and regular; which arouses further doubts, because the patient has not yet been treated with steroids.

With regard to putaminal haemorrhages, surgery and its timing depend upon the clinical status of the patient at the time. Haemorrhages with a statistically favourable expectation based on past experience are usually treated conservatively; those with stationary or slowly worsening clinical pictures are operated in an elective manner; those IPH's with early signs of internal brain herniation are traditionally taken to emergency surgery; and the massive haemorrhages in those patients having a dire general and neurological status (e.g., deep coma, decerebration) are not usually treated surgically (17).

The second form of hemispheric IPH (15-25%) is localized wholly within the white matter. These so-called lobar or subcortical intraparenchymal haemorrhages are linked in one-third of all cases to high blood pressure and in the remaining two-thirds of cases to other causes described previously.

The position of these lobar haemorrhages can be parietal (30%), frontal (20%), occipital (15%) or mixed (35%). In fact, they often occur at the temporo-parietal-occipital junction (Fig. 1.34). Their CT appearance and evolution are very similar or identical to that previously discussed for more "typical" positions of IPH.

Frontal haemorrhages (Fig. 1.35) are usually unilateral (lobar haemorrhages can be bilateral in forms secondary to aneurysm ruptures of the anterior communicating artery). They are round

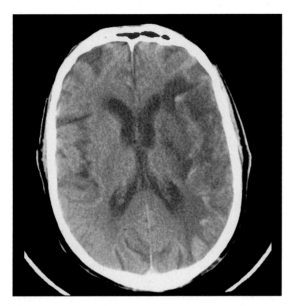

Fig. 1.46 - Haemorrhagic infarct.
An extensive ischaemic infarct that massively affects the territory of the left middle cerebral artery, four days from onset presents an unexpected worsening of clinical conditions.
CT documents irregular circumvolute hyperdensities, which can refer to overlapping bleeding phenomena.

or oval in rostral positions and wedge-shaped (with the apex directed at the ventricles and the base towards the brain surface) if located in a frontal-basal position. Only 20% of lobar haemorrhages rupture into the cerebral ventricular system. At least 50% are life-threatening (22). Those lobar haemorrhages with locations in the temporal lobes are round; they can rupture into the temporal horns and develop early internal transtentorial brain herniation. When they develop within the Sylvian fissure, thus becoming frontal-temporal, they are more likely caused by ruptured aneurysms of the middle cerebral artery. Larger haemorrhages often extend deep into the basal ganglia, although they do not usually cross the internal capsule, an important distinction with regard to subsequent treatment.

Parietal lobar haemorhages (Fig. 1.36) have the most favourable prognosis and often resolve with little or no neurological sequelae, even without surgery.

10% of occipital lobar haemorrhages rupture into the occipital horns of the cerebral ven-

tricles. Nevertheless, these haemorrhages also typically resolve spontaneously in the vast majority of cases, although they often leave some degree of visual deficits.

Cerebellar IPH's account for approximately 8% of the total, which more or less corresponds to the proportion of the space occupied by the cerebellum as compared to the remainder of the brain. Once again, in this position hypertension is by far the most common cause. Hypertensive bleeds are followed, in second place, by vascular malformations that account for 10-15% of the total; these haemorrhages are usually caused by the rupture of cryptic angiomas, which are even more frequent at this location than in the cerebral hemispheres (Fig. 1.38).

Approximately 80% of cerebellar IPH's have lobar origins (Fig. 1.37), initially affecting the dentate nucleus; this is where vessel wall alterations such as Charcot-Bouchard aneurysms as observed in the lenticulostriate arteries in association with basal ganglia haemorrhages are seen pathologically. From here, the haemorrhage can cross the midline, affecting the vermian area to enter the contralateral cerebellar hemisphere; it may also rupture into the 4th ventricle. More infrequently, it can dissect into the brainstem, which more commonly is simply affected by compression or displacement.

Less frequently, IPH's may primarily affect the cerebellar vermis, especially in the case of aneurysm ruptures (Fig. 1.38).

In cases where consciousness is largely unaffected and CT presents an IPH devoid of mass effect with a diameter of less than 3 cm, complete recovery can be expected and surgery is generally not required (Fig. 1.26). However, emergency surgery is usually essential (and must be carried out urgently, in order to be lifesaving), in most of the other cases, especially when there are CT or clinical indications of brainstem and fourth ventricle compression (e.g., contralateral brainstem displacement, distortion and marked brainstem compression with associated obstruction of the 4th ventricle, loss of the basal subarachnoid cisterns, and obstructive supratentorial hydrocephalus) (22) (Fig. 1.37).

With regard to the brainstem, three anatomical and pathological distinctions can be made for

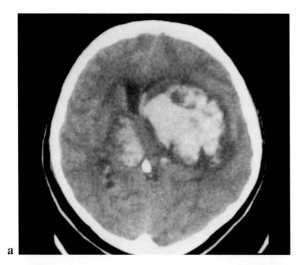

a

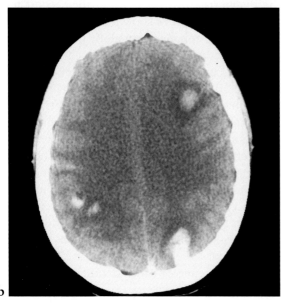

b

Fig. 1.47 - Although rarely, IPH's can also present with bilateral multiple localizations.
In (**a**) an example of a deep form, in (**b**) lobar forms. The haematomas of (**a**) are both putamino-thalamic; that on the left has a non-homogeneous core and, due to its larger dimensions, prevails in the shift effect on the contralateral ventricular chambers. The IPH's in (**b**) are due to the recent bleeding of breast cancer metastases.

non-traumatic parenchymal haemorrhages: 1) those haemorrhages encapsulated within the brainstem parenchyma, 2) large brainstem IPH's with ventricular rupture (Fig. 1.39); 3) petechial brainstem haemorrhages secondary to expanding supratentorial mass effect complicated by internal transtentorial cerebral herniation (22). The

small dimensions of the latter make them difficult to perceive on CT. Pontine haemorrhages have variable appearances and longitudinal extents depending on the size of the vessels from which they originate and the point at which they occur. If bleeding is caused by the rupture of larger arterioles, the haemorrhage is more commonly medial, affecting the base of the pons and the tegmen and spreading to the fourth ventricle. Due to mass effect, in 80% of cases the peribrainstem subarachnoid cisterns are obliterated.

However, in haemorrhages associated with smaller vessels (having a more lateral and tegmental position), the bleeds are usually smaller and unilateral and do not rupture into the fourth ventricle.

CT is invaluable in differentiating pontine haemorrhages from those affecting the adjacent cerebellar peduncles and especially the fourth ventricle; the latter are paramedial, pyramid-shaped (reproducing the form of the ventricle, which is usually dilated), and are often accompanied by hydrocephalus and the presence of blood in the basal subarachnoid cisterns (22).

IPH's rarely occur in the midbrain; when they do they are not usually caused by hypertension but are instead often related to aneurysm ruptures. They rarely spread to the pons or the thalamus (above, Fig. 1.39).

In the majority of cases, CT permits a precise spatial definition of bleeding and its extensions. In certain cases, more accurate information may be required, which is now easily obtainable with CT angiography using 3D reconstructions, especially with the use of computerized postprocessing analysis (10).

Contrast agent use

During the acute phase, paranuclear IPH's do not require enhanced examinations using IV contrast medium administration. This technique is used when the diagnosis is in doubt, if the aetiology of the haemorrhage is uncertain (Fig. 1.42), or in the following conditions:

a) patients under 40;

b) absence of history of high blood pressure documentation;

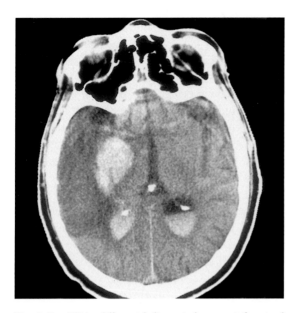

Fig. 1.48 - CT in differential diagnosis between infarct and haemorrhage.
It is rare for ischaemic and haemorrhagic pathologies to present associated. This case serves to demonstrate the difference between the CT pictures for the two.
On the right the sequelae of an extensive infarctual lesion (hypodense), which affects the territory of the middle cerebral artery and, immediately adjacent, a recent rounded formation (hyperdense) of haemorrhagic type, which expands in depth to the basal grey nuclei.

c) progression of neurological deficit over more than 4 hours;

d) history of transitory prodromes;

e) an atypical CT appearance and disproportionate degree of subarachnoid and/or subdural haemorrhage;

f) presence of possible combined pathology, such as proven neoplasia, bacterial endocarditis or arteritis (22).

Contrast agent use is therefore essential in all cases where an IPH potentially caused by other types of pathology is suspected. In fact, in the case of bleeding tumours, contrast agents usually only enhance the solid mass component, which can therefore be better distinguished from the surrounding parenchyma (if isodense) and the haemorrhage (if hyperdense). Enhancement can be nodular, diffuse or ring-shaped (thickened and irregular). The haemorrhage is most frequently found at the interface between the tumour and the surrounding oedematous parenchyma; it can sometimes present

with a pseudo-cystic appearance or appear with a fluid-fluid level of differing densities (22).

During the subacute phase, in other words when the IPH tends to be accompanied by greater degrees of perilesional oedema and consequent greater mass effect, and starts to lose its characteristic hyperdensity, it can sometimes reveal an atypical CT picture, similar to that seen in cases of neoplasia. On the other hand, these IPH's usually have a lobar location, and therefore at onset their symptomatology may be mild and progress slowly; for this reason they may not be seen in hospital until the subacute phase. In such circumstances, the use of IV contrast agents can aid in the determination of the diagnosis (Fig. 1.45). From the second to the sixth week, IPH's show a characteristic but minor ring of enhancement along the margin of the haemorrhagic portion. However, this finding is not constant and in fact does not appear in some 50% of cases (Figs. 1.43, 1.44). This ring enhancement may also be present in the iso- and hypodensity phases of haemorrhage evolution, when the perilesional oedema and mass effect are completely resolved. The enhancing ring is usually thin, approximately 3 mm wide, and of uniform thickness (this appearance of the rim enhancement is therefore different from that which often surrounds neoplastic masses, which is thicker and has uneven dimensions).

In the absence of other definitive differentiating elements between the two conditions, the final diagnosis is possible on the basis of subsequent serial imaging studies, which, in the case of IPH's show a gradual decrease in the contrast enhancing intensity of the rim, together with a further reduction in the diameter and density of the central haemorrhagic component.

There are at least two mechanisms that explain this semeiological aspect of contrast enhancement surrounding benign IPH's: one prevails in the first stage (3-4 weeks from onset of haemorrhage), which depends on the brain-blood barrier breakdown of otherwise normal native vessels and is reduced in degree by the use of steroids (Figs. 1.43, 1.44); the other, which takes place during the later phases, is

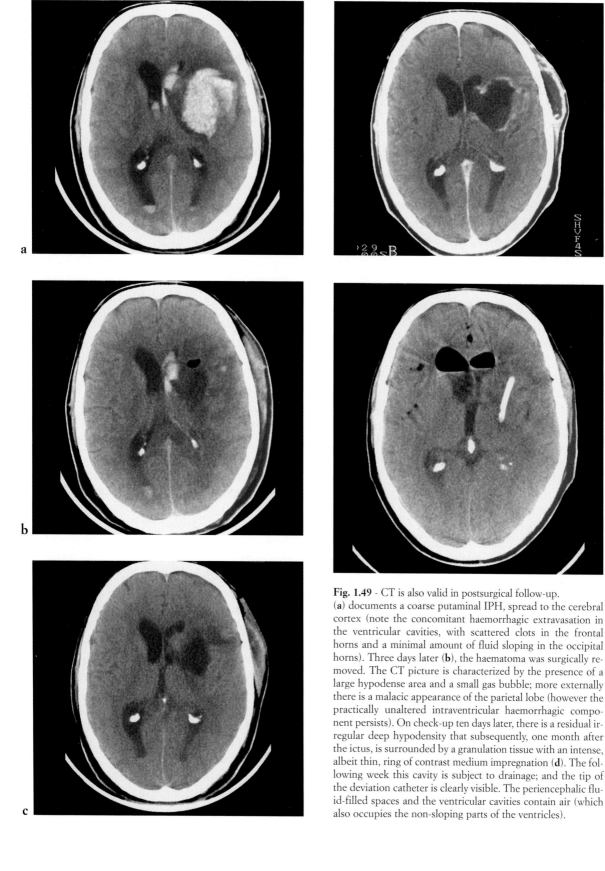

Fig. 1.49 - CT is also valid in postsurgical follow-up.
(a) documents a coarse putaminal IPH, spread to the cerebral cortex (note the concomitant haemorrhagic extravasation in the ventricular cavities, with scattered clots in the frontal horns and a minimal amount of fluid sloping in the occipital horns). Three days later (b), the haematoma was surgically removed. The CT picture is characterized by the presence of a large hypodense area and a small gas bubble; more externally there is a malacic appearance of the parietal lobe (however the practically unaltered intraventricular haemorrhagic component persists). On check-up ten days later, there is a residual irregular deep hypodensity that subsequently, one month after the ictus, is surrounded by a granulation tissue with an intense, albeit thin, ring of contrast medium impregnation (d). The following week this cavity is subject to drainage; and the tip of the deviation catheter is clearly visible. The periencephalic fluid-filled spaces and the ventricular cavities contain air (which also occupies the non-sloping parts of the ventricles).

linked to the hyperneovascularization of the granulation tissue that surrounds the IPH and is not altered by steroid treatment (Fig. 1.45).

It is believed by some researchers that functional recovery is better in cases in which the contrast-enhancing rim is present. Besides IPH and neoplasia (glioma, metastasis, lymphoma), other types of pathology with similar appearances include abscesses (in which the ring enhancement is usually thicker and denser, although regular in its thikness, and is accompanied by nodular daughter components or ring enhancing satellite foci), and thrombosed aneurysms and angiomas (in which calcifications or vascular components that can aid in the correct diagnosis are often found).

PARTICULAR FORMS OF IPH

Haemorrhagic infarction

A haemorrhage may develop within an ischaemic lesion when a lack of oxygen that causes the necrosis of the endothelial cells of the capillaries occurs. In actual fact, infarctions almost always contain a variable haemorrhagic component as determined pathologically, sometimes in the form of small petechial haemorrhages that are not visible on CT. It is therefore the presence or absence of this CT visualized component that indicates or dispels suspicion of haemorrhagic infarction (12). This type of event is most frequently observed as a result of cardiogenic cerebral emboli or anticoagulation treatment. These haemorrhages are usually visible on CT scans performed 4-5 days after the infarct (up to a maximum of 2 weeks) (22) and are often accompanied by a worsening in the patient's clinical condition. Haemorrhagic infarctions occur in 20% of cases of ischaemic cerebral disease (small petechial haemorrhages are present in at least 50% of autopsy findings). The haemorrhages are almost always confined to the cerebral cortex and usually affect the deeper gyri. On CT scans these infarcts appear as a hypodense area that reflects the circulation territory (i.e., watershed) of the affected artery; however, due to the larger degree of accompa-

nying oedema, the low density area has greater dimensions than the actual dimensions of the infarct. These infarcts do not usually have significant mass effect and usually show small hyperdense haemorrhagic components within the infarcted region (Fig. 1.46). Small diapedetic forms are not usually visible with CT, in part due to the limited spatial and contrast resolution of the technique. The most widespread cortical haemorrhages usually have a gyral distribution with convolutional hyperdensity or are only visible in the apex of the infarct area. Intravenous contrast agent administration with CT in the subacute phase results in a classic gyral enhancement pattern.

Intraventricular haemorrhage

Intraventricular haemorrhages can be divided into two categories: one, the more frequent, secondary to the spread of an IPH that dissects through the ependymal lining of the ventricular surface; and two, a primitive type of haemorrhage due to the rupture of vessels of the choroid plexus or the ventricle walls. The most common causes of the latter are connected to regional vascular malformations, haemangiomas of the choroid plexus or, more rarely, malignant neoplasia affecting the paraventricular tissues.

CT is able to establish both the presence as well as the aetiology of the intraventricular bleed with considerable accuracy, showing a hyperdense haemorrhage that forms a cast of the morphology of the ventricular chambers (Figs. 1.25b, 1.29b, 1.33, 1.35). A blood-fluid (i.e., blood-CSF) level can often be observed, in which hyperdense blood due to gravity layers in the occipital horns in supine patients (Figs. 1.33, 1.35). However, in some rare cases the intraventricular blood occupies the temporal horns alone. If the intraventricular haemorrhage is a result of an ipsilateral hemispheric IPH, the ventricular blood may be present in the adjacent lateral ventricle only.

These two conditions, that is IPH versus intraventricular haemorrhage (IVH), can usually be differentiated relatively easily, although, especially if the IPH is particularly small, they may be confused as a single-compartment hyperdense haemorhage due to partial volume averaging effects. In fact, there is no absolute correlation between IPH dimensions and association of IVH; in some cases small haematomas of the caudate nucleus or the thalamus are accompanied by massive intraventricular bleeding.

Certain studies have shown a direct relationship between the volume of intraventricular blood (e.g., presence of blood in the intraventricular space, number of ventricles containing blood, intraventricular extension of hyperdensity from adjacent brain parenchyma) and the prognosis of these patients (20). Within a few days, blood hyperdensity is gradually diluted by the CSF circulation and by the breakdown of haemoglobin products. Due to the effect of CSF flow obstructions at various levels within the ventricular system, partial or total loculations of the ventricular chambers may form over time.

Multiple IPH's

IPH recurrences at the same site are somewhat rare, as are multifocal haemorrhages (Fig. 1.47). These types do not account for more than 3% of all intraparenchymal haemorrhages. The causes of multiple haemorrhages are often the same as those of single ones, although they usually occur in patients with normal blood pressure, and tend to specifically be seen in patients with clotting defects, cerebral metastatic neoplastic disease (Fig. 1.47b), thrombosis of the dural venous sinuses, herpes simplex encephalitis or bacterial endocarditis with cerebral septic emboli. However, even after selective cerebral angiography, it is often difficult to trace the original cause. In two-thirds of cases, the IPH's have bilateral lobar positions, and in the remaining one-third they are lobar-nuclear (basal ganglia nuclei), thalamic-cerebellar, paranuclear-bilateral, etc. (22).

In general this does not pose a diagnostic problem in distinguishing multiple benign IPH's from other multiple spontaneously hyperdense lesions (metastases, multiple meningiomas, rare multifocal angiomas, etc.), all of which significantly enhance on CT with IV contrast agents.

CONCLUSIONS

CT enables the direct visualization of haemorrhagic lesions and assists in the differentiation from other acute cerebrovascular events (Fig. 1.48). CT typically accurately illustrates the site(s), extent and volume of the IPH(s). In the early phases CT is helpful in monitoring morphological and densitometric characteristics as well as for revealing complications such as intraventricular rupture or progressive hydrocephalus.

CT is later useful in identifying spontaneous progression and postsurgical recurrence, in the case of surgical removal (Fig. 1.49). The ease and rapidity with which the examination is performed, its high sensitivity and specific nature make CT the examination of choice for studying this type of pathology. Spiral CT, the latest technological innovation of this technique and one that has proved particularly useful in a number of disease categories (including injuries of polytraumatized patients), has more limited applications in the evaluation of clinical stroke. In reality, its use is not indispensable: traditional CT scans of the cranium are nearly as fast and equally accurate. In this part of the body, there are no problems posed by breathing misrecording, correct contrast agent timing or even motion artefacts caused by long examination times. However, the spiral CT technique may play a role due to its application in multiplanar image reconstruction studies (15).

REFERENCES

1. Andrews BT, Chiles W, Olsen W et al: The effect of intracerebral hematoma location on the risk of brainstem compression and clinical outcome. J Neurosurg 69:518-522, 1988.
2. Bagley LJ: Imaging of neurological emergencies: trauma, hemorrhage, and infections. Semin Roentgenol 34:144-159, 1999.

3. Blankenberg FG, Loh NN, Bracci P et al: Sonography, CT, and MR imaging: a prospective comparison of neonates with suspected intracranial ischemia and hemorrhage. AJNR 21:213-218, 2000.

4. Boulin A: Les affections vasculaires. In: Vignaud J, Boulin A: Tomodensitométrie cranio-encéphalique. Ed Vigot Paris, 1987.

5. Broderick JP, Brott TG, Tomsick T et al: Ultra-early evaluation of the intracerebral hemorrhage. J Neurosurg 72:195-199, 1990.

6. Cirillo S, Simonetti L, Sirabella G et al: Patologia vascolare. In: Dal Pozzo G (ed): Compendio di Tomografia Computerizzata (pp. 127-147). USES Ed. Scientifiche Florence, 1991.

7. Grossman CB: Magnetic resonance imaging and computed tomography of the head and spine (pp. 145-183). Williams & Wilkins Baltimore, 1990.

8. Juvela S, Heiskanen O, Poranen A et al: The treatment of spontaneous intracerebral hemorrhage. J Neurosurg 70:755-758, 1989.

9. Kase C: Diagnosis and treatment of intracerebral hemorrhage. Rev Neurol 29:1330-1337, 1999.

10. Loncaric S, Dhawan AP, Broderick J et al: 3-D imaging analysis of intra-cerebral brain hemorrhage from digitized CT films. Comput Method Programs Biomed 46:207-216, 1995.

11. Mader TJ, Mandel A: A new clinical scoring system fails to differentiate hemorrhagic from ischemic stroke when used in the acute care setting. J Emerg Med 16:9-13, 1998.

12. Masdeu JC, Fine M: Cerebrovascular disorders. In: Gonzalez CF, Grossman CB, Masdeu JC (eds) Head and spine imaging (pp. 283-356). John Wiley & Sons New York, 1985.

13. Miller JH, Warlaw JM, Lammie GA: Intracerebral haemorrhagic and cerebral amyloid angiopathy: CT features with pathological correlation. Clin Radiol 54:422-429, 1999.

14. Modic MT, Weinstein MA: Cerebrovascular disease of the brain. In: Haaga JR, Alfidi RJ (eds) Computed tomography of the brain, head and neck (pp. 136-169). The C.V. Mosby Co. St. Louis, 1985.

15. Novelline RA, Rhea JT, Rao PM et al: Helical CT in emergency radiology. Radiology 213:321-339, 1999.

16. Ross DA, Olsen WL, Ross AM et al: Brain shift, level of consciouness and restoration of consciousness in patients with acute intracranial hematoma. J Neurosurg 71:498-502, 1989.

17. Scarano E, De Falco R, Guarnieri L et al: Classificazione e trattamento delle emorragie cerebrali spontanee. Ricerca Neurochirurgica 1-2:21-32, 1990.

18. Sellier N, Lalande G, Kalifa G: Pathologie vasculaire. In: Montagne JP, Couture A: Tomodensitométrie pédiatrique (pp. 70-90). Ed. Vigot Paris, 1987.

19. Takasugi S, Ueda S, Matsumoto K: Chronological changes in spontaneous intracranial hematoma - an experimental and clinical study. Stroke 16:651, 1985.

20. Tuhrim S, Horowitz DR, Sacher M et al: Volume of ventricular blood is an important determinant of outcome in supratentorial intracerebral hemorrhage. Crit Care Med 27:617-621, 1999.

21. Waga S, Miyazaki M, Okada M et al: Hypertensive putaminal haemorrhage: analysis of 182 patients. Surg Neurol 26:159-166, 1986.

22. Weisberg LA, Nice C: Cerebral computed tomography. A text atlas (pp. 133-162) W.B. Saunders Co. Philadelphia, 1989.

23. Zazulia AR, Diringer MN, Derdeyn CP et al: Progression of mass effect after intracerebral hemorrhage. Stroke 30:1167-1173, 1999.

24. Zhu XL, Chan MS, Poon WS: Spontaneous intracranial hemorrhage: which patients need diagnostic cerebral angiography? A prospective study of 206 cases and review of the literature. Stroke 28:1406-1409, 1997.

1.4

CT USE IN SUBARACHNOID HAEMORRHAGE

N. Zarrelli, L. Pazienza, N. Maggialetti, M. Schiavariello, M. Mariano, A. Stranieri, T. Scarabino

INTRODUCTION

Subarachnoid haemorrhages (SAH's) are the fourth most frequent type of acute cerebrovascular event and account for approximately 8% of the total. In most cases (at least 75%), SAH's are caused by the rupture of aneurysms of the circle of Willis, with the aneurysm itself lying within the subarachnoid space. SAH's affect approximately 11 of every 100,000 inhabitants in the general population. The most critical period is during the first few days after the haemorrhage: 25% of deaths occur on the first day and 50% in the first five days. Remedying this situation calls for rapid and specific diagnosis, which is not possible using clinical data alone.

In recent years SAH survival rates have increased, due in part to progress in intensive care and surgical techniques, but above all thanks to the more precise diagnostic methods that are now available (6). Computerized Tomography (CT) plays a fundamental role (19). From the outset its non-invasive nature and sensitivity have made it an examination technique capable of achieving early diagnosis. More specifically, its sensitivity is given as ranging between 93-100% if performed within the first 12 hours of the onset of symptoms (24, 26). In addition to the observation of subarachnoid bleeding (with the typical hyperdensity of the basal subarach-

noid cisterns and within the cortical sulci), CT is also able to document collateral phenomena and complications such as intraparenchymal, intraventricular and subdural haemorrhages, any mass effect upon the cerebrum, hydrocephalus and cerebral infarcts associated with vasospasm. In some cases, it is possible to establish the more or less precise origin of the haemorrhage from the distribution pattern of blood collection, which is particularly useful in directing subsequent selective angiographic examinations. In the case of multiple aneurysms, the pattern of the blood collection on CT is important in indicating which of them has bled (4). CT allows approximative prognosis assessment (e.g., widespread and massive forms of SAH have a more severe prognosis than smaller ones). Lastly, CT is useful in selecting which patients are to undergo angiography and in determining when it should be performed (28).

SEMEIOTICS

On CT, the more or less pathognomonic appearance of SAH is revealed by the increase in density of the cisternal subarachnoid spaces that appear proportionately denser as a factor of the concentration of blood they contain. Lesser extravasations of blood or those that oc-

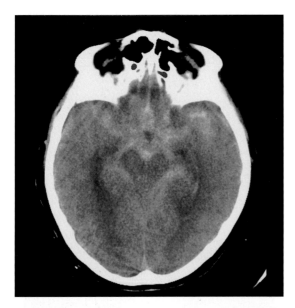

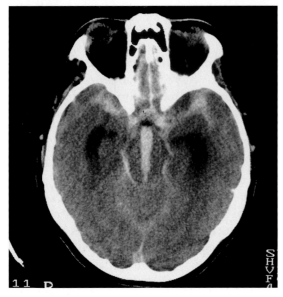

Fig. 1.50 - CT pictures of SAH's subsequent to the rupture of an aneurysm of the anterior cerebral artery, a few hours after the ictus.
a and **b**: in both cases, the widespread haemorrhagic extravasation demarcates the perimesencephalic and supra-sellar cisterns, the initial part of the Sylvian fissures and the interhemispheric fissure with its hyperdensity. In **b** the blood collections are clearly less thick in the perimesencephalic location, but they are accompanied by the blocking of the 3rd ventricle.
Both cause a discreet early ectasia of the ventricular chambers.

form clearly visible and somewhat focal blood collections (6). On average, the density of fresh extravasated blood has a value of approximately 70-80 H.U. (normal CSF = ~10 H.U.).

Generally speaking, abnormal hyperdensity typically involves the suprasellar and perimesencephalic cisterns (or more broadly speaking, the CSF spaces of the basal subarachnoid cisterns), the Sylvian fissures and the cortical sulci. Although infrequent, CT scans performed at the onset of symptoms can prove falsely negative. However, this false negative tendency becomes more frequent the longer the time period is between the initial bleed and the performance of the CT examination. In reality: 1) in the milder clinical forms that may only present clinically at a later stage, the subarachnoid blood will have undergone dilution and dispersal within the native CSF, and therefore detection is understandably more problematic; and, 2) in awake patients with good neurological status, it is probable that bleeding is only minor.

MR using conventional acquisitions is not preferable to CT in patients suspected of having an acute SAH; in fact, in this phase, conventional MR acquisitions may be negative due in part to the slower conversion of oxyhaemoglobin into metahaemaglobin (resulting in relative hyperintensity) within the erythrocytes in the subarachnoid space (the oxygen tension in the subarachnoid space is relatively high, thereby maintaining oxyhaemoglobin for longer periods of time than might otherwise be expected).

As mentioned previously, statistics on CT sensitivity in demonstrating SAH's vary greatly (e.g., from 55 to 100% if we consider data published over the last 20 years). This great variability can be attributed to at least two factors: the first being the time of the CT examination performance, because those performed within 24 hours of the onset of symptoms result in positive rates of 93% - 100% of cases, whereas for those performed on the second day the figures drop to 63-87%; and the second factor being the particular medical centre where the patient is hospitalized, as those with greater experience also treat more serious cases in which

cur in subjects with low haemoglobin counts may be less hyperdense and therefore more difficult to identify. On the contrary, larger SAH's, which tend to clot in contact with the CSF, widespread bleeding is more common and is therefore more easily detected using CT.

With the exception of these findings, the current improvements in sensitivity are due largely to the progress made in the technology with regard to higher spatial and contrast resolution; from the 55% sensitivity of first generation equipment, we have now reached numbers approaching 100% sensitivity for modern day CT appliances (26). It should also be noted that the reduction in the time elapsing between the event and the moment in which the CT scan is performed can be attributed to the greater distribution of equipment throughout the world. Lastly, progress has been made in the interpretation of subtle changes, which are usually caused by more focal blood collections (Fig. 1.51). In stable patients, CT is suitable for de-

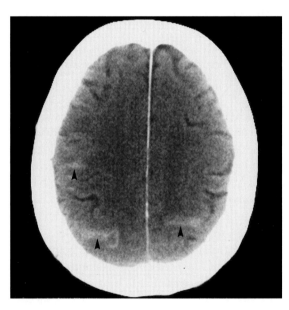

Fig. 1.51 - Curcumscribed SAH signalled by focal blood extravasations in some of the cortical sulci (arrows).

termining not only the presence of extravasated blood in the subarachnoid space (which confirms the clinical suspicion of SAH), but also the dominant site of the haemorrhage, the dimensions of the cerebral ventricular chambers on sequential scans, and the presence of early complications, which may or may not be detected during clinical examinations.

In this acute phase, and depending on the experience and expectations of the surgical staff, CT documentation of SAH may make it unnecessary to perform emergency angiography; this is especially true when early surgery is not planned. However, in the case of a negative CT scan and a clinical picture suggestive of SAH, the definitive diagnosis relies on a diagnostic lumbar puncture. This happens most commonly when CT is carried out late (i.e., more than 12 hours from the ictus) (24, 26) or occasionally very early, within the first few hours (1). The former situation has already been sufficiently discussed, while the second circumstance is somewhat rare. Nevertheless, when the initial CT scan is negative, a diagnostic lumbar puncture is mandated in patients that present with meningeal symptoms (e.g., spontaneous onset of stiff neck), when its main function is to exclude other types of pathology that might be responsible for the clinical signs, such as meningitis.

In patients with poor neurological status, CT should be the first diagnostic imaging investigation performed, considering the possible risk of internal herniation of the cerebellar tonsils posed by a diagnostic lumbar puncture. Subject to emergency angiography, many such cases may require early surgery aimed at addressing complications such as acute hydrocephalus and intraparenchymal haematomas. Such surgery can remove the viscous clots from the basal subarachnoid cisterns and place clips on aneurysms before vasospasm develops (34). The ability of CT to detect such complications in the hyperacute phase, which often prove fatal, makes CT essential in order to define whether surgery is required or whether, for example, conservative monitoring of the intracranial pressure is preferable.

At some point in the patient's clinical course, selective cerebral angiography is almost always recommended in order to establish the nature of the responsible vascular lesion (e.g., aneurysm, arteriovenous malformation) as well as the dimensions, orientation and accessibility of the intracranial vessels and the vascular origin of the anomaly, which are sometimes altered by vasospasm.

Cisternal hyperdensity related to the SAH declines with time as a consequence of clot and red blood cell lysis, in part in proportion to the resorption of haemoglobin and plasma proteins (8). Generally speaking, blood is no longer documented by CT within a week following the ictus, and if hyperdensity does persist beyond this period, it is more likely that it is due to rebleeding. In the subacute phase, typically more than three days after the bleed, and especially in chronic cases, a rapid decline in CT sensitivity is usually mirrored by increasing MRI sensitivity. In certain studies, MR has proved to be 100% accurate in cases studied 3-45 days after the stroke (21); in particular this has been observed in those cases where FLAIR (fluid attenuation inversion recovery) sequences have been used, making it the technique of choice in the subacute phase of SAH.

CAUSES

As mentioned previously, most SAH's are caused by the rupture of aneurysms at the base of the brain. This condition is rather frequent, as aneurysms are found in approximately 1-2% of all routine autopsies. Fortunately, it has also been found that only a small number of all aneurysms subsequently rupture (1 in 17). Aneurysm ruptures are infrequent during childhood and adolescence, and reach a peak between 35 and 65 years of age. Aneurysms are thought to form as a consequence of congenital defects or weaknesses in arterial walls coupled with subsequent degenerative changes associated with aging. Aneurysms statistically prevail in certain families, and there is a considerably higher incidence of such aneurysms in hypertensive patients, those with polycystic kidney disease or coarctation of the thoracic aorta. Approximately 90-95% of aneurysms originate in the anterior half of the circle of Willis. The four most common sites are the anterior communicating artery (30%), the origin of the posterior communicating artery from the internal carotid artery (25%), the middle cerebral artery bifurcation/trifurcation (20%), and the bifurcation of the supraclinoid internal carotid artery into

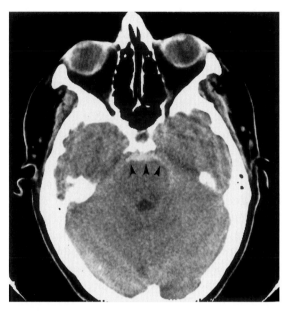

Fig. 1.52 - So-called «sine materia» SAH picture, with exclusive blood localization in the perimesencephalic area (in this case mainly towards the left side, arrows). The angiograph of the 4 vessels is completely negative, both at the time of hospitalization and on a control performed one week later.
The patient, who was awake and in good conditions at onset, recovered completely a few days later.

the middle and anterior cerebral arteries (10%). Other locations are rare; the basilar artery is involved only in 5% of cases. In 20% of cases, aneurysms are multiple, and their dimensions are variable among each other. However, bleeding is more frequent in those aneurysms that are less than 1 cm in diameter, and is most common in those with a diameter of 3-5 mm (Fig. 1.53b). This accounts for the rarity of their being identified using CT, at least when "standard" techniques are employed. Large (i.e., diameter 1-2.5 cm) and giant (i.e., diameter 2.5 cm or larger) aneurysms rarely present with SAH. Instead, they often present with neurological symptoms related to their mass effect (e.g., paralysis of the 3rd cranial nerve due to an aneurysm of the posterior communicating artery in the parasellar area). Other types of aneurysms, including mycotic and atherosclerotic aneurysms, in turn distinguished by their morphology into fusiform, or diffuse globular, only rupture very rarely.

The CT findings of intracranial aneurysms are closely linked to their site and vessel origin. As most aneurysms are small and localized in the base of the brain, identification in the past was hindered by the spatial resolution of the available CT equipment. In most cases, non-thrombosed saccular aneurysms with thin walls present as round or elongated masses, with moderately high CT density, and are not calcified. After IV contrast administration, enhancement of their residual lumen is uniformly hyperdense. Smaller aneurysms are more difficult to visualize, and this is usually only possible when they are located within or next to the subarachnoid spaces. With the advent of spiral CT technology, so-called CT angiography has made detection of these smaller aneurysms much easier. This technique uses three-dimensional reconstructions of the vessels after IV administration of a contrast agent bolus and can provide valuable information for surgical planning (22), sometimes even more so than conventional angiography. In many cases, it is more effective than conventional angiographic techniques in illustrating the neck, shape and dimensions of the aneurysm as well as its position and relationship with surrounding structures (18).

MRI and MR angiography in particular are often even more effective in detecting aneurysms than CT; nevertheless, a conventional selective angiographic investigation remains compulsory (Figs. 1.53b and 1.55b). Despite the fact that uncontrolled use of the latter affects overall medical costs in this condition, it is nevertheless considered essential, especially in surgical planning (14).

We do not intend to prolong this discussion of aneurysms beyond its application in SAH, except to highlight the fact that in recent years a number of studies have been performed to analyse the use of CT and especially MRI in screening for potential occult, asymptomatic aneurysms, particularly when there is a family history of aneurysms (5), and known, non-ruptured aneurysms (33).

Aneurysm rupture usually presents in a dramatic fashion and typically causes sudden, violent headaches, cardio-circulatory collapse, relative conservation of consciousness and a paucity of lateralizing signs (34). The second most frequent cause of SAH after aneurysms (with the exception of traumatic forms, which will be

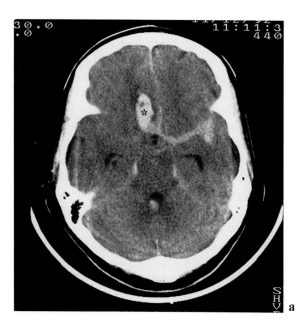

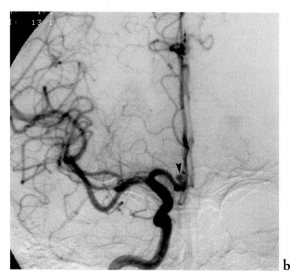

Fig. 1.53 - (**a**) large right frontal haematoma (*) and widespread subarachnoid bleeding mainly at the root of the Sylvian fissure are the most striking aspects of this small aneurysm which ruptured in the stretch between A1 and A2 (**b**). This is accompanied by a small haematic layer in the fourth ventricle and the perimesencephalic cisterns.

dealt with separately) is the rupture of arteriovenous malformations (AVM's), of which some 50% present with haemorrhage (both intraparenchymal and subarachnoid); in a small percentage of cases the patients have prodromic signs such as epileptic disorders. They are most frequent during childhood and are often directly documented by CT, although MRI and selective angiography in particular are yet more sensitive. The latter documents AVM's in accurate anatomical and haemodynamic detail.

Another condition that may be associated with SAH (approx. 12%) is non-specific spontaneous intraparenchymal haemorrhages. Other rarer causes of SAH are blood dyscrasias, intraventricular neoplasia and metastases that are cortically located (especially metastatic melanoma) (8).

Interestingly, in a percentage of cases that ranges from 7 to 28% according to different published studies, SAH's occur without any definable cause. These cases have had completely negative selective angiography, even when the study is repeated some time after the ictus. These cases are termed idiopathic or *sine materia*, indicating the failure to identify the determining cause rather than the actual absence of a pathological cause. Such forms typically present with a specific haemorrhage distribution pattern within the perimesencephalic cisterns, and therefore they are often termed perimesencephalic SAH's (11, 25). In fact, unlike aneurysm ruptures, in which CT shows blood in the basal subarachnoid cisterns that also spreads to the Sylvian and interhemispheric cisterns, these idiopathic cases (Fig. 1.52) generally show a focal blood deposit in the perimesencephalic cistern alone, without spreading to contiguous subarachnoid spaces. These focal haemorrhages are also clearly different from the blood of ruptured aneurysms in the posterior aspect of the circle of Willis, in which CT usually documents massive bleeding into the basal subarachnoid cisterns, and occasionally reveals retrograde haemorrhage into the fourth ventricle. These forms are also sometimes termed "benign" because at onset their clinical conditions are far less dramatic and their eventual clinical outcome is more favourable, in part because these SAH's are much less subject to complications. Although their blood distribution is sufficiently typical, it is common practice to follow CT with selective angiography to study all four vessels. In order to rule out aneurysm rupture altogether, selective angiography must be repeated some time later (9).

With the exception of these forms of SAH, selective angiography can be falsely negative due to: 1) severe vascular spasm that prevents the blood flow from reaching the aneurysm; and 2) the presence of thrombus within the aneurysm lumen that makes it angiographically invisible (34).

Site

As we have already mentioned, CT does not reliably document the presence of aneurysms. Nevertheless, on the basis of the predominant localization of haemorrhagic hyperdensity in particular cisternal areas, CT is often able to define the probable origin of the bleed, and by inference the location of the aneurysm responsible for the haemorrhage. This is possible in up to 52% of cases; the highest accuracy rate is obtained for the rupture of aneurysms of the anterior cerebral and anterior communicating arteries (sensitivity 79%, specificity 96%).

However, CT's ability to accurately forecast the localization of ruptured aneurysms of the middle cerebral artery, the supraclinoid internal carotid artery, and the posterior circulation arteries is far lower (29). Although the association of an intraparenchymal haematoma contributes to determining the location of aneurysms, this factor does not account for more than one-quarter of all SAH's.

Despite these limitations, we will attempt to define the most common findings concerning the various sites of aneurysm rupture.

1) In aneurysm ruptures of the anterior communication artery, hyperdensity prevails in the suprasellar cisterns and the anterior aspect of the interhemispheric fissure, from where it tends to spread to the bifrontal regions. The callosal and cingulate gyri are often "outlined" by blood, which is also frequently present surrounding the brainstem and within the Sylvian fissures; in some cases this haemorrhage is in a somewhat asymmetrical distribution (Fig. 1.54b). Unilateral dominance of the blood therefore does not exclude bleeding from the anterior communicating artery. In the larger haemorrhages, these findings may be accompanied by satellite frontobasal or septal intracere-

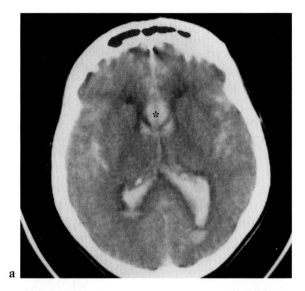

a

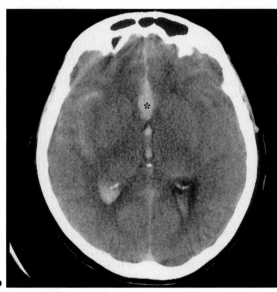

b

Fig. 1.54 - Validity of CT in defining the site of the bleed.
The presence of a haematoma of the septum pellucidum hollow
(*) in its typical midline position between the frontal horns
constitutes an accurate localizing element, as it is almost invariably associated with the rupture of an aneurysm of the anterior
cerebral artery. In (**a**) the following are present: widespread
bleed inside the Sylvian fissures, the cortical sulci and the anterior interhemisperic fissure and massive inundation of the ventricular chambers. In (**b**): a blood collection in the right Sylvian
fissure, blocking of the 3rd ventricle and involvement of the
sloping part of the lateral ventricles.

Failure to demonstrate blood within the anteri-
or interhemispheric fissure militates against the
rupture of an anterior communicating artery
aneurysm (34). It should also be pointed out
that it is important to pay attention to distinguishing the normal falx cerebri from the extravasated blood. The posterior or retrocallosal
falx cerebri can in fact be visualised in 88% of
normal patients, whereas the anterior extent of
the falx is only visible in 38% of cases (35).
Therefore, if interhemispheric hyperdensity
(Figs. 1.50, 1.54, 1.56) does not spread laterally
to the paramedian sulci and does not show evolution in density, volume or extent on subsequent CT examinations, it obviously represents
a normal finding.

2) Aneurysms of the middle cerebral artery
bifurcation/trifurcation (Fig. 1.55) invariably
produce a unilateral bleed within the Sylvian fissure and often in the adjacent suprasellar cistern.
Other possible findings in such cases include
temporal or insular lobe parasylvian intraparenchymal haematomas and rupture into the
temporal horns of the lateral ventricles (usually
only present in cases of lobar haematoma).
Whereas bleeding in the Sylvian cisterns is often caused by an aneurysm of the middle cerebral artery, temporal haematomas can also be
due to other causes, including bleeding from
AVM, neoplasm or more rarely hypertension
(i.e., "spontaneous" form).

3) Aneurysms of the supraclinoid internal
carotid artery and the posterior cerebral artery
may present with a range of haemorrhagic localizations including the suprasellar and interpeduncular cisterns, the medial temporal
lobe, the Sylvian fissure, the anterior interhemispheric fissure and the paranuclear area adjacent to the head of the caudate nucleus.

4) Aneurysms at the tip of the basilar artery
tend to bleed in the interpeduncular, perimesencephalic and suprasellar cisterns, and spread
to the peripeduncular and prepontine ciserns
and the parasylvian regions, with or without
parenchymal brainstem haematoma formation.

5) Aneurysms of the intradural segment of
the distal vertebral or posterior inferior cerebellar artery present with bleeding that mainly
affects the prepontine and pericerebellar cis-

bral haematomas. Haematomas localized in the
cavum septi pellucidi are more or less diagnostic of such aneurysms; however, such findings
are not observed in more than 50% of cases (32).

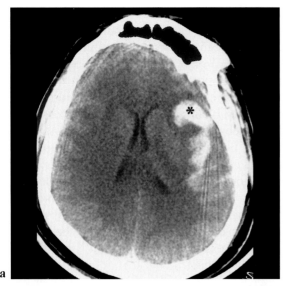

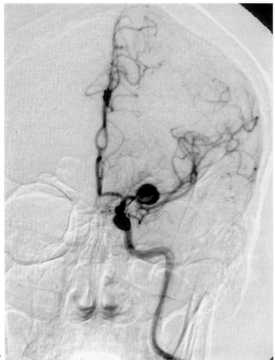

Fig. 1.55 - (**a**) the irregular haemorrhagic collection inside the Sylvian fissure (*) and above all, the presence of an adjacent comma-shaped haematoma suggest the rupture of an aneurysm of the middle cerebral artery. The angiograph (**b**) confirmed the presence of a «giant» aneurysm in this position.

terns; in these cases, obstruction of the outlets of the 4th ventricle may occur.

6) Aneurysms arising from the pericallosal artery are somewhat rare, and when they bleed tend to result in a pathognomonic haemorrhage within the anterior pericallosal cistern. They are also often associated with frontal lobe and callosal intraparenchymal haematomas.

7) In addition to the distribution of blood in the subarachnoid spaces, a further important and accurate topographic criterion is represented by parenchymal haematomas adjacent to the SAH (24). We have already mentioned examples of haematomas of the cavum septi pellucidi (e.g., in anterior communicating artery aneurysms), and temporal lobe and paranuclear bleeds (e.g., in middle and posterior cerebral artery aneurysms). So-called "comma-shaped" haematomas of the Sylvian fissure (Fig. 1.55a) are characteristic of middle cerebral artery aneuryms and can usually be easily differentiated from those of the external capsule in hypertensive patients presenting with spontaneous forms.

8) Finally, it has been observed that in the presence of parenchymal haematomas, the percentage of aneurysms directly visualized on CT after bolus IV contrast administration is estimated to be between 30% and 76% (32).

Size of haemorrhage vs. prognosis

CT enables an overall assessment of the quantity of blood that has extravasated during a SAH. This means that it is possible to utilise CT to estimate patient prognosis at the onset of the ictus (10). The general rule in such cases is: "the more blood, the worse prognosis"; scoring systems have been proposed for SAH evaluation using CT aimed at linking these scores to the patient's clinical evolution, including the occurrence of subsequent sequelae such as rebleeding, vasospasm and cerebral infarction (13). Consideration is given to either the widespread (Figs. 1.50, 1.54a) or focal (Fig. 1.56a) appearance of the bleeding and the size of clots in the cisterns and fissures. These clots can be divided into "thin" and "thick" categories based on their greatest dimension (Fig. 1.56). Generally speaking, a "thin", focal haemorrhage indicates a limited SAH, and is typically accompanied by a milder onset of symptomatology, a more favourable outcome and a reduced probability of complications. The widespread or locally "thick" forms of

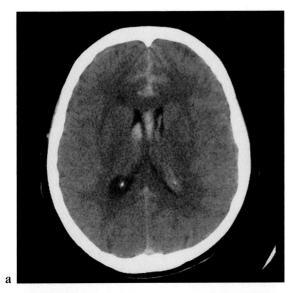

a

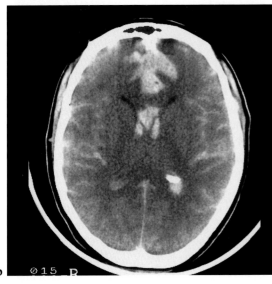

b

Fig. 1.56 - CT's role in the prognostic definition of SAH. CT scans concerning two cases of aneurysm ruptures of the anterior communicating artery. In both the haematoma of the septum pellucidum hollow is typical. The different entity of the bleed is clearly shown by the thickness of hyperdensity in the anterior interhemispheric fissure and in the adjacent cortical sulci (very in **a** thin and thick in **b**), by the diffusion of the bleed (widespread in **b**), by the type of ventricular involvement (in **a** restricted to a clot in the frontal horn, massive in **b**). The patient in case (**a**) was in discreet neurological conditions and was subjected to surgery without subsequent complications. Patient **b** was in a coma when the examination was carried out and died a few hours later.

haemorrhage are commonly seen in patients in more grave clinical condition and with worse prognoses, in whom serious sequelae are likely to occur. Despite the obvious inaccuracy of this approach, it does tend to be relatively valid in forecasting survival and the probability of the development of subsequent neurological symptoms (2).

Contrast agent use

In acute SAH, CT is usually performed without the IV administration of contrast agents, as this does not typically affect patient management. In fact, within the first 72 hours of the ictus it may mask the presence of SAH due to the enhancement of the vessels and even the leptomeninges surrounding the basal subarachmnoid cisterns, a result of the ongoing chemical meningitis related to the SAH. Gross extravasation of contrast material into the subarachnoid space through a ruptured aneurysm during a CT examination is rare, but when observed is associated with an extremely unfavourable prognosis (16). IV contrast agent use in CT sometimes makes it possible to visualize the lumens of smaller aneurysms, although is it easy to confuse the findings with loops within native arteries.

Later, within one to two weeks of the ictus, it is possible to see a subtle widespread or focal enhancement of the basal cisterns and the regional surfaces of the cortical sulci (50-60% of cases). As noted above, this is linked to a chemical meningitis in response to the SAH. This is associated with increased vascularization and a change in vessel permeability of the leptomeninges, which favours the accumulation of contrast material in these regions (20). This is further associated with an increased incidence of delayed hydrocephalus, which may be secondary to the chemical arachnoiditis (27). Finally, contrast agents can be helpful in a limited number of cases in the subacute stage in which the presence of enhancement of the leptomeninges and basal arachnoid cisterns reveals a prior noxious event (i.e., SAH).

COMPLICATIONS

Vasospasm, ischaemia, infarction

Cerebral ischaemia during the acute phase represents the most frequent cause of death and disability in SAH's (6, 12). The incidence of vasospasm as determined from angiography statistics and transcranial echo-Doppler examinations varies from 20 to 75%. In general, vasospasm usually occurs approximately 3-6 days after the ictus and reaches a peak of severity around day ten.

The pathogenesis of vasospasm and its sequelae is not completely clear and a number of contributing factors have been considered. These factors are primarily attributed to the toxic or irritational actions of substances within the clots or the subsequent blood breakdown products.

Vasospasm is usually diagnosed using transcranial Doppler techniques to measure blood flow velocity (2). There is usually a prognostic correlation between the SAH characteristics on the CT study with the subsequent development of a significant vasospasm. If, for example, the amount of SAH blood is minimal as determined by CT, vasospasm only occurs in 8-10% of cases. This correlation is more valid in younger patients; it is well known that vasospasm is somewhat age-dependent and occurs more frequently and to a greater degree in the elderly.

The relationship of vasospasm to rebleeding is important (34). In fact, in the case of a single haemorrhage, cerebral infarction occurs in 22% of cases, while infarction occurs in 41% of cases of rebleeding (12). Vasospasm can be either focal and in proximity to an aneurysm, or diffuse.

Clinically, significant vasospasm always causes a neurological deterioration due to the underlying cerebral ischaemia caused by the vascular narrowing, which tends to be progressive although gradual (a rapid worsening usually indicates rebleeding) (17). CT is obviously not able to show vasospasm, but it does reveal the ischaemic consequences upon the cerebral parenchyma, the most serious of which is infarction.

Even though vasospasm is the most common cause of infarcts following SAH, ischaemic alteration can also be secondary to compression of vessels resulting from the mass effect of a regional intraparenchymal haematoma, or less frequently thrombic emboli originating from vascular flow reduction (20).

In agreement with angiographic findings, delayed ischaemic lesions occur in 22-60% of cases of aneurysms (12). The resolution of the vasospasm is usually accompanied by an improvement in the clinical condition (15).

Hydrocephalus

Hydrocephalus may occur either in the immediate period following the SAH or alternatively from two weeks to six months later. Hydrocephalus results from alterations in normal CSF reabsorption or from mechanical obstruction, both of which are caused by subarachnoid space and intraventricular blood. Many SAH patients develop acute hydrocephalus within the first 48 hours of the initial bleed (one to two cases out of three).

There is a certain correlation between the quantity of blood in the ventricles and the subsequent development of hydrocephalus. The initial CT examination is therefore important in establishing the extent of haemorrhage and the baseline ventricular size for the purpose of monitoring the patient in whom clinical conditions are not critical and do not therefore require immediate shunt placement.

Acute hydrocephalus can be transient, if normal CSF dynamics are restored after reabsorption of the SAH. However, so long as there is blood in the subarachnoid pathways, the formation of adhesions is a risk (i.e., basal arachnoiditis) with the potential of resulting in permanent hydrocephalus of the communicating type (8). In many such patients a shunt may therefore be required. Hydrocephalus and the associated neurological deterioration can benefit by prolonged treatment with tranexamic acid (31).

Rebleeding

The incidence of this complication reaches a peak 7 to 12 days after the initial SAH and occurs in 20 - 25% of cases (34); rebleeding carries with it a mortality rate of approximately 50%. It is accompanied by a worsening in neurological status. Rebleeding remains the most important cause of a seriously worsening prognosis, even in cases that have undergone early surgery (23).

The most important diagnostic criterion of rebleeding is an obvious sequential increase in density of the subarachnoid spaces on CT that follows an initial gradual reduction in the initial haemorrhagic hyperdensity during the first few days after the ictus. It is also important to consider persistent hyperdensity apparent on a CT examination performed more than seven days after the ictus as a probable expression of rebleeding.

Intraparenchymal haematoma (IPH)

IPH occurring adjacent to a ruptured aneurysm is identified on CT in 15% (29) to 27% (8) of cases of SAH. These figures are probably slightly overestimated as they only include the most seriously ill patients, in whom complications are most frequently encountered. IPH's are almost always accompanied by a rapidly progressive deterioration in clinical status (34). The appearance of IPH in these cases is much the same as with other forms of clinical stroke, irrespective of the SAH.

Intraventricular haemorrhage (IVH)

IVH can be observed in association with any ruptured aneurysm, although the distribution of intraventricular blood seldom indicates the origin of the haemorrhage. However, ruptured aneurysms of the AICA (anterior communicating artery) can rupture into the 3rd ventricle and the area of the intraventricular foramen of Monro; and aneurysms of the PICA (posterior inferior cerebellar artery), vertebral artery and basilar trunk often cause reflux of blood into the 3rd and the 4th ventricles, without reaching the lateral ventricles.

Blood in the cerebral ventricles is almost always accompanied by dilation, accounting for the most frequent cause of hydrocephalus in patients with SAH. It has been observed that the dimensions of the ventricular chambers correlate with clinical outcome more accurately than the dimensions of the blood clots they contain. Generally speaking, the more dilated are the ventricles, the worse is the clinical status and the greater is the need for a ventricular shunt (some experts hold that this can cause greater risk of aneurysm rebleeding) (34).

Subdural haematoma (SDH)

SDH's in association with SAH are most commonly caused by ruptures of circle of Willis and middle cerebral artery bifurcation/trifurcation aneurysms. The CT characteristics of these SDH's are not dissimilar to traumatic forms. They are always accompanied by progressive neurological deterioration and usually require surgical drainage.

A progressive worsening of neurological conditions in patients with SAH can be caused by a number of extracerebral causes, such as infections, pulmonary embolism, gastric haemorrhage and myocardial infarcts. In such cases, CT is obviously negative with regard to SDH.

POSTSURGICAL FOLLOW-UP

After surgical aneurysm clipping, the CT accuracy for focal SAH or aneurysm recurrence diminishes due to the imaging artefacts created by the metal clips (Fig. 1.57). Nevertheless, CT remains the imaging technique of choice in cases of worsening of post-surgical condition or when there is a delay in the normally expected timeframe of recovery. CT is particularly suitable for the demonstration or sequential follow-up of infarcted areas caused by post-surgical vasospasm. Vasospasm can also be indirectly presumed from CT in emergent forms where frank cerebral infarction is not evident, especially if the other more frequent postsurgical complications such as hydrocephalus and rebleeding are excluded (34).

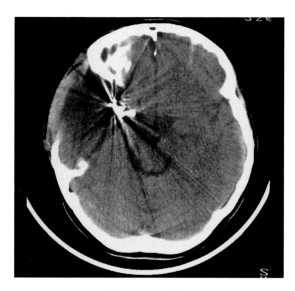

Fig. 1.57 - Postsurgical CT may not always prove accurate due to the overlapping of artefacts produced by the metal clips. It is usually required to distinguish between the main surgical complications (hydrocephalus, vasospasm, rebleeding). In this case there is widespread hypodensity adjacent to the craniotomy, presumably exclusively due to subsequent malacic sequelae.

CONCLUSIONS

CT has had dramatic effects upon the primary diagnosis and management of SAH patients. The rapidity with which it is performed and its overall accuracy make it the imaging technique of choice in all patients with suspected SAH. It is preferable that the CT examination be performed at an early stage as it has been shown that those having CT studies performed later ultimately have the more severe prognoses (7).

Immediately after the stroke, CT provides information on the extent and distribution of bleeding, as well as signs of possible early complications such as hydrocephalus, intraparenchymal haemorrhage, and presence of developing ischaemic areas. The appearance of some of these complications, in particular intracerebral haematomas with mass effect and acute hydrocephalus, is of practical importance as they usually require immediate neurosurgical treatment.

CT findings correlate well with patient status as the imaging observations are usually more striking in those patients with disorders of consciousness or other severe neurological alterations. The role of CT in long-term recovery prognosis is not yet clear (3). However, its ability of early diagnosis undeniably improves overall clinical outcomes.

CT can also demonstrate SAH in patients in whom SAH is not clinically suspected, and positive findings can also exclude the need to perform diagnostic lumbar punctures; the latter are usually only performed in patients whose symptoms suggest SAH but in whom CT is negative (24, 26). With regard to other medical imaging techniques, we have already mentioned that MRI has a limited role to play in the acute and hyperacute phases of SAH; MRI is more suitable than CT in subacute phases, indicating that the two imaging techniques play a complementary roles from a temporal point of view. MRI also plays a role in aneurysm, and particularly AVM, evaluation when combined with MR angiography.

CT has had a considerable effect on the use of selective cerebral angiography in the diagnosis and follow-up of patients with SAH. Surgery can be postponed after the emergent phase, especially in gravely ill patients, until clinical conditions have stabilized. In turn, CT can direct both angiography and surgery towards the more likely area of aneurysm rupture (28). All of these reasons make CT not only the most suitable, but also the most rapidly accessible imaging examination to be performed in patients with acute clinical stroke.

REFERENCES

1. Andrioli G, Cavazzani P: Differential diagnosis of subarachnoid hemorrhage. Minerva Anestesiol 64:141-144, 1998.
2. Boecher-Schwartz HG, Fries G, Mueller-Forell W et al: Cerebral blood flow velocities after subarachnoid haemorrhage in relation to the amount of blood clots in the initial computed tomography. Acta Neurochir 140:573-578, 1998.
3. Botia E, Vivancos J, Leon T et al: Predictive mortality factors and the development of major complications in non-traumatic subarachnoid hemorrhage. Rev Neurol 24:193-198, 1996.
4. Brouwers PJ, Dippel DW, Vermeulen M et al: Amount of blood on computed tomography as an independent predictor after aneurysm rupture. Stroke 24:809-814, 1993.

5. Brown BM, Soldevilla F: MR angiography and surgery for unruptured familiar intracranial aneurysms in persons with a family history of cerebral aneurysms. AJR 173:133-138, 1999.

6. Cesarini KG, Hardemark HG, Persson L: Improved survival after aneurysmal subarachnoid hemorrhage: review of case management during a 12-year period. J Neurosurg 90:664-672, 1999.

7. Chan BS, Dorsch NW: Delayed diagnosis in subarachnoid haemorrhage. Med J Aust 154:509-511, 1991.

8. Cirillo S, Simonetti L, Sirabella G et al: Patologia vascolare. In: Dal Pozzo G: Compendio di Tomografia Computerizzata (pp. 127-147) USES Edizioni Scientifiche Florence, 1991.

9. Duong H, Melancon D, Tampieri D et al: The negative angiogram in subarachnoid haemorrhage. Neuroradiology 38:15-19, 1996.

10. Germanson TP, Lanzino G, Kongable GL et al.: Risk classification after aneurysmal subarachnoid hemorrhage. Surg Neurol 49:155-163, 1998.

11. Gilbert JW, Lee C, Young B: Repeat cerebral panangiography in subarachnoid hemorrage of unknown etiology. Surg Neurol 33:19-21, 1990.

12. Gruber A, Dietrich W, Richling B: Recurrent aneurysmal subarachnoid haemorrhage: bleeding pattern and incidence of posthaemorrhagic ischaemic infarction. Br J Neurosurg 11:121-126, 1997.

13. Hijdra A, van Gijn J, Nagelkerke NJ et al: Prediction of delayed cerebral ischaemia, rebleeding, and outcome after aneurysmal subarachnoid haemorrage. Stroke 19:1250-1256, 1988.

14. Kallmes DF, Kallmes MH: Cost-effectiveness of angiography performed during surgery for ruptured intracranial aneurysms. AJNR 18:1453-1462, 1997.

15. Kassel NF, Sasaki T, Colohan AR et al: Cerebral vasospasm following aneurysmal SAH. Stroke 15:562, 1985.

16. Kingsley DP: Extravasation of contrast-enhanced blood into the subarachnoid space during computed tomography. Neuroradiology 18:259-262, 1979.

17. Kistler JP, Crowell RM, Davis KR: The relation of cerebral vasospasm to the extent and location of subarachnoid blood visualized by CT scan: a prospective study. Neurology 33:424, 1983.

18. Lenhart M, Bretschneider T, Gmeinwieser J et al: Cerebral CT angiography in the diagnosis of acute subarachnoid hemorrhage. Acta Radiol 38:791-796, 1997.

19. Leonardi M: Diagnosis and general assessment of acute subarachnoid hemorrhage. Minerva Anestesiol 64:145-147, 1998.

20. Modic MT, Weinstein MA: Cerebrovascular disease of the brain. In: Haaga JR, Alfidi RJ (eds): Computed tomography of the brain, head and neck (pp. 136-169) The CV Mosby Company St. Louis 1985.

21. Noguchi K, Ogawa T, Seto H et al: Subacute and chronic subarachnoid hemorrhage: diagnosis with fluid attenuated inversion recovery MR imaging. Radiology 203:257-262, 1997.

22. Ohkawa M, Tanabe M, Toyama Y et al: CT angiography with helical CT in the assessment of acute stage of subarachnoid hemorrhage. Radiat Med 16:91-97, 1998.

23. Roos YB, Beenen LF, Goen RJ et al: Timing of surgery in patients with aneurysmal subarachnoid haemorrhage: rebleeding is still the major cause of poor outcome in neurosurgical units that aim at early surgery. J Neurol Neurosurg Psychiatry 63:490-493, 1997.

24. Sames TA, Storrow AB, Finkelstein JA et al: Sensitivity of new-generation computed tomography in subarachnoid hemorrhage. Acad Emerg Med 3:16-20, 1996.

25. Schwartz TH, Solomon RA: Perimesencephalic nonaneurysmal subarachnoid hemorrhage: review of the literature. Neurosurgery 39:433-440, 1996.

26. Sidman R, Connolly E, Lemke T: Subarachnoid hemorrhage diagnosis: lumbar puncture is still needed when the computed tomography scan is normal. Acad Emerg Med 3:827-831, 1996.

27. Sobal D: Cisternal enhancement after subarachnoid hemorrage. AJNR 2:549-552, 1981.

28. Terbrugge KG, Rao KC, Lee SH: Cerebral vascular anomalies. In: Lee SH, Rao KC (eds): Cranial Computed Tomography and MRI (pp. 607-641) Mc Graw- Hill Book Company New York, 1987.

29. van der Jagt M, Hasan D, Bijvoet HW et al: Validity of prediction of the site of ruptured intracranial aneurysms with CT. Neurology 52:34-39, 1999.

30. Vale FL, Bradley EL, Fisher WS: The relationship of subarachnoid hemorrhage and the need for postoperative shunting. J Neurosurgery 86:462-466, 1997.

31. Vermeij FH, Hasan D, Vermeulen M et al: Predictive factors for deterioration from hydrocephalus after subarachnoid hemorrhage. Neurology 44:1851-1855, 1994.

32. Yock DH, Larson DA: Computed Tomography of hemorrage from anterior communicating artery aneurysms with angiographic correlation. Radiology 134:399-407, 1980.

33. Yoshimoto Y, Wakai S: Cost-effectiveness analysis of screening for asymptomatic, unrupted intracranial aneurysms. A mathematical model. Stroke 30:1621-1627, 1999.

34. Weisberg LA, Nice C: Cerebral Computed Tomography: A text atlas (pp. 163-179). WB Saunders Philadelphia, 1989.

35. Zimmerman RD, Yurberg E, Leeds NE: The falx and interhemispheric fissure on axial computed tomography: I. Normal anatomy. AJNR 3:175-180, 1982.

1.5

MRI IN ISCHAEMIA

L. Simonetti, S. Cirillo, R. Agati

INTRODUCTION

Magnetic Resonance Imaging (MRI) has brought about substantial changes in the diagnostic algorithms formulated in almost all aspects of Central Nervous System (CNS) pathology. This has occurred in part secondary to MRI's greater sensitivity to changes in the water content of the tissue examined, and therefore, in demonstrating all categories of CNS pathology.

However, in the particular case of ischaemic cerebral vascular disease, MRI initially had a more limited impact, due mainly to the large preceding experience gained in the treatment of this type of pathology using CT, and therefore the resulting clinical reliance on the CT semeiology (3, 4). This situation has recently undergone profound changes, both with regard to the technical progress made in MRI as well as to the newer treatments that are being introduced, in particular thrombolysis (2, 5, 7, 12-15).

The diagnostic questions a clinician poses with regard to the patient with ischaemic cerebrovascular disease are mainly concerned with the site, extent and time of the ictus, the clinical severity of the ischaemic lesion, the potential reversibility of the damage and the presence or absence of reperfusion. Because it is now

universally recognized that early surgery can potentially improve or even reverse otherwise serious events such as cerebral ischemia, the necessity to respond in the very first minutes and hours following the onset of the neurological deficit has become all the more pressing (1, 6, 8-11, 16).

The responses to such important considerations often surpass the capabilities of traditional neuroradiological imaging techniques to aid in this emergent situation; in the past, CT and MRI only very rarely provided direct diagnostic information during the first six hours from an ischaemic cerebral event. This is predictable given that even from a pathoanatomical point of view "... identification of an ischaemic lesion on human or animal brains cannot be detected by macroscopic examinations less than 24-72 hours from the event" (Davis, 1997).

It therefore follows that, in order to obtain useful diagnostic neuroimaging information in the hyperacute phase, other aspects of ischaemic disease including morphological, macroscopic, submacroscopic, and pathophysiological parameters must be explored.

The rational use of MRI in a way that enhances its intrinsic potential, as well as taking advantages of recent progress in acquisition techniques (e.g., perfusion, diffusion and spectroscopy) have begun to provide answers to the clinical questions posed during the hyperacute phase of cerebral ischaemia. The goal of this chapter is to explore the chronology of the pathophysiological events of acute/hyperacute cerebral ischaemia and consider how these alterations can be investigated using the newer advancements of MRI.

SEMEIOTICS

Arterial occlusion

Generally speaking, the principal cause of cerebral ischaemia is vessel occlusion, in the form of an embolus or a thrombus. It therefore follows that the simplest manner of demonstrating the cause of hyperacute cerebral ischaemia non-invasively is MR angiography to examine the cerebral blood vessels in search of the partially or completely occluded vessel. However, in practice this theoretical observation can be limited by a number of factors:
– the acquisition time required to perform an MR angiographic examination is not compatible with the clinical condition of many patients in the hyperacute phase of cerebrovascular ischaemia, who are often agitated or otherwise uncooperative;
– the poor anatomical definition of the 2nd and 3rd order vascular branches of the cerebral arteries, especially in cases of complete or near complete occlusion;
– the age-related alterations in vascular arboration of the cerebral vasculature in elderly patients results in generalized flow reduction, which can erroneously point to pathology, especially in the presence of flow asymmetries between one hemisphere and the opposite side;
– the presence of clinically silent past vessel stenoses/occlusions.

In short, MR angiography in the hyperacute phase of cerebral ischaemia is a reliable diagnostic technique in young, cooperative patients, a conclusion that is somewhat out of line with the typical profile of the patient presenting with cerebral ischaemia. Although rare in younger age groups, the advantage of MR angiography in the young lies in the fact that it is this category of patient that potentially has the most to gain from prompt, correct diagnosis of vascular events.

Reduction of cerebral perfusion

If prolonged beyond a somewhat unpredictable time period, the reduction in regional cerebral perfusion secondary to arterial stenosis/occlusion leads to the establishment of an ischaemic or frankly infarcted area. This reduction in flow can be studied using MR perfusion.

Generally speaking, there are two main strategies for studying cerebral blood flow: the use of diffusible tracers and the use of strictly intravascular tracers. The use of *diffusible tracers* represents the traditional strategy for studying cerebral perfusion, beginning with Kety's nitrous oxide method, through CT with xenon-133 inhalation, and to PET (positron emission tomography) with $H_2^{15}O$. Although deuterium, fluorine-19 and $H_2^{17}O$ can be used as diffusible tracers in studying brain flow and oxygen consumption with MRI, at present these isotopes are still confined to animal experimentation. In particular, although $H_2^{17}O$ would appear to be very promising, these latter techniques are unlikely to be clinically feasible due to their high cost and to the limited availability of the various isotopes.

Perhaps the most clinically feasible possibilities might include the use of endogenous diffusible tracers such as "arterial" water, whose spins could be marked by the inversion of the MR radiofrequency pulses; if perfected, this technique would have the advantages of being inexpensive, physiological and non-invasive.

The use of endogenous or exogenous *vascular tracers* is currently the most widely employed human brain perfusion study technique. In commonly used experimental models employing this kind of tracer, blood flow is a function of the volume of blood in a tissue and the mean transit time of an ideal instantaneous bolus of the tracer substance passing through the tissue.

MR perfusion images can be obtained either using a bolus of exogenous contrast agent or using methods dependent on the phase contrast of blood flow.

Currently the most common method used employs paramagnetic exogenous contrast agents, in particular gadolinium, which exploits their effects on relaxation times and magnetic susceptibility.

The reduction in T1 relaxation times gained by the IV injection of a gadolinium agent over time is obviously proportionate to the concentration of the contrast agent used, and therefore provides information on tissue perfusion. For example, MR sequences that use inversion pre-pulses (e.g., FLASH, TURBOFLASH) that permit the acquisition of T1-weighted images in less than one second, make it possible to show the hyperaemic areas to be relatively hyperintense as compared to normal brain, while ischaemic areas appear relatively hypointense.

With regard to techniques that exploit the magnetic susceptibility of gadolinium, it should be remembered that magnetic susceptibility results in part in the distortion of the applied magnetic field by the presence of a paramagnetic substance (e.g., gadolinium); this causes artefacts in the MR image, especially if acquired using the pulse sequences referred to above. Such techniques are therefore based on the exploitation of this artefact obtained using long TE sequences, thus obtaining T2*-weighted images. If a series of these pictures are acquired during the injection of a bolus of a paramagnetic contrast agent, it will be possible to evaluate variations in the local blood volume over time. The intravascular passage of a high concentration of the contrast agent through the brain distorts the local magnetic field, thus causing a dephasing of spins in the brain tissue adjacent to the blood vessels and consequentially the artefactual loss of signal due to the effects of magnetic susceptibility and a reduction in T2* relaxation time. This reduction can be measured, and using a complex formula, T2* variation can be correlated to blood volume. Having acquired a series of images that give the mean transit time, we can also obtain a blood volume transit time ratio that corresponds to the cerebral blood flow in traditional vascular tracer models.

The study of animal models and human patients with hyperacute cerebral ischaemia using this technique has demonstrated its validity in illustrating regional hypoperfusion distal to a proximal cerebrovascular occlusion within a few minutes after the vascular blockage. This technique also has the advantage that it can be performed using clinical MRI units fitted to enable the acquisition of serial T2*-weighted images in the brief timeframes referred to above. From this point of view, it is most useful to have access to an MR unit having the capability of ultra-fast echo planar imaging (EPI) acquisitions, which has the advantage of greater temporal definition (i.e., capability of a greater number of images acquired per unit of time) and therefore allows a more accurate discrimination of the relative delay in passage of the contrast media through the ischemic tissue as well as a greater relative degree of sensitivity to magnetic susceptibility artefacts.

Alteration of the Na⁺-K⁺ ion pump

An alteration of the Na^+-K^+ ion pump occurs within 30 minutes of the cerebrovascular occlusion secondary to the consumption and consequent reduction of ATP, which is no longer produced due to the anoxia that blocks the aerobic glycolysis chain. Approximately three minutes after the vascular occlusion, the Na^+-K^+ ion pump dysfunction and the resulting electrolytic alteration it causes, there is an uncontrolled entry of water into the cell, and therefore the establishment of cytotoxic oedema. This intracellular oedema affects various compartments and components of brain tissue (e.g., astrocytes, dendrites, endothelial cells, pericytes, oligodendrocytes); these alterations can be studied using the MR diffusion technique, that demonstrates the "macroscopic" molecular movement of the water. The underlying principle of diffusion-sensitive MR pulse sequences is the addition of a pair of diffusion sensitising pulses to a sequence of otherwise standard imaging pulses that dephases the spins proceeding along the applied diffusion gradient. Due to the signal attenuation caused by the resulting loss of phase coherence, normal diffusion causes a tissue signal loss on images dependent on this parameter. Conversely, tissue areas in which diffusion is reduced (e.g., ischaemia, cytotoxic oedema) appear relatively hyperintense. In vivo diffusion can be quantified using the apparent diffusion coefficient (ADC), which is a function of two parameters: the difference in signal between two differently calibrated diffusion images and a constant known as the "diffusion weighted factor"; in this manner, diffusion weighted images measure variations in the ADC.

Hyperacute ischaemic lesions can appear as areas of reduced diffusion as early as three minutes after occurrence of the embolus/thrombus. It is assumed that the reduction of diffusion in the ischaemic area is connected to the cytotoxic oedema, resulting in part from the alteration of the ion pump, as there is a movement of water from the vast extracellular compartment to the more restricted intracellular compartment. The extent of the area detected at an early stage using diffusion weighted images generally has an excellent correspondence with the actual ischaemic lesion.

Clinically speaking, the largest drawback of MR diffusion imaging techniques is that image quality and sensitivity to variations in the ADC are considerably affected by even the slightest patient movement during the examination, thus restricting its use in acute phase patients who are unable to cooperate fully. Therefore EPI and the possibility it offers of ultrafast acquisitions, is expected to improve the clinical applicability of diffusion weighted imaging.

Lactic acid accumulation

Within ten minutes of cerebrovascular occlusion, intracellular pH drops from approximatey 7.1 to 6.64 due to an increase in lactates secondary to the metabolic shift during hypoxia towards anaerobic glycolysis. This lactic acid increase can multiply fivefold within a very few minutes and contributes to tissue necrosis due to the resulting increase in cellular swelling and the alteration to the blood-brain barrier that it causes; therefore, in cases of ischaemia, hyperglycaemia must be avoided at all costs, as it will only cause an increase in the lactic acid concentration. This metabolic factor can be evaluated using MR spectroscopy; this MRI technique studies the biochemical aspects of brain tissue, not as absolute concentrations of metabolites, but rather as relative concentrations given by the size of the spectroscopic peak corresponding to various molecular species. Proton MR spectroscopy is currently the most widely used technique; this method enables the study of relative concentrations of N-acetyl-aspartate, choline, creatinine and lactate (the lactate peak is almost absent in the normal spectrum). In hyperacute infarcts it is therefore theoretically possible to identify the ischaemic area by the appearance of a noticeable lactate peak in the MR spectrum, which precedes the subsequent drop in N-acetyl-aspartate, a neuron population reduction marker. The main limits to the clinical application of MR spectroscopy are the lengthy acquisition times and the fact that in the area of interest selected the technique requires a voxel size that is generally too large to avoid partial volume effects (i.e., contamination of the sample by relatively normal tissue surrounding the tissue of interest).

Cerebral microcirculation damage

Experiments have shown that within a few minutes after occlusion of the middle cerebral artery, a reduction in flow occurs with the stacking up or stasis of red blood cells in the cerebral microvessels (arterioles, capillaries, venules) and the microcirculation of the nucleus of the ischaemic lesion. This causes a swelling of endothelial cells and perivascular astrocytes and an adhesion between the surface receptors of PMN leucocytes and the corresponding ligands of endothelial cells which brings about a further deterioration of the microcirculation. The mechanical stenosis is

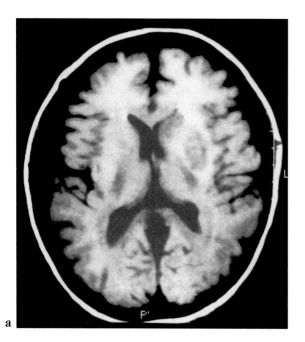

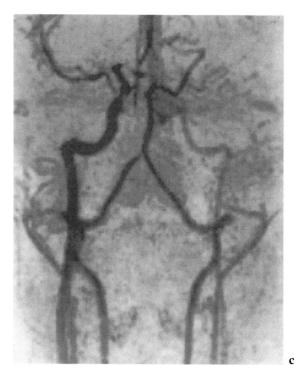

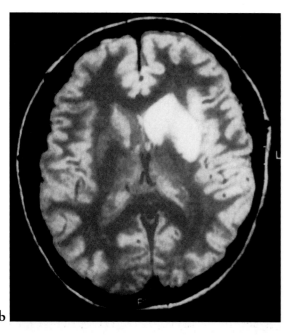

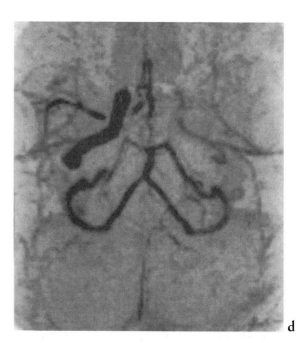

Fig. 1.58 - Acute phase ischaemia (30 hours) in the territory of the left middle cerebral artery in a 20 year-old patient without apparent risk factors. Axial T1- (**a**) a,d PD- (**b**) dependent scans. AP (**c**) and axial (**d**) projections TOF MRA reconstructions. In T1, signal hypointensity in the grey matter of the caudate and left lenticular nuclei, with mass effect on the frontal horn of the homolateral ventricle; signal alteration, as hyperintensity, is clearer in the PD-dependent images. The MRA examination shows a clear reduction in calibre of the left internal carotid artery, from the origin to the siphon, with visualization of the sole M1 tract of the middle cerebral artery, which appears filiform.

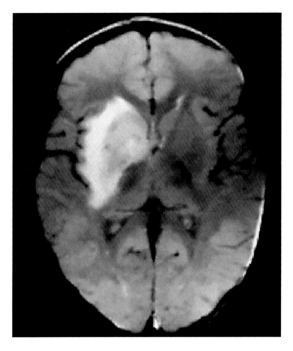

Fig. 1.59 - Acute phase ischaemia in the territory of the perforating arteries. Axial PD-dependent scan. Note the loss of the boundaries of the anatomical structures affected (lenticular nucleus, caudate nucleus, claustrum, internal, external and extreme capsule.

accompanied by a necrotizing effect upon the endothelial cells and the neurons due to the liberation of free radicals. The importance of leukocyte adhesion is shown by the fact that, by administering monoclonal antibodies that prevent leukocyte adhesion, a reduction in the stenosis of the microcircle is obtained, while with administration of interleukin 2 (a leukocyte activator), the clinical status worsens due to an increase in nerve cell damage.

Microcirculation alteration and the consequent congestion and stasis of the local circulation and the pial vessels in hyperacute ischaemia can be studied with MR by the acquisition of T1-dependent images after injection of gadolinium contrast medium. Pathological enhancement of small and medium sized vessels that "mark" the affected area, accompanied by adjacent pial congestion, have been observed within six hours of onset of the ischaemic event. This enhancement is not in any way connected to the extravascular tissue enhancement later observed secondary to blood-brain barrier injury, and is exclusively confined to the vascular compartment.

Oedema

Based on pathoanatomical findings and on micro- and macroscopic clinical, rather than

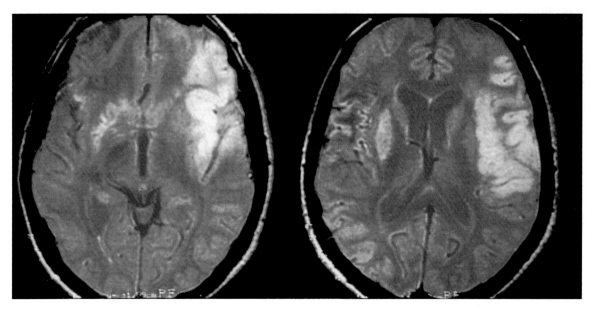

Fig. 1.60 - Acute phase ischaemia (20 hours) in the anterior superficial territory of the left middle cerebral artery. Axial PD-dependent scans: increase in signal of the cortex with increase in volume of the gyri. The white matter is spared.

experimental, features, the development of an types of oedema over time can be broken down as follows:

- 2 hours from vascular occlusion it is possible to observe cytotoxic oedema that commences within a few minutes of the vascular occlusive event;
- 12 hours after the event, cytotoxic oedema can be identified histologically on stained macrosections as a paleness of the affected area; it appears earlier and more obviously in the caudate-putaminal complex than in the cortex;
- after 72-96 hours, the vasogenic oedema results in mass effect;
- in the absence of complications, there is progressive resolution of oedema and mass effect from the 4th day.

It is therefore the cytotoxic oedema that, within 12 hours and occasionally as early as 6 hours from the event, causes the appearance of altered signal areas due to T1- and T2-lengthening (i.e., hypointensity on T1-weighted images, hyperintensity on PD- and T2-weighted images), localized in the cau-

date-putamen complex (Figs. 1.58, 1.59) in ischaemia affecting the perisylvian region. In the subsequent hours, it is still the cytotoxic oedema that appears in much the same fashion in the overlying cortex (Figs. 1.60, 1.61, 1.62).

If studied accurately, CT can also document this pathophysiological situation within the first 12 hours of ictus, seen as disappearance of the normal caudate and putamen hyperdensity as their tissue margins blend into the surrounding white matter. This sign, which indicates vascular occlusion in the territory, is somewhat difficult to perceive (especially if it is not compared with the contralateral putamen), but it is important and has a verified role in early diagnosis as well as in predicting ad unfavourable outcome.

With these CT and MRI signs explained, we will now move from theoretical and experimental neuroradiology to clinical neuroradiology, after concluding that the principal drawback of medical imaging is the large individual variability in appearance times of the findings (from 4 to 12 hours from onset of ictus), a fact

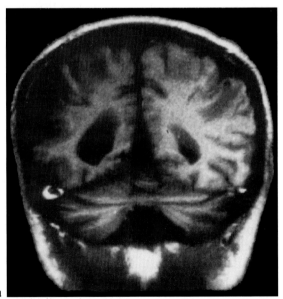 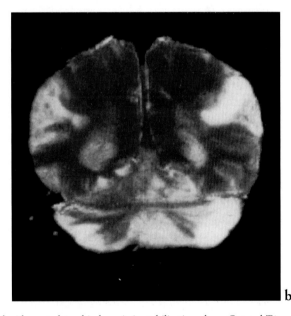

a   b

Fig. 1.61 - Acute phase (36 hours) left parietal ischaemia associated with contralateral ischaemia in stabilization phase. Coronal T1- (**a**) and T2-dependent (**b**) scans. The recent ischaemia appears as a hypodense cortical area in T1, with an increase in volume of the gyrus circumvolution. The finding is less clear in T2, where the difference in signal between acute focus and resolution phase is however evident.

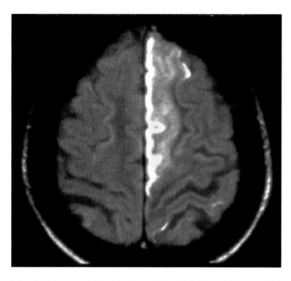

Fig. 1.62 - Acute phase ischaemia in the left anterior cerebral artery territory. Axial PD-dependent scan: note the increase in signal with obliteration of the adjacent cortical sulci.

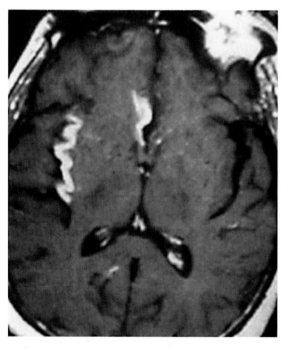

Fig. 1.63 - Hyperintense, haematic rim in T1, in an acute phase ischaemic lesion: note the spiral shape.

that does not always make them suitable for the practical diagnostic evaluation of the patient presenting with clinical evidence of hyperacute cerebral ischaemia.

POSSIBLE USES OF CLINICAL MR IN THE DIAGNOSIS OF EMERGENCY ISCHAEMIA AFTER THE HYPERACUTE PHASE

MRI's greater sensitivity over that of other imaging modalities is useful in identifying parenchymal lesions caused by transient ischaemic attacks (TIA's), where MRI's sensitivity is greater than 70%, compared to approximately 40% for CT.

The clinical course of cerebral infarction can include sudden alteration in the classic progression. Clinical and pathological studies show that such shifts are principally due to the haemorrhagic conversion of the primary ischaemic lesion in the time period between the 2nd and 3rd week; this haemorrhagic incidence can be as high as 80% in infarcts caused by cerebrovascualr embolism. For many years CT contradicted, at least with regard to frequency, the existence of this haemorrhagic phenomenon. However, since the advent of MRI, evidence of haemorrhagic conversion of cerebral infarction is more frequently observed (Fig. 1.63) in MR examinations performed between the 10th and 20th days of the ischaemic ictus; this is especially true in cases arising from embolism or those infarcts located in the vascular territory of the posterior cerebral artery. Such areas were not previously visualized on CT images for a number of reasons, including technical factors, such as partial volume averaging effects and limitations concerning mean attenuation coefficients, and biological factors, such as the relatively rapid evolution of blood products in ischaemic areas. Therefore, in cases of cerebral ischaemia having sudden alterations of clinical status that could be a result of haemorrhagic conversion, the examination of choice is MR rather than CT.

REFERENCES

1. Adams RD, Victor M: Principles of Neurology. McGraw-Hill, Inc., New York: 1985, 508-572.
2. Awad L, Modic M et al: Focal parenchymal lesions in TIA: correlation of CT and MRI. Stroke 17:399-403, 1986.

3. Bastianello S, Brughitta G, Pierallini A et al: Neuroradiological findings in acute cerebral ischemia. In: Ottorino Rossi Award Conference. Zappoli F, Martelli A. (eds). Edizioni del Centauro, Udine, 131-140, 1992.

4. Bozzao L, Angeloni U et al: Early angiographic and CT findings in patients with hemorragic infarction in the distribution of the middle cerebral artery. AJNR, 12:1115-1121, 1991.

5. Brant-Zawadzki M, Pereira B et al: MRI of acute experimental ischemia in rats. AJNR 7:7-11, 1986.

6. Brierley JB: Cerebral hypoxia. In: Blackwood W, Corsellis JAN (eds). "Greenfield's Neuropathology" Chicago: Year Book Medical Publishers 43-85, 1976.

7. Bryan RN, Whitlow WD, Levy LM: Cerebral infarction and ischemic disease. In: Atlas SW (ed). "MRI of brain and spine". New York: Raven Press 411-437, 1991.

8. Duchen LW: General pathology of neurons and neuroglia. In: "Greenfield's neuropathology" Chicago: Year Book Medical Publishers 1-68, 1992.

9. Garcia JH, Anderson ML: Circulatory disorders and their effects on the brain. In: Textbook of Neuropathology. Davis RL & Robertson DL. (eds). William&Wilkins, Baltimore, 1997.

10. Graham DI: Hypoxia and vascular disorders. In: "Greenfield's Neuropathology" Chicago:Year Book Medical Publishers 153-268, 1992.

11. Gullotta F: Vasculopatie cerebrali. In: Schiffer D ed. "Neuropatologia" Roma: Il pensiero scientifico, 1980:155-178.

12. Kendall B: Cerebral ischemia. Rivista di Neuroradiologia 3 (suppl. 2):35-38, 1990.

13. Mathews WP, Witlow WD, Bryan RN: Cerebral Ischemia and Infarction. In: MRI of brain and spine. (ed). Atlas SW Lippincott-Raven, Philadelphia, 1997.

14. Savoiardo M, Sberna M, Grisoli M: RM e patologia vascolare del sistema nervoso centrale. Rivista di Neuroradiologia 1 (suppl. 1):95-100, 1988.

15. Simonetti L, Cirillo S, Menditto M: Hemorrhagic infarcts of arterial origin: physiopathological aspects and MR semeiology. In: Ottorino Rossi Award Conference. Zappoli F, Martelli A. (eds). Edizioni del Centauro, Udine 141-145, 1992.

16. Von Kummer R: Changing role of the neuroradiologist in the investigation of acute ischemic stroke. In: Syllabus of 7th Advanced Course of the ESNR. Byrne JW. (ed). Edizioni del Centauro, Udine 41-44, 1997.

1.6

FUNCTIONAL MRI IN ISCHAEMIA

T. Scarabino, G.M. Giannatempo, T. Popolizio, M. Armillotta,

INTRODUCTION

The performance and capabilities of magnetic resonance imaging (MRI) equipment have recently been greatly improved by innovations to both the hardware (e.g., magnets, gradients and coils) and software (e.g., image acquisition sequences and data processing). These enhancements have made MRI more powerful and versatile than previously. This progress has translated into beneficial reductions in the overall examination times with regard to static imaging studies that are essential for primary diagnosis, and also the practical implementation of functional imaging, offering the promise of an increase the diagnostic power of MRI in terms of both sensitivity and specificity. These functional studies are increasingly being used together with conventional MR to obtain a more complete pathophysiological and prognostic picture of the CNS pathology in question. In addition, these MR techniques provide information on the movement of water molecules caused by thermal agitation (i.e., diffusion), microvascular haemodynamics (i.e., perfusion) and cerebral metabolism (i.e., spectroscopy).

In cases of cerebrovascular disease, these types of examinations permit very early and accurate diagnosis, and are capble of indicating the optimal treatment programme to be adopted (9). In addition to detecting irreversibly damaged tissue, they also point out areas at risk of infarction that could benefit from further treatment. In the particular case of hyperacute cerebral ischaemia, in which conventional T2-weighted MRI can be negative or ambiguous (1), diffusion weighted imaging is nearly always positive, clearly revealing the areas of infarction. Surrounding the ischaemic core, most cerebral infarctions also include a peripheral zone that is ischaemic but uninfarcted, the so-called ischaemic penumbra, which could potentially progress to frank infarction; this penumbra can be distinguished using perfusion MRI and/or spectroscopy.

The information obtained using such techniques can be expressed with qualitative data in the form of variations in MR signal intensity, or with quantitative data, thus making it possible to interpret the results in a somewhat unbiased manner, irrespective of the reader.

DIFFUSION MRI

Diffusion MRI (DWI) examinations have found a concrete application in clinical practice. DWI studies the diffusion potential of water, or rather the proclivity of water molecules to undergo random microscopic movement, driven in part by the thermal energy generated by the body. According to the variations in this physiological motion, the molecular motion of water in different tissues can be characterized in just a few seconds by means of DWI.

Technique

DWI uses spin echo sequences acquired ideally using the echoplanar technique, to which diffusion weighting is layered, thus making the resulting image sensitive to the movement of water. This characteristic is made possible by the use of two powerful bipolar diffusion gradients applied symmetrically to the 180° radiofrequency pulse. The application of these gradients causes the dephasing and subsequent rephasing of the protons in water, which varies according to the diffusion potential of the water molecules in different regions of the brain, which in turn translates into variations in MRI signal intensity. The water molecules that diffuse freely during or after the application of the dephasing gradients are not completely brought back into phase by the rephasing gradient, which does not happen for normal tissues. Following the 180° pulse, the protons that diffuse more slowly will be in a different phase than those that diffuse more quickly and will therefore have a different signal than the latter. Therefore, relatively high diffusion areas (such as normal brain) will show comparably lower signal than will slow diffusion areas (such as hyperacute infarction), which are characterized by a relatively higher signal. It is for this reason that DWI provides the key clinical information required in stroke cases: what tissue is undergoing hyperacute infarction.

Gradients of different strength can also be used to obtain a quantitative analysis of variations in water diffusion potential. The parameter used to quantify the in vivo results of DWI is the apparent diffusion coefficient (ADC), which can also be expressed in the form of a map in which high diffusion areas are relatively hyperintense and low diffusion areas are relatively hypointense. However, the fact that ADC maps require complex and timely postprocessing and because they are less well spatially defined than is DWI, makes them nonessential in the emergent examination of clinical stroke cases.

Applications

DWI is principally used to assess hyperacute ischaemic cerebral lesions (11, 14). In this hyperacute phase, there is a reduction in blood supply to the cerebral tissues, which makes the oxygen that is essential for cerebral metabolism unavailable; this in turn causes a reduction in adenosine triphosphate (ATP), damage to the sodium-potassium ion pump that in part maintains cellular homeostasis, a flow of Na+, Ca++ and Cl- ions from the extracellular to the intracellular space and a passive influx of water molecules from the extracellular compartment to the intracellular space (i.e., cytotoxic oedema). This restricts the diffusion capabilities of water molecules in the intracellular space, revealing the pathological tissue as an area of hyperintensity on DWI in comparison to normal brain (Fig. 1.64). Underlying these semeiotics, and within minutes after the onset of the clinical stroke, there is a sudden drop in ADC values which decrease over time by 30-60%; these changes occur at a time when conventional MRI is still negative. These ADC values tend to normalize within 5-10 days after onset of the stroke in part due to the appearance of vasogenic oedema. During the hyperacute phase, the ischaemic focus is characterized by a core of tissue having markedly reduced ADC values, surrounded by a layer of brain in which this reduction is less severe. Subsequent further reduction in the ADC values within the peripheral area would indicate irreversible impairment of the tissue in the ischaemic penumbra with an enlargement of the final extent of the infarction. The evaluation of the changes in ADC values over time is therefore important with regard to forecasting the evolution and ultimate volume of the infarct (11).

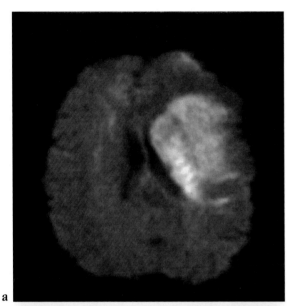

a

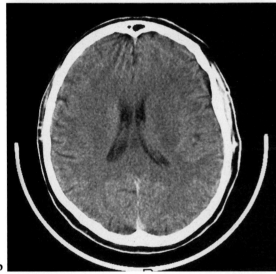

b

Fig. 1.64 - Hyperacute ischaemia in the supply territory of the left middle cerebral artery. Diffusion weighted MR images show (**a**) the pathological hyperintensity of the ischaemic area; CT (**b**) findings were negative.

Quantitative and qualitative diffusion studies are both highly sensitive as well as specific for infarction. The earlier the examination is performed and the longer the duration of the syntomatology, the greater is this degree of sensitivity and specificity (within the first 6 hours following the acute event).

Negative diffusion studies do not necessarily exclude the diagnosis of cerebral ischaemia (Fig. 1.65) (12). An alteration in DWI diffusion

signal is not universal to all patients with typical strokes, and in certain cases patients with clinical symptoms compatible with TIA's completely recover (10); in other cases, the DWI examination may be performed before the ischaemia has developed into a frank infarct; and in others, the site of the ischaemic lesion (e.g., in the posterior fossa) or the small dimensions of the infarct focus may lead to non-visualization. In reality, however, the spatial definition of DWI is usually sufficient to allow documentation of lesions only measuring a few millimetres (Fig. 1.66).

DWI also makes it possible to determine the age of mixed duration ischaemic lesions, and therefore declare which lesion(s) is responsible for the current signs and symptoms. When two or more cerebral lesions present are hyperintense on conventional T2-weighted MRI, it is possible to distinguish chronic lesions (i.e., isointense on DWI) from recent ones (i.e., hyperintense on DWI) (Figs. 1.67, 1.68).

The hyperintense pathological area on DWI can remain stable in its dimensions and ultimately undergo necrosis; it can shrink or disappear completely, depending on the duration of the occlusion or on the response to treatment; or it can increase due to repeated episodes of ischaemia (13).

In addition to serially monitoring an infarct's temporal and spatial evolution, DWI proves also useful in monitoring the effects and response of treatment. In cases where patient conditions allow repeated examinations, tailored thrombolytic and/or neuroprotective treatment programmes can be individually devised for each patient. However, the beneficial effects of this kind of management can be reduced by the occurrence of haemorrhagic complications, which therefore calls for more critical patient analysis using a combination of diffusion and perfusion imaging (2, 3).

PERFUSION MRI

Perfusion MR, a potentially valuable element in the assessment of acute cerebral ischaemia, studies microvascular haemodynamics.

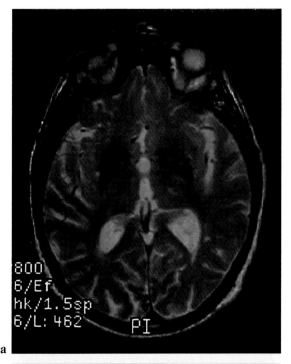

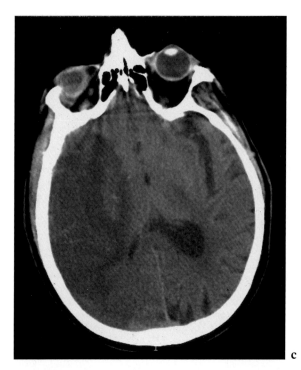

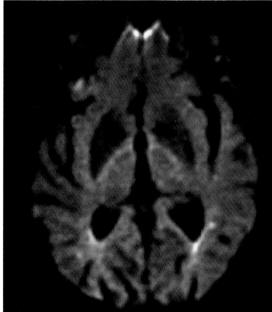

Fig. 1.65 - Acute ischaemia of the right middle cerebral artery territory. At clinical onset, the conventional (T2-weighted FSE sequence) (**a**) and diffusion (**b**) MR findings were negative. CT (**c**), performed 3 days later, showed a vast cortical-subcortical hypodensity with associated mass effect.

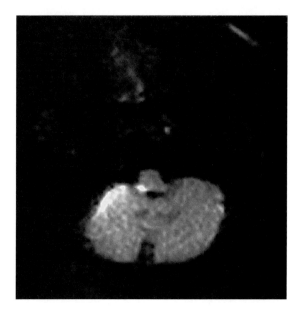

Fig. 1.66 - Lacunar ischaemia (millimetric dimensions) of the right lower cerebellar peduncle.

Technique

There are a number of ways in which to perform studies of brain perfusion (4). The most commonly used methods involve the intravenous administration of gadolinium, a paramagnetic contrast medium, and the utilization

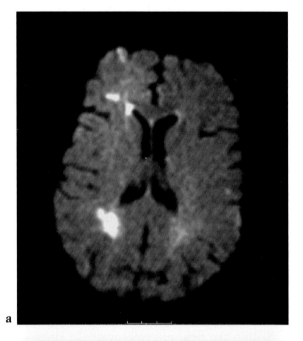

a

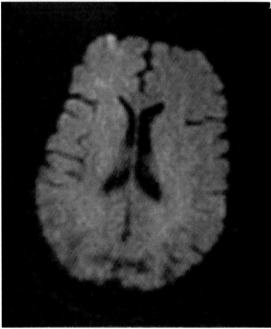

b

Fig. 1.67 - Previous multiple lacunar infarcts in the periventricular, bi-hemispheric white matter. The lesions appear hyperintense in the EPI-FLAIR sequence (**a**), whilst the weighted diffusion images (**b**) are isointense.

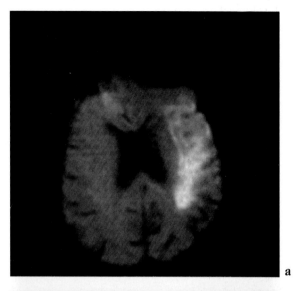

a

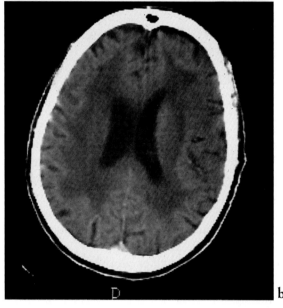

b

Fig. 1.68 - Hyperacute ischaemia of the left middle cerebral artery territory visible only in the weighted diffusion MR images (**a**) and not in CT (**b**) or EPI-FLAIR sequence (**c**) in which it is possible to see a chronic paraventricular vascular sufferance sustained with hypodensity and hyperintesity, respectively.

of ultrafast sequences (e.g., echoplanar sequences), which are able to simultaneously acquire a number of sections having a temporal resolution of approximately one second. As an alternative to this MRI technique, certain investigators employ selective radiofrequency (RF) pulses for labelling arterial spins (phase labelling) (5).

Alternatives to MRI exist for analysis of cerebral perfusion. One example is SPECT using signal/time curves, can be used. The degree of signal reduction in such curves is directly proportional to the tissue concentration of the contrast agent, which is in turn proportional to the regional cerebral blood flow (rCBF), as well as to the regional cerebral blood volume (rCBV). This makes it possible to obtain regional cerebral perfusion maps from the data gained from the perfusion MR. Further analysis of the concentration/time curve provides information from which to calculate additional parameters of perfusion such as the mean transit time (MTT), the time required to pass through the tissue and the peak time (PT), or the time required to reach peak perfusion.

Applications

Within the field of cerebrovascular disease, the most important applications of perfusion MR are related to cerebral ischaemia; however, its usefulness is not in the hyperacute phase as with diffusion, but rather in the hours that follow. Principally, perfusion is valuable for the assessment of the ischaemic penumbra, or the ischaemic area surrounding the core of the infarction. The perfusion of this penumbra and neuronal vitality within this tissue depend on the severity of the regional ischaemia and the collateral circulation.

In the presence of hyperacute cerebral ischaemia caused by the occlusion of a given vessel, the rCBV map will show a reduction in the MR signal intensity in the ischaemic area. Moreover, by using comparative region of interest (ROI) calculations in the contralateral homologous areas of the cerebrum, it is possible to observe the delay in or reduction of signal loss, and therefore the differential in the peak time. It is possible in this way to distinguish the areas destined to infarction from the areas of the ischaemic penumbra. The penumbra is the target of fibrinolytic treatment, within the area of hypoperfusion and therefore forecasts the final infarct territory. In fact, by examining the time/intensity curve, one can see three different curves reflecting a decrease in signal intensity that is variable in relation to the

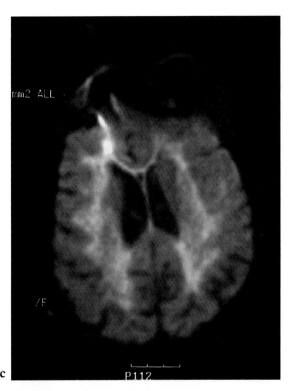

c

Fig. 1.68 - (*Cont.*).

(single photon emission computerized tomography); however, perfusion MR by comparison is more sensitive and specific and has the added advantage of greater spatial definition. It can also be performed at the same time as conventional MR examinations, with consequential reductions in cost and time.

In the same manner as diffusion imaging, the results obtained with MR perfusion can be both qualitative and quantitative. Qualitative evaluation uses variations or asymmetries of signal intensity viewed using cine-loop display. In normal conditions of cerebral perfusion, the gadolinium passage through the cerebral capillary bed causes a drop in T2 signal intensity, not only in the vessels but also in the perfused brain itself. If, however, the perfusion of a specific region of the brain is impaired, there will be a delay or an attenuation of the loss of signal intensity that varies in relation to the degree of reduction in the blood flow. In certain cases qualitative evaluations alone are insufficient for an accurate study of perfusion, and for this reason quantitative data, especially that cerebral perfusion of the ischaemic core (no decrease in signal intensity due to an absence of perfusion), of the area of ischaemic penumbra (reduction in signal intensity due to reduced perfusion), of the surrounding intact parenchyma (normal decrease in signal intensity caused by normal perfusion) (Fig. 1.69) (6).

The distribution of the perfusion deficit therefore permits the identification of potentially reversible ischaemic brain tissue, the selection of patients for various treatment protocols and the formulation of an early prognostic evaluation.

Diffusion/perfusion MR

The combined use of diffusion/perfusion MR can be more informative than the results obtained using a single examination alone, especially with regard to predicting the evolution of the cerebral infarction and clinical outcome. For these reasons, the two studies together may be more helpful in determining important treatment decisions (3, 16). It is possible to identify at least six different imaging patterns using diffusion and perfusion MR in combination (2):

1) Visualized ischaemic area is greater in perfusion than in diffusion. This is the most common situation (approx. 55-77% of cases), especially when the imaging examination is performed within 6 hours from the onset of the ischaemic event. In this case, the hyperacute phase shows the lesions of both the rCBV and the ADC to be relatively minor, but still positive, despite the negative CT and MR findings. However, in DWI the area of reduced ADC is generally smaller than the area demonstrated on the rCBV in the perfusion study, which includes both the area of frank infarction as well as the penumbra area. From a prognostic point of view, the early lesions visualized on the perfusion MR examination represent the maximum potential dimension of infarction and indicate the worst probable clinical outcome in the absence of further vascular occlusions or disruption of collateral circulation. Generally speaking, in DWI the size of the infarction

tends to grow over time, but with regard to perfusion MR, the volume of ischaemic tissue tends to shrink.

2) Visualized ischaemic area in perfusion MR is the same as the ischaemic region demonstrated in DWI.

3) Visualized ischaemic area in perfusion is less than in DWI. In this case reperfusion probably occurs in the interim between the start of irreversible tissue damage and the MR examination. The interim appearance of collateral circulation or the enlargement of the ischaemic area beyond the initial perfusion deficit may also be considered as causes of this imaging picture.

4) Presence of a DWI deficit without a perfusion abnormality.

5) Presence of a perfusion deficit without a DWI abnormality (associated with a transient neurological deficit).

6) Absence of a visualized lesion in both DWI and perfusion MR, despite a positive clinical picture.

The observation of an early deficit in perfusion MR that is greater than the volume of the abnormality seen in diffusion (patterns 1 and 5) indicates the presence of tissue "at risk" in the ischaemic penumbra, which can therefore potentially be saved by forms of reperfusion

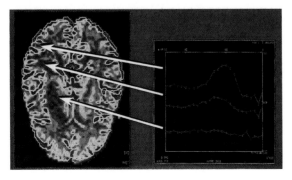

Fig. 1.69 - Perfusion study of an acute ischaemia. The intensity/time graph shows 3 different curves indicating a drop in signal intensity that varies with the entity of the cerebral perfusion of the ischaemic core (absence of drop in signal intensity due to the absence of perfusion), of the ischaemic penumbra area (reduction of the drop in signal intensity due to reduced perfusion), of the intact surrounding parenchyma (normal reduction in signal intensity due to normal perfusion).

treatment. When the perfusion deficits on MRI are absent or smaller than those in diffusion (patterns 2, 3, and 4), treatment involving neuroprotective drugs is felt to be more suitable.

MR SPECTROSCOPY

MR spectroscopy is a real time non-invasive study of some of the biochemical elements involved in cerebral metabolism.

Technique

The technique of spectroscopy is based on the physical principle of the so-called "chemical shift" that reflects the variation in frequency of resonance of the nuclei of different molecules; this variation is influenced by the magnetic field that is generated by the cloud of electrons that surrounds these nuclei, as well as by the electrons of nearby atoms. Therefore, the same atom can exhibit different degrees of chemical shift depending on the environment in which it finds itself, and on the basis of this it is possible to identify the molecule containing the atom in question.

We usually speak of *proton* spectroscopy, because the nucleus typically chosen to study, and for which to calibrate the MR unit, is the hydrogen proton. This choice is in part made because the hydrogen proton is particularly plentiful in organic structures.

Proton spectroscopy provides metabolic information concerning molecules having a low molecular weight that are present in relatively high concentrations (0.1-1 mM); these include N-acetyl-aspartate (NAA), choline (Cho), creatine (Cr), phosphocreatine (PCr), myoinositol (mI), lactate (Lac), lipids (Lip), glutamine and glutamate (Glx). The concentration of these metabolites is detected in the form of spectra in which each peak in a given position (expressed in parts per million; ppm) represents a particular metabolite.

Normally in adults, NAA has the highest peak among the expected metabolites, where it is localized to about 2 ppm. This metabolite is only found in the central nervous system, and in particular is detected in neurons and, to a lesser extent, in certain glial precursor cells. For this reason it is considered a neuronal marker. Its presence is more or less equal in the white and grey matter, so that it is also considered an axonal marker.

NAA concentration is depressed or non-detectable in certain types of brain pathology. Cho, with a peak of approximately 3.2 ppm, contains composites containing choline principally represented by membrane lipids; it is therefore considered a membrane marker. It is seen to increase in diseases characterized by an elevation in cellular turnover, an increase in the number of cells or by membrane damage/degeneration. Cr and PCr can be observed with a single peak at 3.02 ppm. These metabolites are derived from the high energy phosphate pool involved in metabolism. Being a stable peak, it can be used as a control value even in the presence of pathology. MI, which is a specific marker for glial cells, is localized at 3.3-3.6 ppm.

When present, Lac has an unusual "doublet" peak at 1.32 ppm. When present, it indicates the production of energy in conditions of insufficient oxygen supply. An example of when this situation can occur is when incomplete vascular occlusion results in the activation of the enzymatic pathway that leads to anaerobic glycolysis. It can also accumulate due to the infiltration of macrophages that contain lactate, or because the production of lactate is trapped by the ongoing pathological process and is not removed from the tissue under study.

Lipids, which can be observed in necrotic processes, produce peaks of 0.8, 1.2, 1.5 ppm. Glx is represented by peaks at 2.1, 2.5 and at 3.6-3.8 ppm and includes the signal from the neurotransmitters glutamate and glutamine.

These metabolites can be studied using two localization techniques: 1) the single volume technique, with which it is possible to acquire spectra from specific regions of the brain, and 2) the spectroscopic imaging technique, with which one can simultaneously obtain spectra from tissue volumes acquired from one or more imaging sections in order to obtain the spatial distribution of the metabolites under examination.

Applications

Spectroscopy can be used for the early detection and better characterization of ischaemic lesions, for monitoring the effects of treatment, and most importantly, for distinguishing the infarct focus from the area of surrounding ischaemic penumbra (6, 15). The area of cellular necrosis is characterized by a depression of NAA (50% within the first 6 hours), whereas the ischaemic penumbra is characterized by the presence of an increase in the peak of lactic acid in the absence of significant NAA alterations (Fig. 1.70).

A serious NAA depression and a marked increase in lactate in the acute phase have proved to be prognostic indexes of more marked ischemic lesion (7, 8).

CONCLUSIONS

The various functional MR examination techniques (diffusion, perfusion, spectroscopy) are essential to the meaningful, productive therapeutic management of acute stroke patients.

The goal of fibrinolytic treatment is to safeguard the ischaemic tissue that has suffered reversible damage so that it can be properly reperfused, together with the prevention of reperfusion of irreversibly damaged, non-vital tissue. This requires diagnostic techniques capable of distinguishing vital ischaemic tissue from that which is frankly infarcted, where there is a risk of damage from reperfusion resulting in haemorrhagic complications.

Diffusion MR examinations are able to provide immediate and simple demonstration of hyperacute cerebral ischaemia, before the appearance of signal changes in MRI and/or density changes in CT; however, it is not able to distinguish between ischaemic penumbra, which could therefore benefit from recanalization treatment, and irreversibly ischaemically damaged tissue.

MR spectroscopy and, in particular, spectroscopic imaging can be of use in this sense, however it requires relatively long examination times. Perfusion MR studies provide direct information on the status of cerebral parenchyma perfusion (depending on the adequacy of collateral circulation) and on tissue vitality and reversibility that is required for a

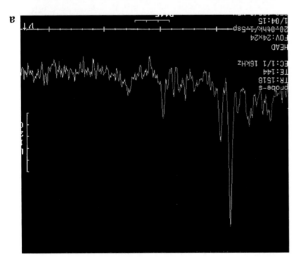

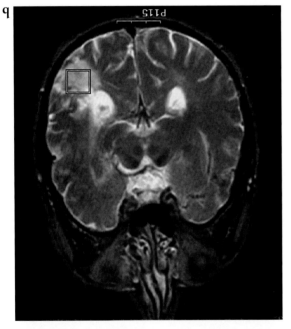

Fig. 1.70 - Spectroscopic study (a) of subacute ischaemia with morphological MRI (T2-W FSE). The drastic reduction of NAA concentration is evident.

suitable selection of patients for thrombolytic treatment.

It therefore follows that a multimodal solution is required to solve the problem of acute cerebral ischaemia and to appropriately guide treatment choices. The key to interpreting acute phase ischaemia is to combine different MR and spectroscopic acquisition sequences. Diffusion/perfusion integration in particular enables accurate mapping, more precise grading and more efficient treatment planning of cases of cerebral ischaemia. These studies also have the advantage of being generally rapid to perform in association with basic MR examinations.

REFERENCES

1. Baird AE, Warach S: Magnetic resonance imaging of acute stroke. J Cereb Blood Flow Metabolism 18:583-609, 1998.
2. Barber PA, Darby DG, Desmond PM et al: Prediction of stroke outcome with echoplanar perfusion and diffusion weighted MRI. Neurology 51:418-426, 1998.
3. De Boer JA, Folkers PJM: MR perfusion and diffusion imaging in ischaemic brain disease. Medica Mundi 41:20, 1997.
4. Detre JA, Leigh JS, Williams DS et al: Perfusion imaging. Magn Reson Med 23:37-45, 1992.
5. Edelman RR, Siewert B, Darby DG et al: Quantitative mapping of cerebral blood flow and functional localization with echo-planar MR imaging and signal targeting with alternating radio-frequency. Radiology 192:513-520, 1994.
6. Graham GD, Blamire AM, Howseman AM et al: Proton magnetic resonance spectroscopy of cerebral lactate and other metabolites in stroke patients. Stroke 23:333-340, 1992.
7. Federico F, Simone IL: Prognostic significance of metabolic changes detected by proton magnetic resonance spectroscopy in ischaemic stroke. J Neurol 243:241-247, 1996.
8. Federico F, Simone IL: Prognostic value of proton magnetic resonance spectroscopy in ischaemic stroke. Arch Neurol 55:489-494, 1998.
9. Hacke W, Kaste M, Fieschi C et al: Intravenous thrombolysis with recombinant tissue plasminogen activator for acute hemispheric stroke. The European Cooperative Acute Stroke Study (ECASS). JAMA 274:1017-1025, 1995.
10. Kidwell CS, Alger JR, Di Salle F et al: Diffusion MRI in patients with transient ischemia attacks. Stroke 30(6):1174-1180, 1999.
11. Li TQ, Chen ZG, Hindmarsh T: Diffusion-weighted MR imaging of acute cerebral ischemia. Acta Radiologica 39:460-473, 1998.
12. Lovblad KO, Laubach HJ, Baird AE et al: Clinical experience with diffusion-weighted MR in patients with acute stroke. AJNR 19:1061-1066, 1998.
13. Lovblad KO, Baird AE, Schlaug G: Ischemic lesion volumes in acute stroke by diffusion-weighted magnetic resonance imaging correlate with clinical outcome. Ann Neurol 42:164-170, 1997.
14. Lutsep HL, Albers GW, DeCrespigny A et al: Clinical utility of diffusion-weighted magnetic resonance imaging in the assessment of ischemic stroke. Ann Neurol 41:574-580, 1997.
15. Mathews VP, Barker PB, Blackband SJ et al: Cerebral metabolites in patients with acute and subacute strokes: a serial MR and proton MR spectroscopy study. AJR 165:633-638, 1995.
16. Ueda T, Yuh WT, Taoka T: Clinical application of perfusion and diffusion MR imaging in acute ischemic stroke. J Magn Reson Imaging 10(3):305-309, 1999.

1.7

MRI IN HAEMORRHAGE

L. Simonetti, S. Cirillo, R. Agati

INTRODUCTION

Intracranial haemorrhages account for approximately 20% of all cerebral ictuses related to vascular disease, with a higher prevalence of intraaxial localizations (15%) as compared to those principally within the subarachnoid space (5%) (1, 6, 9). Although MRI is highly specific with regard to haemorrhagic lesions, CT remains the examination of choice, especially in emergencies, in part due to the difficulty in managing acutely ill patients within the MR scanning unit.

Any physician who acquired an MRI unit in its early stages of clinical application will remember the sense of confusion experienced with the first acute intracerebral haematoma patient, as initially diagnosed on MRI. In such cases, the lesion MR signal was "ambiguous", nearly devoid of the specific characterizations seen on CT in patients with haemorrage. In the early stages haemorrhage could appear quite similar to an ischaemic ictus, being differentiated when possible by the differing topography and morphology.

This impact conditioned the attitude of neuroradiologists against the use of MRI in acute haemorrhagic pathology for some years, and this instinctive wariness has only partly been re-conditioned by a clear working knowledge of the evolution of the MR signal of parenchymal haemorrhagic collections (13, 15-18).

In this chapter, we will analyse the information that can be deduced from intracranial haemorrhages using MRI, making a distinction between intraaxial and subarachnoid forms due to the difference in the anatomopathological and biochemical environment in which the phenomena that influence the haemorrhagic MRI signal occur.

SEMEIOTICS

Intraaxial haemorrhage

Intraaxial cerebral haemorrhages are serious clinical events characterized by a variable alteration in the state of consciousness, an often severe neurological deficit and by the possible association with meningeal signs. Alongside this more common presentation, there are more serious clinical forms such as sudden decerebration as well as milder forms with relatively minor effects on the state of consciousness and a less serious clinical deficit.

The most frequent cause of intraaxial haemorrhage, which accounts for more than 50% of cases, is systemic hypertension associated with intracranial atherosclerotic vessel alterations. Other causes, in order of frequency, are the rupture of vascular malformations, coagulation disorders, intratumoral haemorrhages (especially neoplastic metastases and malignant gliomas), trauma and postsurgical/iatrogenic causes.

Evolution-based semeiology

Neuroradiological semeiology based on the time elapsed since the onset of the intraaxial bleeding is complex (2, 7, 8, 14, 19): with regard to CT, the observations are linked above all to the macroscopic and sub-macroscopic anatomopathological alterations of the haemorrhagic focus, while with MR the imaging findings of haemorrhage must be integrated with varying biochemical factors.

The various steps that take the haematic collection from the hyperacute phase, with a prevalence of oxyhaemoglobin, to the outcome and reparation phase, in which the final breakdown components such as haemosiderin prevail, and the consequent variations in the MR signal are now well understood and categorized. It should be remembered that it was precisely the need to explain the dynamic behaviour of the MR signal of the haematoma that prompted the reconsideration, proper correlation and accurate categorization of the stages of haemoglobin metabolism outside the vascular bed. It goes without saying that the state of the haemoglobin within the haemorrhagic focus is of little importance from a diagnostic and therapeutic point of view, but it nevertheless provides a very real stimulus for the neuroradiologist to understand clearly this physiological process in order to properly interpret the images.

The temporal evolution of the MR characteristics of blood is caused both by alterations of the erythrocytes as well as the haemoglobin present under several differing conditions. As far as the red blood cells are concerned, membrane integrity, guaranteed under normal conditions by the ATPase/Na-K units dependent on the membrane and powered by glycolytic energy, is of great importance. Haemoglobin alterations are influenced by various factors, including: pH, conditions of osmolarity, temperature, partial oxgen pressure (pO2) and the metabolic microenvironment along with the concentration of the oxidizable sublayers. Both oxygenated and deoxygenated haemoglobin circulate inside red blood cells; in such forms of haemoglobin, the heme contains bivalent iron. If the iron group is oxidized to form trivalent iron, the molecule (metahaemoglobin) loses its ability to bond oxygen; for this reason, through the pentoso-phosphate pathway, a considerable percentage (10%) of the red blood cell's catabolic energy is used to form reducing agents (NADPH and reduced glutathione) capable of preventing or correcting haemoglobin oxidation. The same reducing agents also perform the important role of controlling the peroxidation of the membrane lipids that would otherwise increase the osmotic fragility of the erythrocytes. The remaining 90% of the glycidic catabolism of red blood cells follows the glycolytic pathway, which produces the ATP used to fuel the Na-K dependent ATPase structures. The proper functioning of these membrane pumps is indispensable for the maintenance of erythrocyte osmolarity and thus the normal biconcave cellular shape. A sufficient glucose supply is therefore required for several purposes: to maintain cellular osmolarity, to keep the haemoglobin properly reduced and to avoid the peroxidation of membrane lipids.

In the light of this, it is easier to interpret the blood's relaxation parameter alterations using MRI. In the hyperacute phase, in other words in the first 12 hours from onset, intraparenchymal haemorrhagic foci are composed of intact red blood cells with high oxygen saturation and therefore containing oxyhaemoglobin. In the absence of paramagnetic molecules or structures, the MR relaxation times are longer than those of the surrounding tissue due to the local alteration in free water content and protein concentration. The resulting oxyhaemoglobin-dominant haemorrhagic lesion on MRI (Fig. 1.71) is complex but includes: relative (as compared to normal brain tissue) minor hypoisoin-

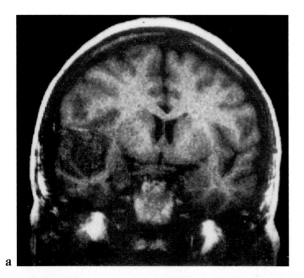

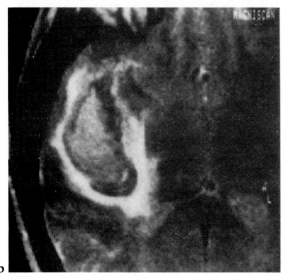

a

b

Fig. 1.71 - Hyperacute phase right intracerebral sub-Sylvian haemorrhage (12 hours). Coronal T1-dependent scan (a) and axial T2-dependent scan (b). The lesion presents as hypointense in T1 and non-homogeneously hyperintense in T2, where the notably hyperintense oedema halo in formation is also visible.

tensity on the T1-weighted images, minor hyperintensity on PD-weighted images, and minor hyperintensity on the T2-weighted images (in truth, the relative intensity differentials as compared to normal brain are quite small in all routine MR acquisition sequences).

In the oxygen-dependent acute phase (12 hours - 2 days), the pO2 within the extravasated blood starts to drop fairly quickly, and consequently there is a reduction in the haemoglo-

bin's oxygen saturation, with the eventual formation of deoxyhaemoglobin. Deoxyhaemoglobin, characterized by high magnetic susceptibility and enclosed in the finite intracellular space of the erythrocyte, causes non-homogeneity of the local magnetic field, thus resulting in a loss of phase coherence of the resident protons. This translates into a preferential field strength -dependent enhancement of T2 relaxation. Although deoxyhaemoglobin is paramagnetic, it does not influence T1 relaxation because its heme groups are contained in apolar pockets that prevent contact with water protons. The presence of deoxyhaemoglobin in the haemorrhagic lesion translates into (Figs. 1.72, 1.73): relative hypo-isointensity on T1-weighted images, iso-hypointensity on PD-weighted images and rather marked hypointensity on T2-weighted images.

The subacute, glucose-dependent phase (2-14 days) is characterized by two events that occur in parallel but slightly out of phase with one another, partly sharing the same pathogenic mechanisms: the formation of metahaemoglo-

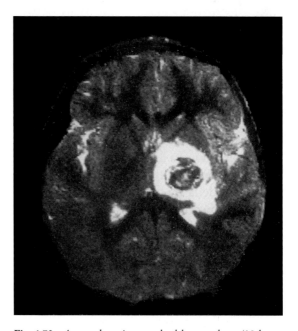

Fig. 1.72 - Acute phase intracerebral haemorrhage (38 hours from onset) in a left thalamo-capsular location. Axial PD (a) and T2 scans: the lesion presents as non-homogeneously hypointense with a vast oedematous halo.

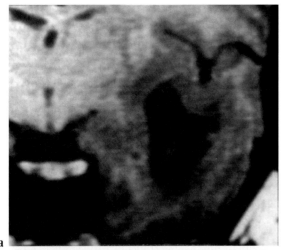

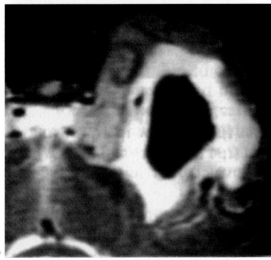

Fig. 1.73 - Acute phase intracerebral haemorrhage in left temporal location: coronal T1- (a) and T2-dependent (b) scans: note the marked hypointensity of the lesion and the perilesional oedema.

bin (methaemoglobin: 2-7 days) and erythrocyte lysis (7-14 days).

Methaemoglobinization presupposes the exhaustion of the oxide-reducing homeostasis of the erythrocyte systems due to a regional reduction in glucose concentration, the blockage of the catabolitic pentose-phosphate pathway and the progressive reduction of NADPH and reduced glutathione. In addition to an extremely reduced concentration of glucose, haemoglobin oxidation to methaemoglobin is also conditioned by a given pO_2 of about 20 mm Hg.

The pathogenesis of red blood cell lysis includes: the exhaustion of erythrocyte ATP reserves with the stoppage of the Na-K dependent membrane pumps and the osmotic swelling of the erythrocytes, the peroxidation of membrane lipids and the catabolization of the membrane phospholipids by tissue phospholipases.

Being intensely paramagnetic, methaemoglobin causes a reduction in T1 relaxation due to the dipole-dipole interaction between the external shell electrons of the methaemoglobin and water protons. The influence of methaemoglobin on T2 relaxation is identical to that described for deoxyhaemoglobin. Once erythrocyte lysis has taken place, a loss of T2 relaxation enhancement occurs, as methaemoglobin assumes a homogeneous distribution, which translates into hyperintensity of the MR signal on T2-weighted images. At the same time, the intensity on T1-weighted images increases due to the greater T1 relaxation effects of the free methaemoglobin as compared to intracellular methaemoglobin.

To summarize, in the first week of this phase (intact membrane methaemoglobinization), the MR signal characteristics of the intracellular methaemoglobin dominance within the haemorrhagic lesion can be classified as follows: relative hyperintensity on T1-weighted images, hyperintensity on PD-weighted images and hypointensity on T2-weighted images. In contrast to this, once erythrocyte lysis has taken place, the extracellular methaemoglobin dominance within the haemorrhage demonstrates: relative hyperintensity on T1-weighted images, hyperintensity on PD-dependent images and hyperintensity on T2-weighted images.

For purposes of completeness, we will now describe MR signal alterations in chronic-phase intraparenchymal haematomas (more than two weeks), although, strictly speaking, this goes slightly beyond the temporal limits of this discussion. The chronic phase of haematoma evolution is characterized by the phagocytosis of erythrocyte lysis products by microphages around periphery of the haemorrhagic collection. Within the macrophages heme iron accumulates primarily within lysosome vacuoles in the form of haemosiderin. The presence of haemosiderin causes increased T2 relaxation and therefore hypointensity on T2-weighted images within the peripheral rim of the haemorrhagic lesion that persists indefinitely. In

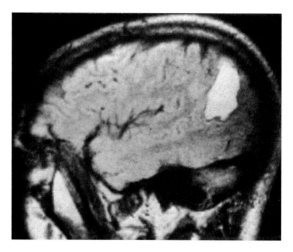

Fig. 1.75 - Sagittal PD-dependent MRI scan: note the thin hypointense rim that surrounds the lesion, due to the presence of haemosiderin.

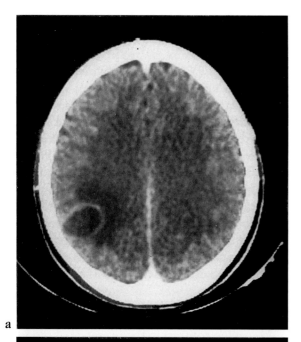

a

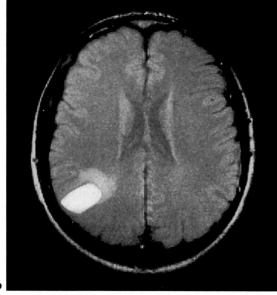

b

Fig. 1.74 - Left parietal haemorrhage in chronic phase (28 days). Axial CT scan after contrast agent (**a**): hypodense lesion with thin hyperdense rim. Axial PD-dependent MR scan: the lesion shows the characteristic hyperintense haematic signal.

the meantime, methaemoglobin within the haemorrhagic collection continues to cause MR signal hyperintensity on the T1- and T2-weighted images. Subsequently, as months pass, methaemoglobin breaks down into derivatives that do not have T1 relaxation effects (Figs. 1.74, 1.75).

Bleeding cause-based semeiology

In addition to the diagnosis of the presence of an intraaxial haemorrhage, MRI can also sometimes provide information that indicates the underlying cause of the bleeding. Apart from arterial hypertension, and excluding trauma, intracerebral bleeding typically is caused by vascular malformations or richly vascularized intracerebral neoplasias. In such cases the site, morphology, structure and number of blood collections can vary. Therefore, using this information together with the clinical picture, the neuroradiologist is able to suggest the likely cause(s) of bleeding.

a) Site

The localization of intraaxial haematomas is represented, in order, by:
- Nucleo-capsular haemorrhages (between the basal ganglia nuclei and the internal cap-

sule: 50%). Nucleo-capsular haematomas can be subdivided into capsulo-lenticular (between the internal capsule and the lenticular nucleus [globus pallidus plus putamen]), capsulo-thalamic (between the internal capsule and the thalamus) and capsulo-caudate (between the internal capsule and the caudate nucleus) haematomas. In most cases the haematomas in this position are considered spontaneous, and are linked to arterial hypertension both as a cause of the induced chronic vascular alterations as well as the triggering cause of the acute haemorrhage. Acute hypertensive crises can also lead to haemorrhages at these locations. Small capsulo-caudate haematomas are an exception, as the rupture of small periventricular arteriovenous malformations more often causes them than does hypertension.

– Lobar haemorrhages (35%). These haemorrhages are rarely spontaneous. Temporal and occipital lobe haematomas are usually secondary to arteriovenous malformations or haemorrhagic infarcts, mainly due to venous ischaemia. Frontal haematomas are generally caused by ruptures of aneurysms associated with the anterior communicating artery or anterior cerebral artery. All lobar haemorrhages can have a neoplastic origin.

– Infratentorial haemorrhages (10%). These haemorrhages can be subdivided into brainstem and cerebellar bleeds. The former are frequently caused by vascular malformation ruptures, most commonly cavernous angiomas; the latter are more typically associated with tumoural bleeding or, less frequently, with aneurysm ruptures.

– Intraventricular haemorrhages (5%). Isolated intraventricular haemorrhages devoid of signs of intraaxial haematoma formation are rare. They are generally secondary to the rupture of small paraventricular or choroid plexus arteriovenous malformations.

b) Morphology and structure

Intraaxial haematomas can be round or oval, with well-defined margins, or alternatively irregular with dendritic margins or even with completely irregular boundaries having a somewhat map-like appearance. Haematoma morphology can be linked to either a vascular malformation/aneurysm or a spontaneous aetiology, however, haematomas with irregular margins are more commonly encountered in patients with blood dyscrasias.

The appearance of the haemorrhage can be homogeneous or heterogeneous, occasionally manifesting a horizontal fluid-fluid level in haemorrhages due to variations in the makeup of the blood clot.

c) Number

Intraaxial blood collections tend to be single in number. The finding of multiple haemorrhagic foci, usually in a superficial lobar position (excluding those of traumatic origin), point in the direction of a diagnosis of a blood disorder (including iatrogenic anticoagulation), multiple haemorrhagic neoplastic metastases (including melanoma) or dural venous sinus thrombosis with venous infarcts/haemorrhages.

Semeiotics based on technical MR parameters

MR tissue contrast in the presence of blood depends to a great extent on the parameters of the image acquisition sequence used. In gradient-recalled echo (GRE) sequences, the sensitivity to paramagnetic constituents is very high. However, this sensitivity requires attention to magnetic susceptibility "border" artefacts at the interface of the petrous bones and the paranasal sinuses with the brain parenchyma.

Fast Spin-echo (FSE) sequences differ from conventional SE sequences in that they use a train of 180° radiofrequency pulses, which generate a set of echoes that are individually coded in the space of a single TR. The implications in brain examinations are that the effects of magnetic susceptibility dephasing are removed and the effects of diffusion-induced signal loss are reduced. T2-dependent FSE sequences therefore have a lower sensitivity to magnetically susceptible blood products than do the corresponding conventional spin echo images. The use of supplementary GRE sequences or T2-weighted conventional spin echo imaging sequences is recommended in cases where clinical history suggests possible cranial haemorrhage. Echoplanar Imaging (EPI) sequences are becoming increasingly suitable for routine clinical applications. They are very sensitive to magnetic susceptibility in both conventional spin echo and GRE sequences.

Closing comments

The importance of understanding the MR signal characteristics of intraaxial haematomas within the framework of the evolutional phase of the individual blood collections should be underlined: this knowledge is in part intended to provide a means of interpreting MR images in patients with an acute clinical ictus (stroke) who have been inadvertently sent to MRI instead of CT. The greater diagnostic contribution of MRI in patients with intracranial haemorrhage is in the subacute and chronic phases. We refer here to those cases in which the initial clinical and CT findings are ambiguous, thus creating problems of differential diagnosis. In such instances the performance of an MR examination that shows the MR signal characteristics specific for the various evolving blood products dispels diagnostic doubts.

One piece of additional information that can be gleaned from MRI as compared to CT is the ability of the former to link many "non-spontaneous" haemorrhages with the underlying pathological condition responsible for the bleed. The better relative sensitivity of MRI in diagnosing vascular malformations (Fig. 1.76), even in the presence of a haematoma, is well known. However, it is less well understood that, in order to be visible when haemorrhage is present, the vascular malformation must be of a rather considerable size. In the presence of acute or subacute haematomas, small vascular malformations are easily overlooked on routine MR images, in part due to the distortion caused by the magnetic field; this applies for both conventional MR as well for MR angiography examinations (Fig. 1.77). And, although MR angiography is an important contribution to pa-

tient treatment planning, it should be complemented with a conventional angiographic examination in the pretreatment phase of patient analysis.

Subarachnoid haemorrhage

Haemorrhage into the subarachnoid space (subarachnoid haemorrhage: SAH) has a sudden clinical onset with headache, nausea, vomiting, varying degress of disturbance of consciousness, widespread cutaneous hyperaesthesia and severe meningeal signs. Clinical variations can range from more subtle forms where the meningeal syndrome alone is present, to mixed cerebromeningeal forms associated with clinical symptomatology of the neurological deficit type to more serious forms characterized by coma.

The most frequent cause of SAH is aneurysm rupture, followed, in order of frequency by the rupture of brainstem or cerebral arteriovenous malformations, trauma, blood clotting disorders and, lastly, acute haemorrhagic necrosis of the pituitary gland (5).

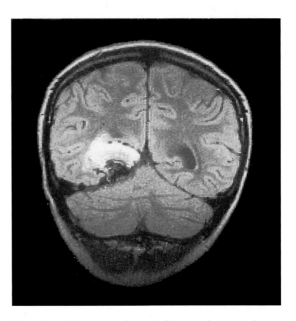

Fig. 1.76 - Right temporal-occipital haemorrhage in subacute phase with arteriovenous malformation. Coronal PD-dependent scan: the haemorrhagic lesion is very clear, as is the malformation nidus with its characteristic signal void.

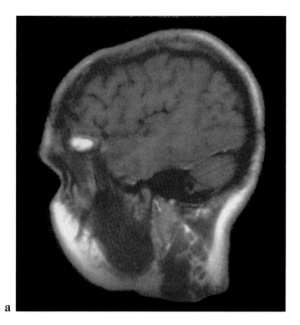

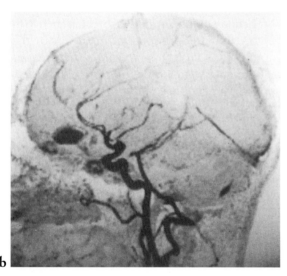

Fig. 1.77 - Small left frontal intraparenchymal haemorrhage. Sagittal T1-dependent scan (**a**) TOF MRA (**b**). The image concerning the haematoma is obvious on the MRA reconstruction: this would prevent the visualization of any small arteriovenous malformation present.

Semeiology and variations based on time

MR semeiology of SAH is made all the more complex by the continuous alterations being undergone by the blood with relationship to the biological parameters of the subarachnoid space (pH, pO2, glucose concentration). The variation of these parameters follows different rules that are less easily codified than those that characterize intraparenchymal blood collections (3, 4). For this reason, MRI generally finds little place in the evaluation of acute phase SAH, given CT's greater sensitivity and rapidity, and its ease of access 24 hours a day. The interpretation of MR images in patients with non-traumatic SAH is doubtlessly more straightforward in the subacute and chronic phases, and its contribution grows with the passing of time since the "acute" moment of the bleed as the diagnostic efficiency of CT dwindles. In reality however, even during the acute phase a well-planned and executed MR examination can also allow a demonstration of the characteristic signs of SAH.

Variations in the relaxation parameters that distinguish the evolutional phases of haemorrhagic collections are linked to the structural and functional variations of erythrocytes and the consequent conditions of haemoglobin oxidation and oxygenation.

In the subarachnoid space, erythrocyte and haemoglobin alterations follow different dynamics than those observed in intraparenchymal haemorrhages, in part due to the different biochemical-metabolic microenvironment. This makes it somewhat difficult to pinpoint the temporal limits of the phases of evolution of SAH.

In the hyperacute phase, there is no lengthening of proton density relaxation times in comparison to the surrounding CSF, but rather a slight shortening of T1 relaxation times due to the increase in protein content; this subtle change is often not detected due to the long relaxation times of the CSF, which mask the theoretical effects of the fresh blood, and consequently the T1-weighted MR images are usually interpreted as being negative.

In the acute phase it is difficult to perceive the reduction of T2 relaxation times characteristic to parenchymal blood collections, given that the CSF environment is an open system in which the focal variations of pO2 are slowed (relatively higher levels of pO2 are maintained as compared to the cerebral parenchyma). And, as noted in the preceding paragraph, it is difficult to evaluate small variations in relaxation times in the environment of the CSF, and as a result the T2-weighted MRI tends to be negative.

During the acute phase it is sometimes possible to find some linear hyperintensity on T1-weighted images in an intrafissural location. Such observations, which indicate SAH, are interpreted to be clotting of the extravasated blood within the subarachnoid space. Contact with the CSF is a sufficient stimulus to cause clotting of the blood present in the subarachnoid spaces. If we then add the fact that the retraction of the clot causes dramatic variations in red blood cell concentration and fibrin structure, we can then explain how it is possible even in an acute phase to visualize SAH in some instances. Clotting is therefore the key to visualizing blood in the early phases of SAH when using conventional MR sequences. The limit of this semeiological element lies in the temporal, quantitative and topographic variability of clotting processes, the percentage of blood in the CSF, the functionality of the clotting mechanisms, the site of the bleed and the biochemical composition of the CSF microenvironment.

In the subacute phase, a reduction in T1 relaxation (hyperintensity on T2-weighted images) caused by the presence of methaemoglobin is clearly visible. In the subarachnoid space, the reduction in glucose concentration, required for methaemoglobinization and erythrocyte lysis, also takes place at a slower pace than that observed in parenchymal blood collections. This phase represents the period in which MRI reaches its peak sensitivity for SAH; this is made all the more important if we consider that in this period, the CT density of the extravasated blood tends to decrease, thus consonantly reducing the sensitivity of this technique.

In recent years, we have started to examine SAH with MRI using FLAIR (fluid-attenuated inversion recovery) sequences (10, 11). FLAIR images are obtained using an inversion recovery (IR) sequence that has long TI (time to inversion) and TE (time to echo). These sequences suppress the CSF signal, and they produce images that are very heavily T2-weighted. This makes FLAIR particularly useful in identifying lesions on the surface of the hemispheres (and overlying subarachnoid spaces), within the basal subarachnoid cisterns, around the brainstem and at the grey-white matter junction. On the basis of these characteristics it is usually possible to detect SAH. SAH presents as high signal areas on FLAIR images and any associated intraventricular haemorrhage is also clearly visible. FLAIR is also useful in detecting acute SAH in the posterior fossa, which is difficult to study using CT due to the presence of scatter artefacts. FLAIR images have been shown to visualize SAH up to 45 days beyond the acute episode.

In the same manner as that mentioned in the preceding section on intraparenchymal collections, MRI can play an important role in the early recognition of the vascular pathology responsible for the SAH.

Closing comments

Given the numerous variables linked to MRI, CT remains the examination of choice in acute phase SAH diagnosis (12). However, in the subacute and chronic phases, the decreasing sensitivity of CT corresponds with increasing sensitivity of MRI for haemoglobin breakdown products; in particular, chronic leptomeningeal haemosiderin deposits can be recognized even years after bleeding (superficial siderosis).

And, MRI can play an important role in the early recognition of the vascular pathology responsible for the bleed. The continuous progress made in MR angiography has recently led to a greater diagnostic reliability. In certain cases, MR angiographic examinations are currently being proposed as the only presurgical vascular evaluation in aneurysms responsible for SAH. However, more experience and further technical progress in MRI are required before it becomes a routine procedure in order to prove the validity and efficacy of the method in this area of diagnosis.

REFERENCES

1. Adams RD, Victor M: Principles of Neurology. New York: McGraw-Hill, Inc. 508-572, 1985.
2. Brott T, Broderick J et al: Early hemorrhage growth in patients with intracerebral hemorrhage. Stroke 28(1):1-5, 1997.
3. Cirillo S, Di Salle F, Simonetti L et al: La RM nell'emorragia sub-aracnoidea: I. Studio in vitro. Rivista di Neuroradiologia 2:211-217, 1989.
4. Cirillo S, Simonetti L, Di Salle F et al: La RM nell'emorragia sub-aracnoidea: II. Studio in vivo. Rivista di Neuroradiologia 2:219-225, 1989.
5. Davis JM, Davis KR, Cromwell RM: SAE secondary to ruptured of intracranial aneurysms. AJNR (1):17-21, 1980.
6. Gardeur D: Pathologie vasculaire. Ellipse, Paris, 1982.
7. Gomori JM, Grossman RI et al: Variable appearances of sub-acute intracranial hematomas on high fields SE MR. AJR 150:171-178, 1985.
8. Gomori JM, Grossman RI et al: Intracranial hematomas imaging by high field MR. Radiology 157:87-93, 1985.
9. Gullotta F: Vasculopatie cerebrali. In: Schiffer D (ed). "Neuropatologia" Roma: Il pensiero scientifico 155-178, 1980.
10. Noguchi K, Ogawa T et al: Subacute and chronic subarachnoid hemorrhage: diagnosis with fluid-attenuated in-version-recovery MR imaging. Radiology 203(1):257-62, 1997.
11. Noguchi K, Ogawa T, Inugami et al: Acute subarachnoid hemorrhage: MR imaging with fluid-attenuated inversion recovery pulse sequences. Radiology 1963:773-777, 1995.
12. Ogawa T, Inugami A, Fujita H et al: MR diagnosis of subacute and chronic subarachnoid hemorrhage: comparison with CT. AJR 165(5):1257-1262, 1995.
13. Osborne AG: Diagnostic Neuroradiology. Chapter 10. Mosby-Year Book, St. Louis, 1994.
14. Patel MR, Edelman RR, Warach S: Detection of hyperacute primary intraparenchymal hemorrhage by magnetic resonance imaging. Stroke 27(12):2321-2324, 1996.
15. Savoiardo M, Sberna M, Grisoli M: RM e patologia vascolare del sistema nervoso centrale. Rivista di Neuroradiologia 1 (suppl. 1):95-100, 1988.
16. Thulborn KR, Atlas SW: Intracranial hemorrage. In: Atlas SW (ed). "MRI of brain and spine". II Edition. Lippincott-Raven Publishers. Philadelphia, 265-313, 1996.
17. Triulzi F: Cerebral hemorrage: CT and MRI. Rivista di Neuroradiologia 3 (suppl.2): 39-44, 1990.
18. Vignaud J, Buolin A: Tomodensitometrie cranio-encefalique. Ed Vigot Paris, 1987.
19. Zimmerman RA, Leeds NE, Naidich TP: Ring blush associated with cerebral hematoma. Radiology 122:707-711, 1977.

1.8

ULTRASOUND

M. Impagliatelli, M. Pacilli, F. Nemore, S. Lorusso, M. Maiorano, T. Scarabino

INTRODUCTION

Some 80% of all cerebrovascular accidents are caused by cerebral ischaemia and the remaining 20% by cerebral haemorrhage (3). Most cases of ischaemia are brought on by thromboembolic complications within the large extracranial supraaortic vessels (only 20% are caused by cardiac embolism), and 90% of them affect the internal carotid, middle cerebral or vertebral arteries (with a ratio of 10:5:2).

Consequential neurological deficits can be complete with possibilities of death, partial with permanent disability (25%) or transitory. In this last case, the risk of a second ischaemic episode is very high, however the probability of death or disability can be considerably reduced by antiaggregation treatment.

In ischaemic cerebrovascular events, ultrasound is highly sensitive and specific with regard to both pathogenetic mechanism and site, findings that can be easily documented using this method. In contrast to cerebral haemorrhage, where ultrasound is not diagnostic, it is fundamental to patients with transient neurological deficit in determining the strategy of primary and secondary prevention of subsequent ischaemic cerebrovascular accidents (2, 4, 6, 8).

PATHOPHYSIOLOGY

Vascular brain function impairment presents clinically with a wide spectrum of signs and symptoms and is usually characterized by a relatively close correlation between the clinical observations and the ultrasound findings of the extracranial carotid vascular system.

Symptomatology of cerebral insufficiency can be divided into four stages:
- Stage I: stenosis or compensated occlusion; the patient is asymptomatic.
- Stage II: stenosis or not completely compensated occlusion; the patient is symptomatic with a transient cerebrovascular insufficiency (TIA, RIND).
- Stage III: multiple stenoses or total progressive occlusion; the patient is symptomatic with a progressive stroke syndrome.
- Stage IV: multiple stenoses or complete occlusion; the patient is symptomatic with a complete stroke.

Ultrasound examinations are usually able to establish the type and site of the extracranial vascular lesion responsible for the neurological picture; that is, ischaemia caused by thrombosis or embolism and whether the latter originates from an atherosclerotic plaque or the heart (in this last case an echocardiographic examination must be performed).

Clinical and medical imaging correlations can be either positive (cerebral neurological symptomatology corresponds to a vascular lesion demonstrated by ultrasound) or negative (no symptoms with a positive ultrasound examination). This clinical presence of signs and symptoms is in part based upon the presence or absence of anterograde cerebral blood flow and the competency of the collateral vascular pathways (which in turn depend on such variables as systemic blood pressure, pCO_2, pO_2 and packed cell volume).

The importance of the collateral vascular circuits lies in the fact that they underlie a number of different types of symptoms, even in the presence of morphologically similar obstructing lesions. These circuits usually develop progressively, and for this reason sudden vascular occlusions cause more serious consequences than gradually developing ones.

The most important anastomotic network is the vascular circle of Willis. The posterior vertebrobasilar vascular circuit compensates for deficits in the two anterior carotid circuits by means of the posterior communicating arteries and vice versa. The anterior communicating artery on the other hand, connects the anterior circulation via this anastomosis between the two cerebral hemispheres.

In certain cases, due to vascular variations in the circle of Willis, the collateral circulation of this network will not be complete due to developmental atresia of one or more of the communicating arteries. This anatomical variation constitutes an unfavourable prognostic factor in cases of acquired cerebrovascular occlusion.

Other pertinent collateral circuits include:
– the orbital branches of the external carotid artery anastomosing with the ophthalmic artery which in turn anastomoses with the internal carotid artery;
– the branches of the external carotid artery such as the muscular branches of the occipital artery, anastomosing with muscular branches of the vertebral artery;
– the anastomotic branches between the subclavian artery and the external carotid artery on the side of unilateral internal carotid occlusion and the patent internal carotid artery on the contralateral side;
– the leptomeningeal anastomoses between the terminal branches of the principal cerebral arteries (flowing from patent vessels through their respective leptomeningeal connections in a retrograde direction into the occluded vascular network);
– the anastomosis of vessels of the dura mater connecting branches of the external carotid artery with the internal carotid arteries and the vertebral arteries;
– the intraparenchymal anastomoses between vessels within the basal ganglia; and
– the anastomoses between the anterior and posterior choroidal arteries.

The formation of an efficient collateral network is naturally negatively influenced by anterograde cerebral vascular flow sustained by adequate systemic arterial pressure as well as by some degree of patency in the remaining vascular circuit.

The haemodynamic rule is that cerebral flow remains constant so long as mean arterial pressure is above 60-70 mm Hg. For lower arterial pressure values the blood flow drops, in part because the cerebral vascular bed loses its self-regulation capacity. In chronic hypertensive subjects, the threshold values below which cerebral flow starts to drop are higher than those in normotensive subjects.

In the regulation of cerebral flow, important roles are also played by pCO_2 (e.g., flow increases with hypercapnia), pO_2 (e.g., its reduction causes a drop in arterial oxygen saturation that results in an increase in cerebral flow and the extraction of oxygen from the blood). It is also inversely proportionate to packed cell volume, as a high packed cell volume reduces the brain's oxygen needs and the cerebral flow regulates itself as a consequence.

TECHNIQUES

Ultrasound examinations of the vascular system can be divided into two techniques:
– B-Mode echotomography: gives a picture of the vessel and its walls; high frequency trans-

ducers (7.5-10 MHz) and high definition are used.

– Doppler-effect echotomography: dedicated to the analysis of endovascular haemodynamic phenomena.

This second group can be subdivided into equipment with continuous emission of the ultrasound band (CW or Continuous Wave) and pulsating emission (PW or Pulsed Wave). CW is a technique in which the transducer functions simultaneously as an emitting and receiving probe and PW is a technique in which the transducer functions alternatively as an emitting and receiving probe with a pulse repetition frequency (PRF) that can be regulated by the operator.

CW equipment has the property that while it easily identifies all vessels on the pathway of the ultrasound emitted by the exploring probe, it cannot separate the signals from the various vessels, unless by means of technical intervention (e.g., when an artery and a vein superimpose upon one another, the compression pressure exerted by the probe operator with the intrument interrupts the venous flow and permits the isolation of the arterial Doppler signal); moreover, with CW is not possible to discriminate the depth from which the reflected signals originate.

PW appliances include:

– *Echo-Doppler* (*Duplex*): in such appliances, the positioning of the sample volume takes place using the echotomography image as a guide. The transducers of these electronic probes (convex, linear, sectorial) act in the same way as do normal transducers used in B-mode ultrasound on all lines of vision with the exception of one which functions alternatively as an emitter and a receiver. In this, at a depth chosen by the operator, the sample volume is positioned (within the vessel to be examined) and velocitometric analysis is performed (spectral analysis). This takes place in real time and appears on the monitor by means of a system of Cartesian axes in which the time variable is on the abscissa, whereas the various frequencies (speeds) appear on the ordinate. What is visualized is the number of red blood cells that flow at any speed, corresponding to the width of the

Doppler signal. The flow moving towards the transducer is shown by the position of the spectrum above the base line, whereas the flow moving away from the transducer is written below the base line.

– *Echo-Colour-Doppler* (*ECD*): This is a further innovative development of Duplex techniques. With this type of appliance, flow information is obtained from numerous sample volumes positioned throughout all or part of the area explored, along each line of vision of the image (not on one line alone). The Doppler signals gathered are subsequently correlated by the computer with the colour code that will indicate the flow direction on red and blue chromatic scales: conventionally approaching flow is coded in red and the flow moving away is coded in blue. By selecting a precise line of vision and sample volume one can obtain the flow spectrum simultaneously.

– *Power-Doppler* (*PD*): This represents the latest development of the Colour-Doppler; it shows the width of the signal given by the density of the blood cells in movement irrespective of the angle of incidence of the ultrasound band and flow direction (Fig. 1.84).

A further, innovative aid to ECD and PD investigations are the recently introduced ultrasound contrast media (e.g., galactose microbubble suspension administered endovenously), which have the property of enhancing the echo-reflectivity of the surrounding blood. They are currently frequently used in the evaluation of the intracranial vessels (transcranial ECD and PD) with the possibility of performing three-dimensional reconstructions of the intracranial vasculature using lastest generation appliances (5).

Ultrasound exploration of blood vessels can be either direct or indirect. In direct explorations, the probe is placed over the vessel to be explored and the information received concerns that vessel. The vessels that can be examined in the neck are the common carotid, external carotid, internal carotid, subclavian and vertebral arteries, where it is possible to detect obstructions, stenoses, ectasias and alterations such as kinking and coiling.

Information obtained from indirect explorations does not only concern the vessel explored with the probe, but also haemodynamic variations that take place up- and downstream of it. Indirectly, using compression manoeuvres, it is possible to evaluate the condition of the circle of Willis and of the intracranial segment of the internal carotid artery. In particular, it is also possible to explore, for example, the condition of the anterior communicating

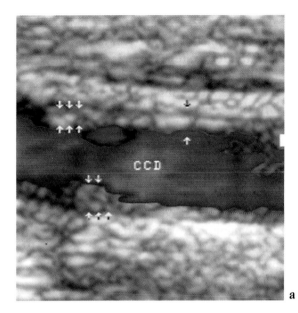

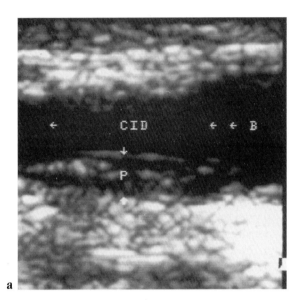

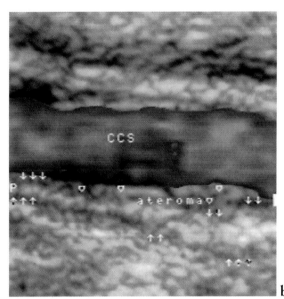

Fig. 1.79 - 79 year-old man with hypertension, diabetes and fibrillation. Severely atheromasic common carotids with plaques bulging into the lumen and marked wall alterations (**a-b**).

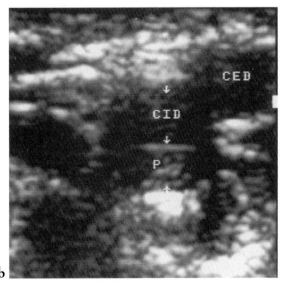

Fig. 1.78 - 65 year-old male patient with hemiplegia of the left side with acute onset. Fibroatheromasic plaque at the origin of the right internal carotid artery (**a**) with reduction in the vessel diameter of more than 50% (**b** - short axis).

artery (probe on the extracranial internal carotid with simultaneous compression of the contralateral common carotid artery) and the posterior communicating artery (probe on the distal vertebral artery with compression of the ipsilateral common carotid artery).

Using special indices (such as CR: carotid ratio; PPI: Perfusion Pressure Index; RI; resistance index, etc) it is also possible to obtain

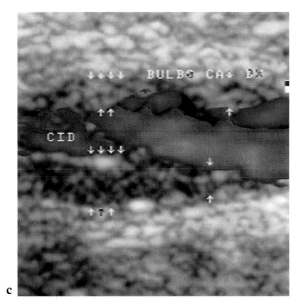

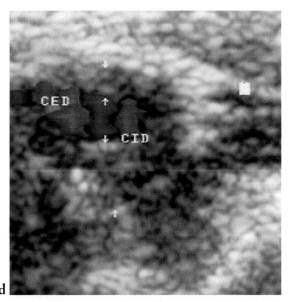

c

d

Fig. 1.79 - (*cont.*) Fibroatheromasic plaque with irregular surfaces in the right carotid bulb and the right internal carotid along the entire extracranial stretch explored with max. reduction in the vessel diameter greater than 65% (**c** - long axis, **d** - short axis).

functional information on the degree of stenosis, the state of resistance of the cerebral vascular bed and the degree of elasticity of the carotid tree as a whole.

In Doppler diagnosis of cerebrovascular emergencies, particular attention is paid to the diastolic speed (velocity) of the common carotid artery, analysed comparatively on the

two sides. In fact, a slight asymmetry of *systolic* velocity can be a normal expression of a difference in calibre of the two common carotid arteries. However, asymmetry of the *diastolic* velocity is always pathological and it alone is sufficient to diagnose an obstruction of the inter-

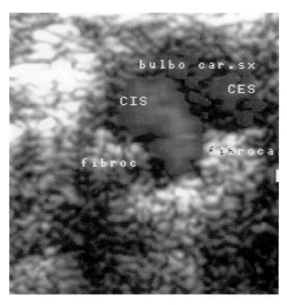

Fig. 1.80 - 70 year-old male hypertensive patient, with dizziness following fall. Cerebral CT: left hemisphere ischaemic lacunae. Ulcerated fibrocalcific plaque on the rear wall of the left carotid bifurcation.

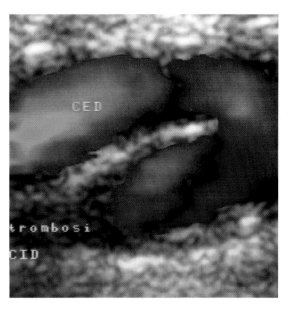

Fig. 1.81 - 45 year-old male patient with left-side hemiplegia. Thrombosis of the right internal carotid artery.

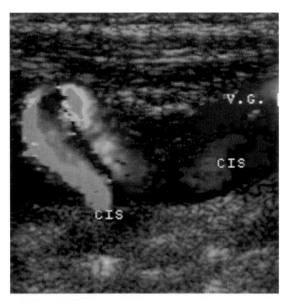

Fig. 1.82 - 68 year-old female patient with left side hemiparesis and dizziness. Kinking of the left internal carotid artery with velocitometric acceleration findings both in the internal carotid artery and downstream (left supraorbital artery).

nal carotid artery. Low diastolic velocity of the two common carotids can be an indirect sign of an aortic insufficiency or an expression of the arteriocapillary resistance downstream due to either a reduced parietal compliance (such as is observed in diabetic patients or in cases of atherosclerosis) or to global vascular compression (such as in cerebral oedema).

CLINICAL APPLICATIONS

Although the ECD technique was principally developed in the previous decade, when faced with a cerebrovascular emergency it is a good rule to begin the exploration using a CW Doppler and complete it with a pulsed Doppler, including in some cases use of the B-mode technique (2, 4, 6, 8).

A CW Doppler examination gives an accurate functional vascular analysis of haemodynamically significant stenosing lesions (stenosis equal to or greater than 70%) and of the occlusions of the supraaortic and the endorbital vascular structures. The reliability of this method is very high, with a sensitivity of approximately 92% and specificity of approximately 82%.

One particular application of the pulsed Doppler technique is the transcranial Doppler (including transcranial ECD and PD, Fig. 1.85) (1), with which it is often possible to penetrate the bony barrier of the skull to explore the large arteries of the circle of Willis. This is done by using compression manoeuvres to evaluate the intra- and extracranial collateral circuits. It can also register severe intracranial vascular spasm even when it is asymptomatic and can follow the course of arterial narrowing with serial recordings; in this manner, invasive selective angiography may be avoided and surgery can be undertaken in the critical phase of high flow velocity. Bilateral recordings of the flow velocity in the anterior, middle and posterior cerebral arteries can also aid in the comprehension of flow modes in the collateral arteries and in stenoses and occlusions of the intra- and extracranial carotid arteries.

With a simple echotomography or one combined with a pulsed or Colour Doppler, the examination is more localized and is restricted to the extracranial vessels (7). This simultaneously allows the collection of functional blood velocity data as well as informa-

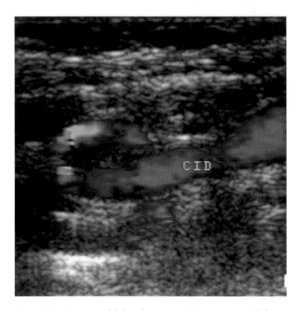

Fig. 1.83 - 78 year-old female patient, hypertensive, diabetic with left side hemiparesis with a duration of a few seconds. Coiling of the right internal carotid artery.

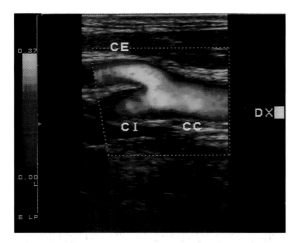

Fig. 1.84 - Power Doppler of the carotid bifurcation.

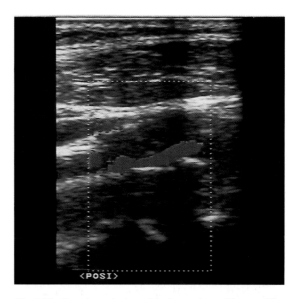

Fig. 1.86 - Pseudo-occlusion of the internal carotid artery. The Power Doppler is able to show a slight flow at an extremely reduced speed.

tion on the morphology of the vessel wall. It can identify both the surface of flat, non-haemodynamically significant atheromatous plaques (Fig. 1.78), and complicated plaques (haemorrhagic, ulcerated, calcified) (Figs. 1.79, 1.80), which are usually stenosing and associated with occlusive and preocclusive thrombus formation (Fig. 1.81). In this last case, PD has a higher sensitivity, specificity and diagnostic accuracy than does ECD, as it is able to detect the presence of a still accessible lumen, even with an extremely slowed flow that cannot be detected by ECD (Fig. 1.86). ECD therefore provides detailed evalu-

ations of the morphological alterations of the wall due to small and complicated plaques, and, on the basis of the alterations in echogenicity, it contributes to the definition of their atheromatous, fibrous and/or calcific nature (in particular, cholesterine deposits and haemorrhagic lesions of vessel walls are hyperechoic due to their low density, whereas fibrocalcific plaques are much more reflective). It also makes it possible to directly visualize any anomalies of the extracranial vessels, such as kinking or coiling (Figs. 1.82, 1.83).

ECD permits a correct diagnosis of lesions in 96% of cases and consequently has greater sensitivity than conventional selective angiography in identifying moderately stenotic lesions and in understanding their nature. It also enables the recognition of subintimal haemorrhages that are not shown on angiography as well as small ulcerated plaques that sometimes are also difficult to visualize.

CONCLUSIONS

From a certain sense, ED is to a vasculopathic patient what the electrocardiogram is to

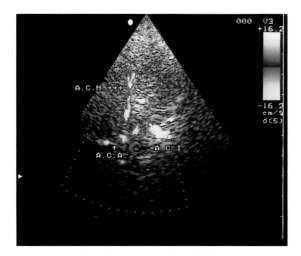

Fig. 1.85 - Transcranial Echo-Colour-Doppler. Intracranial circulation viewed through the temporal window.

the cardiopathic patient, that is, it is the first examination to be performed upon the onset of ischemic signs and symptoms. When faced with a cerebrovascular emergency, once CT has distinguished between haemorrhage and ischaemia, ED is a reliable choice of primary imaging modalities for determining the type and site of extracranial vascular stenotic lesions and for guiding subsequent therapy.

The three ultrasonographic techniques (CW, ECD and PD) are complementary to one another and very useful, in part due to their non-invasive nature. They are not however considered a substitute for angiography, which at present remains essential for the definitive study of the intracranial blood vessels, especially a focused therapeutic approach where intravascular treatment is an option.

REFERENCES

1. Bazzocchi M, Quaia E, Zuiani C et al: Transcranial Doppler: state of the art. Eur J Radiol 27:141-148, 1998.
2. Bendick PJ, Brown OW, Hernandez D et al: Three-Dimensional Vascular Imaging using Doppler Ultrasound. Am J Sur 176:183-7, 1998.
3. Bonita R: Epidemiologia dell'ictus. The Lancet 9:387-390, 1992.
4. Dauzat M: Pratique de l'ultrasonographie vasculaire. Ed. Vigot Paris, 1986.
5. Postert T, Braun B, Pfundtner N et al: Echo contrast-enhanced three-dimensional Power Doppler of intracranial arteries. Ultrasound Med Biol 7:953-956, 1998.
6. Rabbia C, De Lucchi R, Cirillo R: Eco-Color-Doppler Vascolare. Ed. Minerva Medica, 91-94, 1995.
7. Steinke W, Meairs S, Ries S, Hennerici M: Sonographic Assesment of Carotid Artery Stenosis, comparison of Power Doppler Imaging and Color Doppler Imaging. Stroke 27(1):91-4, 1996.
8. Tonarelli A: Diagnostica per Immagini della carotide extracranica: Ecografia ed Eco-Doppler. Rivista di Neuroradiologia 9 (suppl. 2):11-26, 1996.

1.9

MR ANGIOGRAPHY

A. Carella, P. D'Aprile, A. Tarantino

INTRODUCTION

The development of neuroimaging techniques has in part been driven by the need to discover and perfect methods for more rapid and accurate diagnosis of suspected cerebrovascular pathology. As a result, in recent years diagnostic and therapeutic protocols have changed by virtue of theses recent innovations. In addition, progress in the understanding of cerebral ischaemic pathology has clearified many of the physiopathological mechanisms associated with ischaemic tissue damage, which in turn have made it possible to develop more specific and effective treatment options. The neuroradiological diagnostic techniques available in clinical practice today permit a non-invasive and definitive diagnostic evaluation as early as the hyperacute phase of ischaemic stroke, in order to properly select those patients that may best be amenable to treatment with thrombolytic agents (24).

In the neuroimaging diagnostic field, MRI plays a priority role given its many applications and higher sensitivity (82%) as compared to CT (60%) in the early detection of tissue changes caused by an ischaemic event (15). That said, CT still plays a fundamental diagnostic and screening role in hyperacute stroke

patients given that it is more sensitive that MRI in demonstrating the presence of haemorrhagic foci.

With the perfusion, diffusion, spectroscopy and MR angiographic techniques, MRI represents an important arsenal for studying ischaemic stroke (within the first six hours) and the tissue changes caused by an occlusive thromboembolic event. The rational integration of the various MRI methods available permits a non-invasive, rapidly acquired diagnostic analysis of the patient presenting with signs of cerebral ischaemia, especially when it is aimed at optimally selecting patients for a specific treatment such as thrombolysis (24, 26).

MR angiography (MRA) in particular has won itself a well-defined role in diagnostic protocols evaluating cerebral ischaemia not only as a screening method, but also as an alternative to selective digital subtractive angiography (DSA) of the brachiocephalic and cerebral vessels. At present MRA constitutes an indispensable diagnostic method, which when integrated with basic MRI is the means of choice for studying the cerebral vessels with the aim of locating the site of vascular stenoses and occlusions as well as their effects upon the underlying brain tissue. Collectively the various MRI techniques are currently able to acquire high quality images of the intra- and extracranial cerebral blood vessels that not only supply qualitative data, but also yield information on the relative velocity and direction of the blood flow.

TECHNIQUES

The techniques used are unenhanced time of flight (TOF) and phase contrast (PC) 2D and 3D (two and three dimensional) MR angiography and contrast enhanced MR angiography (CE-MRA).

Time of flight (TOF)

The techniques based on the principles of TOF MR angiography are widespread and are easily performed at the same time as the basic MR scan. They are based on "inflow" phenomena capable of creating good flow-related contrast enhancement between the signal of stationary tissues and that of blood protons (i.e., blood) in movement. On entering the imaging volume under examination, the protons have not yet been subject to spatially selective radiofrequency pulses and they produce a much higher signal than that given by stationary protons within the imaging volume, which are partially saturated by previous radiofrequency (RF) pulses.

The degree of increase in flow signal depends on many parameters that are partly specific to the tissues examined (T1 relaxation time) and partly dependent on the acquisition parameters used (TR, TE, flip angle, etc.), the type of flow (velocity, turbulence, etc.) and on the geometry of the acquisition volume in comparison with the direction of the blood flow (1).

The 3D TOF technique is especially useful in studying the arterial circulation, whereas the 2D technique, which has a lower spatial definition than 3D, is particularly useful in studying slow (venous) flow. TOF techniques can be supplemented by techniques able to improve the suppression of stationary background tissue signal, thus increasing the relative contrast of

the flow signal using an additional "off resonance" RF pulse that acts on the stationary protons, saturating them selectively in comparison to those in movement that do not react to this pulse (Magnetization Transfer Contrast: MTC) (4, 6). Other possibilities of accomplishing this are to reduce intravoxel dephasing and saturation of the spins with the tilted optimized non saturation excitation (TONE) and multiple overlapping thin slab acquisition (MOTSA) techniques. In the TONE method, the flip angle is gradually increased as the flow proceeds towards the centre of the acquisition volume in order to compensate for the reduction in longitudinal magnetization of the spins in movement, whereas the MOTSA technique uses an acquisition of multiple volumes that interleave with one another (7, 16-18).

TOF techniques have limitations that are mainly characterized by two situations: the first source of error is caused by the presence in the acquisition volume of stationary tissues that can appear hyperintense (e.g., gadolinium enhancement, meta-haemoglobin, fat and oily subarachnoid contrast media) and that can therefore be wrongly interpreted as blood flow signal; the second source of error considers the possibility that vascular structures may appear isointense and therefore not emit blood flow signal using certain acquisition parameters. This latter situation can depend on a series of technical factors (e.g., TE, TR, flip angle, direction of blood flow, thickness of the acquisition layer and acquisition volume). For example, the inadvertent use of a high TE value can be one of the main causes of a lack of vascular signal; fortunately, many MR systems only allow a variation in TE values within narrow limits.

It should also be stressed that in 3D-TOF acquisitions, the anatomical structure of interest must be correctly positioned within the acquisition volume, in other words in the lower third of the slab (where the inflow effect is highest).

Phase Contrast (PC)

This technique capitalizes upon the phase effects that occur when protons move along the direction of a magnetic field gradient. PC MR angiography techniques allow the quantification of flow velocity and volume as well as the direction of the blood flow. In general, this method entails long acquisition times with wide fields of view, and it is therefore the technique of choice in the study of arteriovenous fistulas and AVM's. In fact, PC and TOF MR angiography are complementary and provide for a more accurate diagnosis when combined.

Contrast Enhancement (CE)

Dynamic MR angiographic techniques use the intravascular phase of a bolus of paramagnetic contrast medium (e.g., gadolinium) injected intravenously, in association with the acquisition of ultrafast sequences dependent on T1 relaxation times (9, 19, 22). The use of intravenous contrast medium causes a significant reduction in the T1 relaxation time of the blood with a considerable increase in the intensity of the blood flow signal as well as the relative contrast between blood and the stationary tissues. It goes without saying that in order for the contrast medium to have a maximum effect, it requires an optimal choice of the time interval between the intravenous injection of the contrast medium bolus and image acquisition.

The main drawback of this technique is an increase in stationary tissue signal and the simultaneous opacification of the veins. However, this limitation can be reduced by the use of very short scanning times (e.g., a partial K space technique as in "key-hole" sequences) and by rapidly administering the contrast medium as a bolus during data acquisition in order to acquire the images when the contrast medium reaches its greatest intravascular concentration.

MR ANGIOGRAPHY OF THE SUPRAAORTIC VESSELS

Technique

In recent years MRA has enabled an accurate and non-invasive diagnostic analysis of the supraaortic vessels, which together with Doppler ultrasound studies in the presurgical phase has limited the use of invasive conventional DSA to selected cases.

Although PC MR angiography can be utilized to examine the supraaortic vessels, TOF techniques are more commonly employed. Generally speaking, for studies of the carotid bifurcation a transverse acquisition plane with a 3D-TOF technique is used to reduce the saturation effects, however, this technique has certain limitations due to its long acquisition times and consequently the associated motion artefacts (14). The proposal made by Prince in 1994 (19) was therefore accepted with enthusiasm; the proposal involved using contrast-enhanced 3D MR angiography to capture the passage of a bolus of paramagnetic contrast material through the inaging volume in order to study the supraaortic vessels. This led to the perfection of a technique capable of examining the extracranial vessels including the aortic arch, the origins of the supraaortic vessels and the neck vessels (13, 23). In particular, extremely fast volumetric acquisitions are used directly in the coronal plane during the injection of the contrast medium bolus, over acquisition times of approximately 15-30 seconds. In this technique, given that the signal is produced mainly by the administered contrast agent, it is mandatory to synchronize the image acquisition with the injection of the contrast agent in order to obtain maximum arterial filling during the central portion of acquisition. The advantage of this method lies in the speed of the examination and in the possibility of now covering the entire length of the brachiochephalic vessels from their origins through their proximal intracranial segments (Figs. 1.87, 1.88).

Clinical applications

The cervical carotid and vertebral arteries were the first vascular segments for the application of MR angiography. Numerous studies of MRA show its high sensitivity in detecting carotid stenoses, 92-100%, with a specificity of 64-100% (2, 5, 14).

Slow and turbulent flow can cause a signal drop-out within the vessel under study, with a consequent overestimation of the degree of stenosis. This represents an important limitation in the use of standard 2D- and 3D-TOF MR angiographic techniques.

The recent introduction of CE 3D-TOF MRA has resolved certain problems concerning the correct estimation of the degree of vascular stenosis and the evaluation of the origins of the supraaortic vessels (Fig. 1.89). Recent studies have shown the CE 3D-TOF technique to be more accurate than standard 2D- and 3D-TOF acquisitions (14, 23).

Stenotic-occlusive atheromatous pathology

The 3D-TOF MR angiographic technique is currently considered the best available method for defining the morphology of stenotic-occlusive lesions of the carotid and vertebral arteries.

To avoid problems with the progressive saturation of the spins when using 2D- and 3D-TOF techniques, one should preferably use an acquisition plane perpendicular to the longitudinal axis of the vessel being examined; consequently, both the carotid and the vertebral arteries must be examined in the axial plane (Fig. 1.90). The 3D-TOF technique can also be used with a bolus injection of a contrast agent (gadolinium), using rapid volumetric acquisitions in the coronal plane (Fig. 1.91). The disadvantage of this technique is in its slightly invasive nature (linked to the intravascular administration of gadolinium) and in its limited spatial resolution as compared to the traditional 3D-TOF method utilizing a transverse plane acquisition.

For stenoses greater than 70%, a signal dropout at the stenotic segment is described in both the 2D- and 3D-TOF MR angiographic techniques. In cases of preocclusive high grade

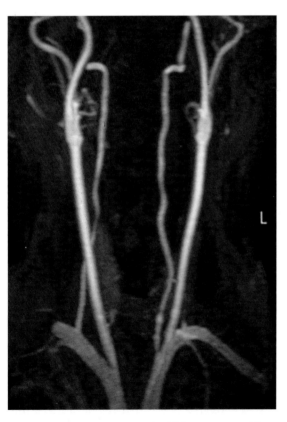
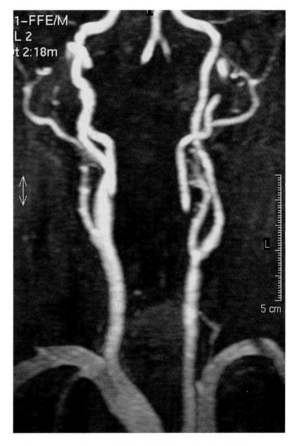

Figs. 1.87-1.88 - Dynamic MRA scan of the epiaortic vessels acquired in the coronal plane with high definition ultrafast T1 sequences (AT: 28 seconds); note the excellent demarcation from the emergence of the epiaortic vessels.

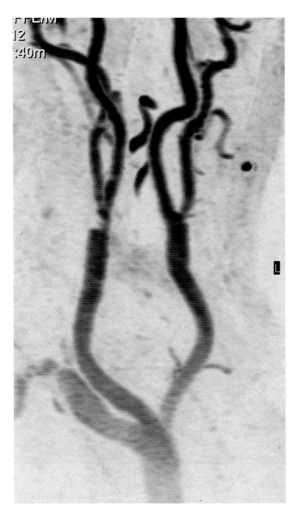

Fig. 1.89 - Dynamic CE MRA: presents a serrated stenosis of the right subclavian artery and a stenosis on the bifurcation of the right carotid artery.

stenosis, the 2D-TOF technique may prove more effective than the 3D because its sensitivity to slow flow makes it possible to identify residual flow distal to the narrowing, whereas the 3D technique can give an erroneous picture of occlusion with a complete absence of distal flow signal.

Vascular dissections

Stenotic-occlusive pathology of the internal carotid artery and the vertebrobasilar vessels is being increasingly seen as cases presenting as neurological and neuroradiological emergencies. With regard to ischaemic strokes, particular attention must be paid to the role of dissection of the cervical arteries. These dissections are often under recognized as they typically affect young patients who commonly lack the usual vascular risk factors (2%).

Increased diagnostic suspicion is often suggested by the appearance of headache, stiff neck, neck pain, Horner's syndrome and dizziness in the dissection of the vertebral artery. Carotid and vertebral dissections can be diagnosed with relative ease using simple MR and MRA acquisitions (Fig. 1.92) (20). Levy et al (12) reported a sensitivity and specificity of 95% and 98%, respectively, for the detection of cervical internal carotid dissection.

Both T1- and T2-weighted spin echo (SE) images and the single partitions of 3D-TOF MRA permit the detection of the characteristic findings of vascular dissection, including the presence of a flow void in the residual lumen and haemoglobin hyperintensity within the subintimal haematoma. An alternative to the TOF method is a combination of PC MRA and a comparative T1-weighted SE study with suppression of the fat signal for the effective visualization of the intramural thrombus.

With regard to dissections of the vertebral artery, although MR angiography is less sensitive than that of the internal carotid artery, it is felt to be preferable to invasive selective conventional DSA as the double lumen caused by the subintimal dissection can cause the detachment of emboli in patients undergoing catheterization.

MR angiography plays an important role in the follow-up of these lesions, which usually successfully heal after treatment with anticoagulants.

INTRACRANIAL VESSELS

Technique

The most frequently used technique for studying the intracranial vessels is 3D-TOF MRA. The acquisition volume is oriented transversally and covers the vessels of the circle of Willis and the proximal segments of the major

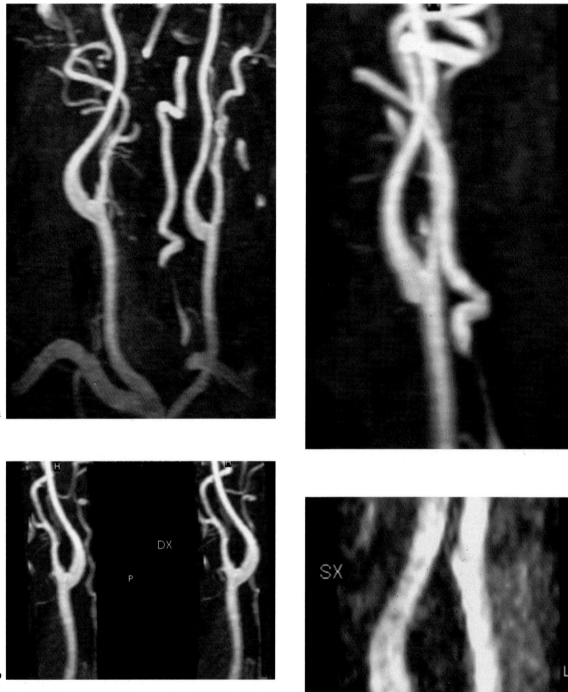

Fig. 1.90 - Dynamic MRA: **a)** panoramic study of the epiaortic vessels; **b)** selective reconstruction of the left carotid bifurcation, which appears normal; **c)** selective reconstruction of the right carotid bifurcation in which one can observe the presence of an atheromasic plaque at the beginning of the right internal carotid artery. **d)** comparative study of the right carotid bifurcation with 3D-TOF technique and axial acquisitions: note a reduction in flow signal by the plaque; echo-Doppler finding: soft stenosing plaque at the origin of the right internal carotid artery.

cerebral arteries; in order to obtain good spatial and contrast resolution, the thickness of the individual scans must be relatively small (0.8 - 1.5 mm). Optimal intravascular contrast is obtained using the variable flip angle technique

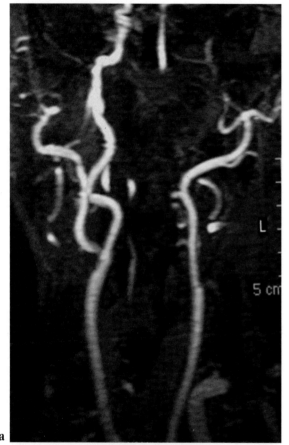

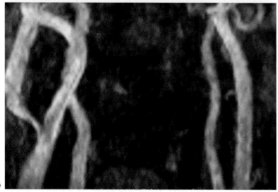

Fig. 1.91 - Dynamic MRA scan of the epiaortic vessels: **a)** stenosis on the bifurcation of the right carotid artery and occlusion at the start of the left internal carotid artery; **b)** the specific study using the 3D-TOF technique better demarcates the presence and entity of the stenosis at the start of the right external carotid artery.

(TONE) coupled with transverse magnetization transfer (MTC) overlay for better suppression of the perivascular stationary tissue signal (4, 16). For the separate study of the arterial and venous systems, it is necessary to correctly position prespatial saturation bands proximal to the flow signal to be eliminated.

In general, contrast agents are not used for studying the cerebral vessels, with the exception of certain cases where the intracranial pathology demands that intravascular contrast material be specifically used for the study of slow vascular flow.

CLINICAL APPLICATIONS

Stenotic-occlusive pathology

In recent years the development and clinical application of MRI in the study of ischaemic stroke patients has provided much information on cerebral perfusion (perfusion MR), metabolic integrity (spectroscopy MR), variations in cerebral diffusion coefficients (DWI) and information on the morphology of the intra- and extracranial vessels using MR angiography (2, 25).

In cases of ischaemic stroke, MR angiography plays a potentially important role. In the hyperacute phase of cerebral ischaemia, integrating the morphological and metabolic imaging information in cases of vascular stenosis or occlusion provides all the data required to make specific therapeutic choices (Figs. 1.93, 1.94).

MR angiography provides a good representation of the first and second order vessels of the circle of Willis, but has limitations in the study of smaller vessels (Figs. 1.95, 1.96, 1.97, 1.98). In addition to spatial definition, limitations include an accurate estimation of the degree of high grade stenoses and the accurate distinction between high grade stenoses and frank occlusions (8, 11).

The carotid siphon can benefit from an MR angiographic evaluation, although care must be taken to avoid errors in overestimation of the pathological changes due to the reduction in flow signal as a result of turbulence. Another problem is posed in some cases by the flow tur-

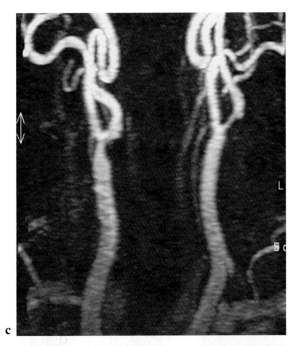

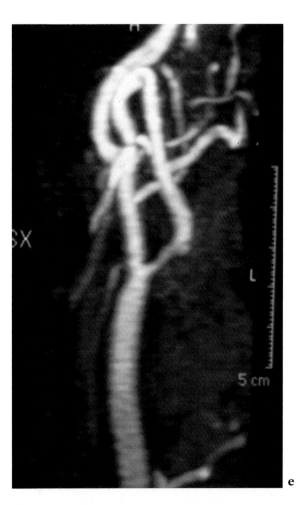

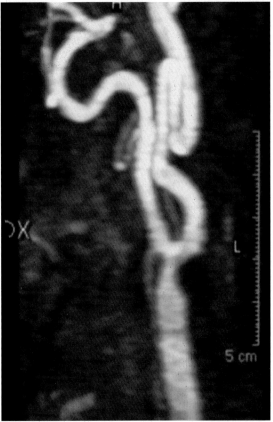

Fig. 1.91 - (*cont.*) – **c**) Another case, medium grade stenosis on the right carotid bifurcation and serrated stenosis with presence of plaque at the beginning of the left internal carotid artery; **d** and **e**) selective reconstruction of the carotid bifurcations.

bulence present at vascular bifurcations, which can erroneously be interpreted as stenoses. The administration of contrast media (gadolinium) has been used to resolve these problems of partial signal loss.

Collateral pathways to the circle of Willis can be evaluated using the 3D-TOF technique by means of an appropriate arrangement of the selective prespatial saturation pulse; an alternative is the PC method that provides information on the direction of blood flow (25).

Occlusive venous pathology

With suspected venous thrombosis, MR venography is the diagnostic examination of choice. This technique is used together with the conventional SE MR scan, which permits the detection of associated parenchymal abnormalities (e.g., venous infarction) as well as the abnormal signal of vascular thrombosis or the ab-

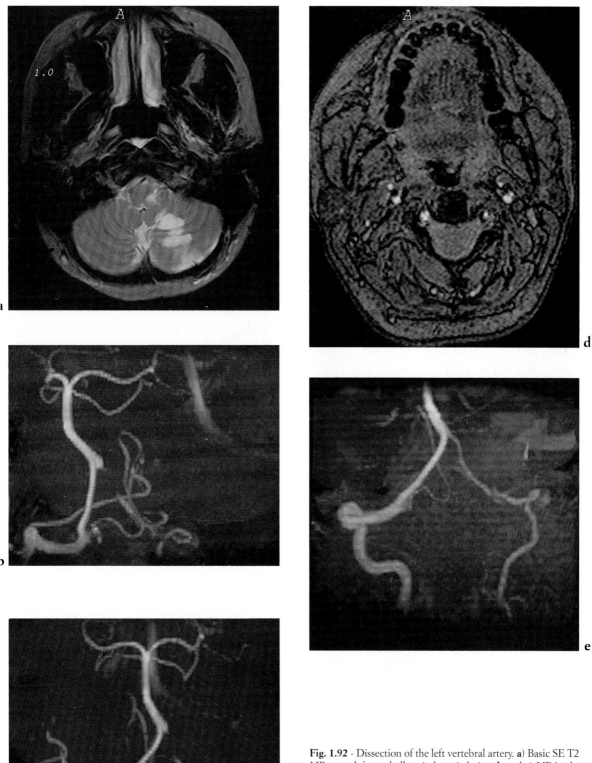

Fig. 1.92 - Dissection of the left vertebral artery. **a)** Basic SE T2 MR scan: left cerebellum ischaemic lesion; **b** and **c)** MRA: absence of signal in the last stretch of the left vertebral artery; **d)** single base partition: presence of hypointense parietal thrombus, in acute phase, at the vertebral artery; **e)** check-up MRA (15 days later): partial recanalization of the vessel.

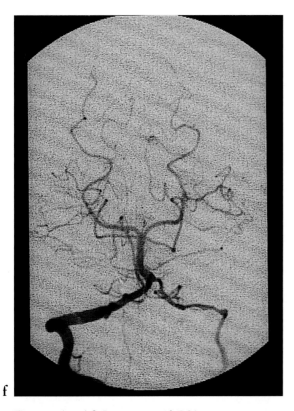

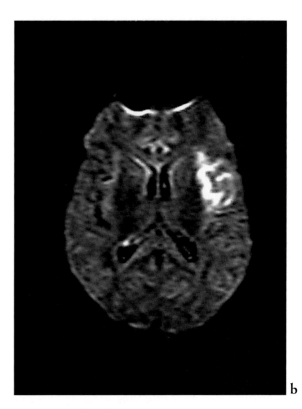

f

Fig. 1.92 - (*cont.*) **f**) Comparison with DSA.

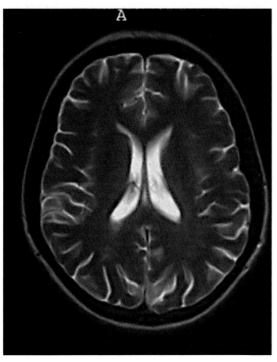

a

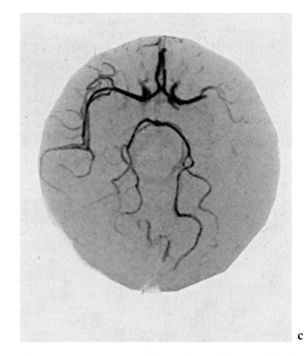

c

Fig. 1.93 - Hyperacute phase ischaemia. **a**) Basic SE T2 MRI: negative finding; **b**) DW MR image; ischaemic lesion in left insular-parietal location; **c**) MRA of the vessels of the circle of Willis: occlusion of the bifurcation of the left Sylvian artery.

sence of normal signal void within the dural venous sinuses. Toward this same aim, T2-weighted SE images acquired perpendicular to the dural venous sinuses are recommended for a more accurate supplemental study.

In MR angiography, the high signal of the thrombus can give false negative results; in such cases a comparative study using T1- and T2-weighted SE images and the application of presaturation bands, as well as use of the PC tech-

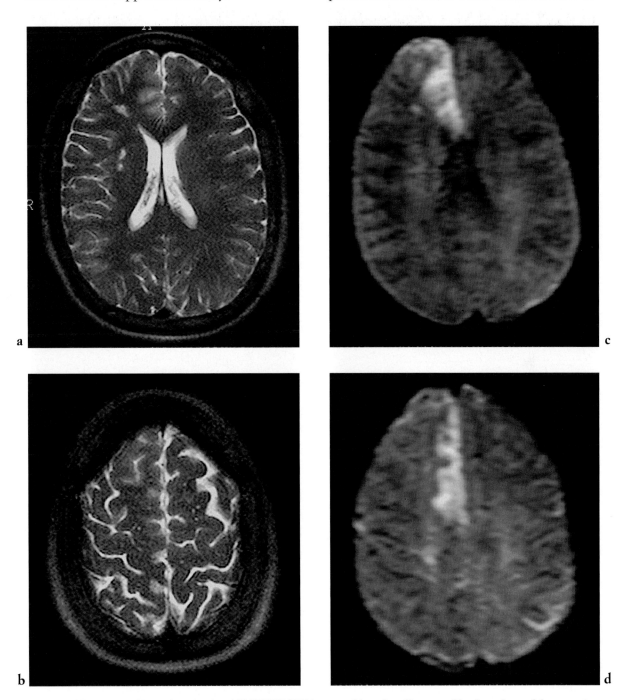

Fig. 1.94 - Hyperacute phase ischaemia. **a**) and **b**) TSE-HASTE images, a blurred swelling caused by the oedema of the cortex in a right parasagittal frontal position with small hyperintensities near the signal; **c** and **d**) DW images: widespread ischaemic focus in the territory of the right anterior cerebral artery.

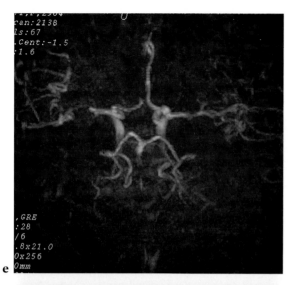

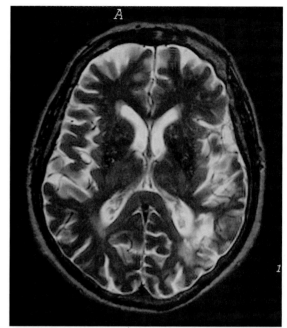

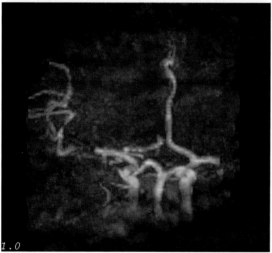

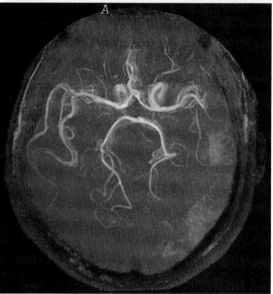

Fig. 1.94 - (*cont.*) **e** and **f**) MRA of the vessels of the circle of Willis: occlusion at the start of the right anterior cerebral artery and serrated stenosis in segment M2 of the right Sylvian artery.

nique are in combination typically able to dispel diagnostic doubts (17).

Aneurysms

In the acute stage of subarachnoid haemorrhage, the examination of choice is CT, followed by invasive conventional selective DSA to reveal the presence of one or more aneurysms and to visualize the anatomy of the individual aneurysms; MRI and MRA have secondary roles during this acute phase.

MRA is the examination technique of choice for screening patients with family histories of

Fig. 1.95 - Left insular-temporal-parietal ischaemic lesion: **a**) basic SE T2 MRI; **b**) 3D-TOF MRA of the vessels of the circle of Willis; occlusion in segment M2 of the left Sylvian artery.

such potentially heritable pathology as the aneurysms associated with polycystic kidney disease, or in cases where there is a relatively high association of aneurysms such as aortic coarctation (21). Studies performed thus far show that MRA is able to detect 3-4 mm aneurysms with approximately 86-90% sensitivity, and with 100% specificity (3, 10) (Fig.

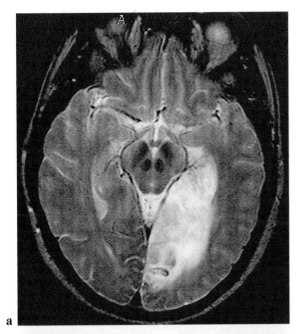

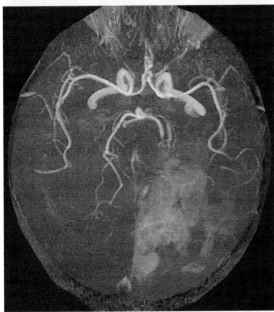

Fig. 1.96 - Left temporooccipital ischaemia: **a)** basic SE T2 MRI; **b)** MRA of the vessels of the circle of Willis: occlusion in the P1 segment of the left posterior cerebral artery.

underestimation of the dimensions of the lumen of the aneurysm.

3D-TOF MRA has recently been used in studying aneurysms treated with Guglielmi's

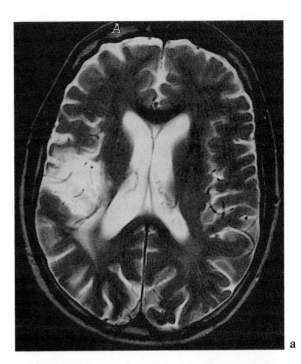

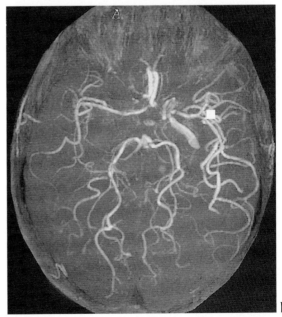

Fig. 1.97 - Right parietal ischaemia: **a)** basic SE T2 MRI; **b)** 3D-TOF MRA of the vessels of the circle of Willis: absence of flow signal in the right carotid siphon with partial revascularization of the right Sylvian artery through the circle vessels.

1.99). Smaller aneurysms are often not visible due to MR angiography's limited spatial resolution and because of the irregular flow dynamics within small aneurysms. And, when studying giant aneurysms the slow and turbulent flow can reduce the intraluminal signal and cause an

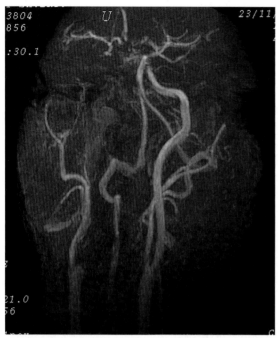

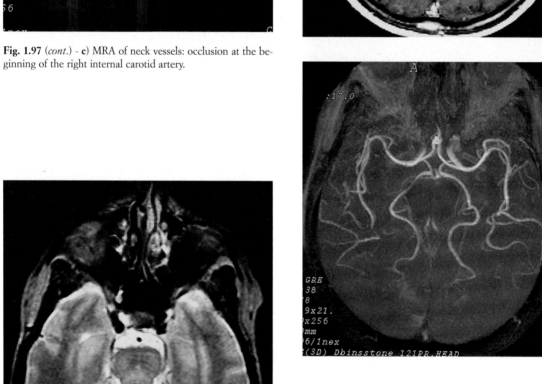

Fig. 1.97 (*cont.*) - **c**) MRA of neck vessels: occlusion at the beginning of the right internal carotid artery.

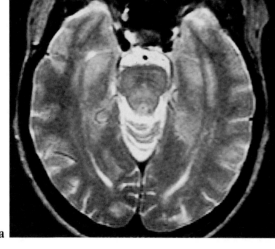

Fig. 1.98 - **a**) Basic SE T2 MRI; blurred signal hyperintensity in right occipital location; **b**) SE T1 image after gadolinium: nonhomogeneous contrast enhancement due to blood-brain barrier damage caused by the presence of an acute ischaemic area; **c**) MRA of the vessels of the circle of Willis: stenosis in the proximal segment of the right posterior cerebral artery.

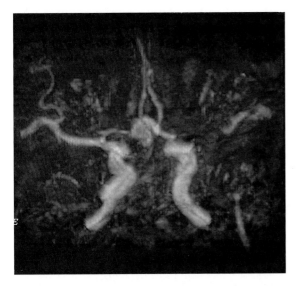

Fig. 1.99 - 3D TOF MRA of the vessels of the circle of Willis: presence of an aneurysm on the anterior communicating artery.

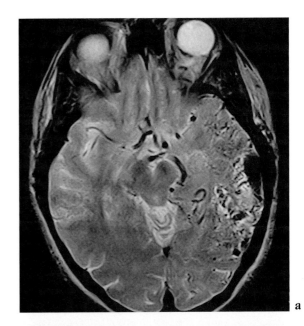
a

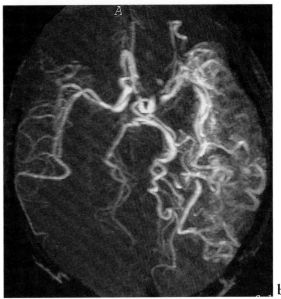
b

detachable embolization coils. This has shown a good correspondence between MRA and selective DSA with regard to the evaluation of aneurysms occluded with coils. It has in fact been possible to evaluate any residual aneurysm neck and flow within the residual aneurysmatic sack if present. However, to be fair, certain vascular details are obviously less easy to evaluate in the single MRA partitions.

Arteriovenous malformations

Generally speaking, MRA used in combination with MRI is sufficient for the detection of most cerebral arteriovenous malformations. The TOF MRA technique gives good documentation of the major arterial feeding arteries (Fig. 1.100). Venous drainage and the central nidus are better studied using PC MRA. The use of intravenous gadolinium improves visualization of the venous vascular components of AVM's.

MRA also permits in-depth studies of the nidus, its dimensions and its relationship with the surrounding neural tissue, which are important elements for treatment planning. This technique is also useful during follow-up after therapy; invasive selective DSA is nevertheless required in order to obtain precise images of the exact anatomical architecture and the dynamic aspects of the AVM.

Fig. 1.100 - AVM: **a)** basic SE T2 MRI: numerous serpigenous images with signal void in the left temporoparietal region; **b)** 3D TOF MRA: presence of a large AVM, supplied by branches originating from the Sylvian artery and left posterior cerebral artery.

CONCLUSIONS

MRA is an important non-invasive method for studying the brachiocephalic and cerebral blood vessels. Its main application in neuroradiological emergencies is for the evaluation of cerebral circulation in suspected cases of ischaemic stroke or thrombosis of the dural venous sinuses. In such cases, MRA can be performed together with conventional MRI aimed at obtaining a rapid and complete diagnostic analysis of the problem, thereby allowing optimal specific treatment choices to be made. It is also widely used to screen for cerebral aneurysms in high risk groups, and more recently to monitor aneurysms following treatment with Gugielmi's detachable embolization coils.

It is important to underline the importance of having access to high performance MRI systems that allow the rapid execution of both the static conventional imaging as well as the angiographic acquisitions.

REFERENCES

1. Anderson CM, Edelman RR, Turki PA: Clinical Magnetic Resonance Angiography. Raven Press New York, 1993.
2. Atlas SW: MR angiography in neurologic disease. Radiology 193:1-6, 1994.
3. Atlas SW, Sheppard L, Godberg HI et al: Intracranial aneurysms: detection and characterization with MR angiography with use of an advanced post-processing technique in a blinded-reader study. Radiology 203:807-814, 1997.
4. Atkinson D, Brant-Zawadzki M, Gilliam G et al.: Improved MR angiography: magnetization transfer suppression with variable flip angle excitation and increased resolution. Radiology 190:890-894, 1994.
5. Bowen BC, Quencer RM, Margosian P et al.: MR angiography of occlusive disease of the arteries in the head and neck: current concepts. AJR 162: 9-18, 1994.
6. Edelman RR, Ahn SS, Chien D et al.: Improved time-of-fligth MR angiography of the brain with magnetization transfer contrast. Radiology 184: 395-399, 1992
7. Furst G, Hofer M, Steinmetz H et al.: Intracranial stenoocclusive disease: MR angiography with magnetization transfer and variable flip angle. AJNR 17:1749-1757, 1996.
8. Heiserman JE, Drayer BP, Keller PJ et al.: Intracranial vascular stenosis and occlusion: evaluation with tree-dimensional time-of-flight MR angiography. Radiology 185:667-673, 1992.
9. Kim JK, Farb RI, Wright GA: Test bolus examination in the carotid artery at dynamic gadolinium-enhanced MR angiography. Radiology 206:283-289, 1998.
10. Korogi Y, Takahashi M, Mabuchi N: Intracranial aneurysms: diagnostic accuracy of MR angiography with evaluation of maximum intensity projection and surce images. Radiology 199:199-207, 1996.
11. Korogi Y, Takahaski M, Nakagawa T et al.: Intracranial vascular stenosis and occlusion: MR angiography findings. AJNR 18:135-143, 1997.
12. Levy C, Laissy JP, Raveau V: Carotid and vertebral artery dissections: three dimensional time of fligth MR angiography and MR versus conventional angiography. Radiology 190:97-103, 1994.
13. Levy RA, Prince MR: Arterial-phase three-dimensional contrast-enhanced MR angiography of the carotid arteries. AJR 167:211-215, 1996.
14. Litt AW, Eidelman EM, Pinto RS et al.: Diagnosis of carotid artery stenosis: comparison of 2D time of fligth MR angiography with contrast angiography in 50 patients. AJNR 12:149-154, 1991.
15. Mathews VP, Elster AD, King JC et al: Combined effects of magnetization transfer and gadolinium in cranial MR imaging and MRA. AJR 164:167-172, 1995.
16. Mattle HP, Wentz KU et al: Cerebral venography with MR. Radiology 178:453-458, 1991.
17. Mohr JP, Biller J, Hilal SK et al: Magnetic resonance imaging in acute stroke. Stroke 26:807-812, 1995.
18. Parker DL, Blatter DD: Multiple thin slab magnetic resonance angiography. Neuroimag Clin North AM 2:677-692, 1992.
19. Provenzale JM: Dissection of the internal carotid and vertebral arteries: imaging features. AJR 165:1099-1104, 1995.
20. Prince MR, Grist TM, Bebatin JE et al: 3D contrast MR angiography. Springer-Verlag (New-York) 1997.
21. Ruggeri PM, Poulos N, Masaryk TJ et al: Occult intracranial aneurysms in polycystic kidney disease: screening with MR angiography. Radiology 191:33-39, 1994.
22. Sardanelli F, Zandrino F et al: MR angiography of internal-carotid arteries:breath-hold gd-enhanced 3D fast imaging with steady-state precession versus unenhanced 2D and 3D time-of-fligth techniques. J Cat 23:208-215, 1999.
23. Scarabino T, Carriero A et al: MR angiography in carotid stenosis: a comparison of three techniques. Eur J Radiol 28:117-125, 1998.
24. Sorensen AG, Buonanno FS, Gonzales RG et al: Hyperacute stroke: evaluation with combined multisection diffusion-weighted and hemodynamically weighted echoplanar MR imaging. Radiology 199:991-401, 1996.
25. Stock KW, Wetzel S, Kirsch E et al: Anatomic evaluation of the circle of Willis: MR angiography versus intraarterial digital subtraction angiography. AJNR 17:1495-1499, 1996.
26. Warach S, Gaa J et al: Acute human stroke studied by whole brain echo planar diffusion-weithted magnetic resonance imaging. Ann Neurol 37:231-241, 1995.

1.10

CONVENTIONAL ANGIOGRAPHY

F. Florio, M. Nardella, S. Balzano, V. Strizzi, T. Scarabino

INTRODUCTION

The relatively recent advent of sophisticated imaging techniques such as CT and MR has dramatically reduced the demand for conventional invasive selective cerebral angiography in radiological diagnosis. Despite the fact that conventional angiography is now considered complementary to other techniques in neurological emergencies, it has been shown not to be completely replaceable because there are certain questions that angiography alone can answer.

In recent years, there has been a return to the use of angiography based on the improvement in the technique's safety, speed and sophistication (e.g., hard- and software improvements, atraumatic catheterization materials, and new low osmolarity contrast agents), and on the progressively increasing experience of vascular interventional radiology treatment techniques (8). This last factor has led to angiography being considered as having a dual purpose: an instrument used in both diagnosis and therapy.

CLINICAL INDICATIONS

The clinical indications for emergency angiography are cerebral ischaemia and haemorrhage, as well as some forms of cranial trauma and thrombotic pathology of the venous structures. The initial diagnostic evaluation is nevertheless left to non-invasive methods such as CT, MR and Doppler ultrasound, which are now able to satisfy the most urgent diagnostic requirements. Generally speaking, angiography is presently used in those cases in which non-invasive techniques have exhausted their usefulness, and, above all, when treatment using endovascular techniques is being considered.

Cerebral ischaemia

In cerebral ischaemia, depending on whether it manifests itself as TIA or frank infarction, angiography is not routinely used except in specific cases during certain time periods following the ischaemic ictus.

a) *Transient ischaemic attacks*: TIA's do not usually constitute an angiographic emergency; patients with TIA's are typically subjected to angiography only after a certain period of time during which the clinical evolution and the less invasive diagnostic techniques (e.g., ultrasound) have indicated the presence of a vascular lesion that might be amenable to surgery. Although in-

frequently encountered, angiographic examina
tions can be mandatory in patients suffering
from repeated ischaemic attacks and having a
non-invasive imaging diagnosis of subtotal occlusion of one of the cervicocranial vessels; in
such cases urgent surgery or angioplasty may be
able to prevent total vascular thrombosis.

b) *Cerebral infarction*: Angiography is rarely
used today in cases of frank cerebral infarction,
and is in any case usually delayed until partial
functional clinical recovery is observed.

Trends recently have pointed towards utilizing very early angiographic examinations, within hours following the acute ischaemic event,
when the clinical syndrome can be attributed to
an arterial occlusion that may be susceptible to
treatment using transcatheter fibrinolysis. This
is one of the more recent innovations of interventional neuroradiology, although its real clinical efficacy merits further investigation (2).

Cerebral haemorrhage

Angiography plays a more important role in
cases of cerebral haemorrhage.

a) *Parenchymal haemorrhages* do not usually
require angiographic analysis when the origin
of the haemorrhage is thought to be spontaneous (i.e., elderly patient with hypertension).
However, when clinical and anatomical conditions favour a different aetiology for the haemorrhage (e.g., relatively young patient, normotensive, atypical position, etc.), angiography
becomes mandatory and should be performed
urgently, especially when the haemorrhage demands emergency surgery.

b) In cases of epidural/subdural haemorrages emergency angiography has varying diagnostic importance. It is unusual for posttraumatic epidural/subdural haemorrages to gain
diagnostic benefit from angiography. Angiography can only be justified when associated lesions of the cerebral vessels are suspected (e.g.,
dissection or rupture of a vessel wall, posttraumatic aneurysms, arteriovenous malforma-
tions/fistulae).

c) Angiography has a different importance
in the case of *subarachnoid haemorrhage*. With
its often abrupt onset and typical clinical picture, subarachnoid haemorrhage is the most
frequently encountered of the potential neurological angiographic emergencies.

Thrombosis of the cerebral veins and dural venous sinuses

This type of pathology, now somewhat rare,
can require emergency angiography when intracranial hypertension dominates the clinical
picture. In such cases, angiography is used to
confirm the clinicoradiological suspicions.
However, while the cranial dural venous sinuses are more critically assessed angiographically,
digital subtraction angiography (DSA) is only
capable of providing indirect information on
the thrombosis of cortical venous structures
(e.g., slow arterial and venous circulation, areas
of paucity of venous vessels, presence of collateral venous circulation).

TECHNIQUES

Angiography performed in emergency conditions is relatively difficult and requires a certain degree of experience as it is almost always
performed in less than ideal circumstances.
This difficulty is due both to the patient's state
of consciousness and ability to cooperate as
well as to the gravity of the clinical picture,
which requires the utmost rapidity of angiographic examination execution and immediate
interpretation. The use of conventional angiography has been much improved by the advent
of modern DSA appliances with high spatial
definition (1024 x 1024 matrix). DSA allows,
above all, reduced examination times, while the
marked simplification of the radiographic technique has made it possible to limit the total
amount of contrast medium required for each
individual injection. In addition, the use of low
concentration, low osmolarity, non-ionic contrast agents has reduced the potential contrast
agent toxicity risk. In short, DSA has evolved
into the a much simpler imaging modality with
less risk to the patient.

The only drawback of DSA is its sensitivity to even the slightest patient motion; this requires complete patient immobilization, which is typically only possible with deep sedation or general anaesthesia. If there are no specific contraindications, such as underlying cerebral haemorrhage, minimal heparinization can be undertaken. With these exceptions, no other particular patient preparation is usually required.

Patient vital functions and neurological status should be monitored constantly during the examination, and the patient should be kept under observation for 12-24 hours after the procedure. In the absence of contraindications, the angiogram is performed through transfemoral access. Other routes of access (e.g., axillary, common carotid arteries) have a higher risk of local complications. Preliminary arch aortography used to explore the large supra-aortic arterial branches is preferable in general and specifically indispensable for identifying vacular variations and ostial/proximal atherosclerotic lesions. In order to study the aortic arch and its branches, the left anterior oblique projection is used with an angulation of 15-20 degrees; generally speaking, 20-25 ml of contrast medium are required with a flow rate of 10-15 ml/sec delivered over 1-2 seconds (total contrast volume: 25-50 ml). Studies of the carotid bifurcation require both oblique projections in order to project the internal carotid free from the external carotid artery, as well as to study the walls and lumen of the vascular structures circumferentially. Although panoramic imaging of the cranial vasculature can be useful as a preliminary approach to locating major lesions and to analyse overall haemodynamic balance of flow between the cerebral hemispheres, selective catheterization of the cerebral vessels is almost always essential. Each arterial injection examined requires at least the two orthogonal projections during DSA; in many cases oblique projection imaging also needs to be performed in order to properly define the pathology. Each individual injection usually requires not more than 6-9 ml of contrast medium delivered at a rate of 6 ml per second (more in

cases of arteriovenous malformation or large arteriovenous fistula). In latest generation angiographic appliances, the examination is facilitated by improvements such as rotational angiography or even 3D angiography (20).

APPLICATIONS

We will examine the dual diagnostic and therapeutic role of angiography in ischaemic and haemorrhagic pathology, and omit trauma and thrombotic pathology of the venous structures, which are more rarely observed at emergency diagnostic cerebral angiography.

Diagnostic role

In cases of ischaemia and haemorrhage, angiography is usually principally responsible for identifying the vascular lesion(s) responsible for the clinical syndrome and for definitively determining the plan for therapy.

a) Cerebral ischaemia: Regardless of whether it involves transient ischaemic attacks or frank infarction, the principle role of DSA is simply to identify the vascular lesion(s) responsible for the ischaemia. Further goals include the analysis of the degree of the stenotic/occlusive pathology and an estimation of its haemodynamic significance, exclusion of the presence of other lesions that could affect treatment and provision of a complete picture of cerebral haemodynamics. Another important factor is the characterization of such lesions: whether they are atherosclerotic, dysplastic (e.g., fibromuscular dysplasia) or related to trauma (e.g., arterial dissection); and whether there are associated complications (e.g., intraluminal thrombus, ulceration of atherosclerotic plaques) (Fig. 1.101). In actual fact, today there are a number of examination techniques available (Echo-Colour-Doppler, MR angiography, CT angiography and SPECT), which alongside angiography contribute to this global evaluation and finally to the formulation of treatment choices.

b) Cerebral Haemorrhage: In the presence of haemorrhages, cerebral angiography plays a

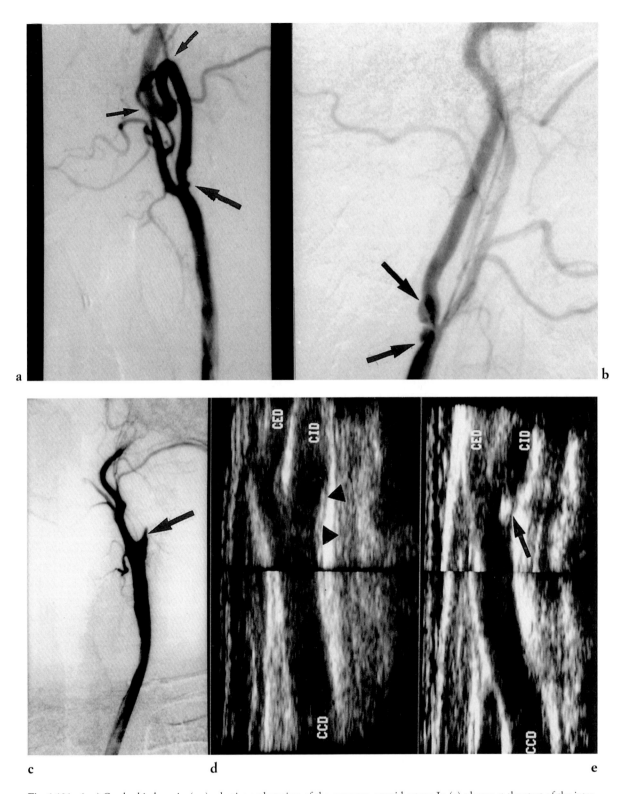

Fig. 1.101 - (**a-e**) Cerebral ischaemia. (**a-c**) selective catheterism of the common carotid artery. In (**a**) plaque at the start of the internal carotid artery, with "rose thorn" image due to ulcer (arrow); kinking in the precranial stretch (small arrows); in **b**) irregular plaque (ulcerated). (**d-e**) Ultrasound of the carotid bifurcation. In (**d**) marked intimal thickening with flat plaques (arrowhead); in (**e**) coarse sclerocalcific plaque (arrow).

more complex role. Nevertheless, in cases of intraparenchymal haemorrhage, when performed correctly using proper techniques, angiography is able to identify or exclude the existence of associated underlying aneurysms or vascular malformations.

With AVM's, utmost attention must be paid to determining the arterial feeders, venous drainage and other singular anatomical and haemodynamic characteristics of the malformation (Fig. 1.102). This information is essential for treatment planning and for optimally choosing between surgery and transcatheter embolic therapy.

The recent interest in intraoperative angiography made possible by the new portable and manageable DSA appliances have allowed to conduct angiographic examinations directly on the operating table. This approach could prove invaluable in immediate preoperative, intraoperative and postoperative evaluations of vascular malformations in patients with intraparenchymal haemorrhage.

In the presence of subarachnoid haemorrhage the use of angiography is even more important and is essential in most cases to determine the optimal surgical approach. Angiography is the most suitable method for directly demonstrating the cause of the bleed (e.g., aneurysm or malformation) in such cases. At present, MR angiography and CT angiography can identify large and many of the smaller aneurysms; however, in patients with subarachnoid haemorrhage, negative MR angiography does not rule out the presence of an underlying aneurysm or vascular malformation. Therefore, although invasive selective angiography is not completely devoid of risks, at the present time it remains the most sensitive angiographic technique. Selecting the time at which to perform the examination is particularly difficult, and is much dependent upon the presence or absence of arterial vasospasm and the timing of surgery. Performing angiography in the period during which vasospasm is most likely to be present (3-10 days after the bleed) can lead to a masking of the presence of the aneurysm sack due to non-filling. The decision as to whether to perform

angiography either in the early phase (day one) following subarachnoid haemorrhage or later (two weeks) depends upon the decision of the surgical team and the patient's clinical condition. This examination requires experience and diligence, paying particular attention to detail. It should also be pointed out that in certain situations, despite the utmost care in angiographic examination execution and interpretation, the study can be negative due to partial or total thrombotic occlusion of the aneurysmal lumen or to the persistence of the arterial vasospasm (18). Angiography permits an evaluation of the size of the aneurysm, its shape and its neck (Fig. 1.103). Angiography is also required to evaluate the entire cerebral arterial system both to search for other possible aneurysms as well as to perform a complete presurgical haemodynamic assessment. To this end, it can be useful to perform cross-compression of the contralateral cervical carotid artery during carotid injections in order to study the cross-filling, and therefore the collateral circulatory capacity, of the elements of the circle of Willis.

Therapeutic role

The interest and utility of interventional radiology is increasing in the neuroradiological field, especially in certain emergency situations where it can provide support for or even replacement of traditional therapeutic approaches.

Cerebral ischaemia: In cerebral ischaemia, the principal therapeutic use of angiography is selective intraarterial fibrinolysis and percutaneous angioplasty.

a) For some years now, selective intraarterial fibrinolysis has been used in treating acute ischaemia of the lower extremities as well as other regions of the body (e.g., renal, mesenteric, coronary ischaemia). This has occurred primarily because of the introduction of new, efficient fibrinolytic drugs that are easy to handle and have low incidence of untoward side effects. Its use in the treatment of cerebral ischaemia, which in industrialized countries accounts for the third largest cause of death and is the most common cause of lifetime disability, is now available in many centres worldwide.

Treatment must be begun within 6-8 hours from onset of the ischaemic ictus, once angiography has demonstrated the obstructive nature of the ischaemia. A microcatheter is introduced via the transfemoral route into the occluded artery; the distal tip of the catheter is positioned in contact with the thrombus and injecting from 200,000 to 1,000,000 Urokinase; 1/3 of the total amount of the dose is administered as a bolus, and the remainder as a continuous infusion over the subsequent 1-2 hours. The main hindrance to the wider use of this technique is the extreme sensitivity of the cerebral tissue to anoxia, which leaves a very small time margin between onset and the start of treatment, and the potential risk of peripheral non-cerebral and cere-

bral haemorrhagic complications (Fig. 1.104). The procedure requires a high degree of specific physician experience and a high level of organization of the medical and paramedical team involved. It is therefore typically only performed in highly specialized centres and in selected patients. However, statistics reveal encouraging figures for this technique. By respecting rigid patient selection criteria, recanalization of the occluded vessel varies from 44% to 100% of cases, and partial or total regression of the clinical picture is observed in 31% - 100% of cases (3, 7, 22).

b) Until recently, percutaneous angioplasty, has found fertile ground in areas of the body outside the brachiocephalic region. The continuous technical evolution of the materials used (e.g., small calibre PTA catheters, thinner guide wires and flexible stents), the experience gained in other body regions and the

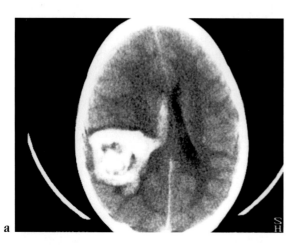

a

Fig. 1.102 - (**a-c**) Intraparenchymal haemorrhage. **a**) CT: voluminous intraparenchymal haematoma in right temporoparietal position of recent onset, with intraventricular expansion. (**b-c**) Selective catheterism of the right internal carotid artery, early and late arteriographic phase of same case: arteriovenous malformation (arrow) sustained by branches of the middle cerebral artery and the rear choroid arteries, with venous drain through ascending superficial veins (arrowheads).

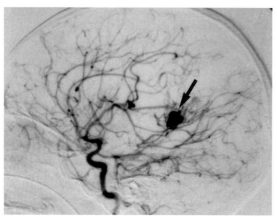

b

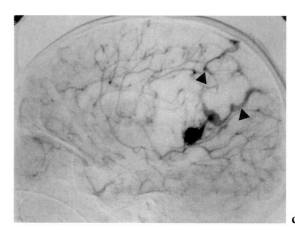

c

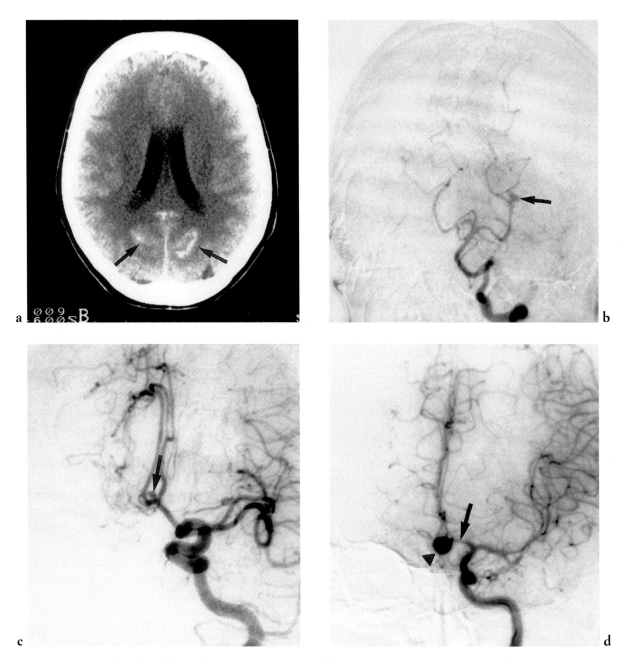

Fig. 1.103 - (**a-d**) Subarachnoid haemorrhage. **a**) CT: subarachnoid blood expansion, at the occipital region of the cortical sulci (arrows). **b**) selective catheterism of the left vertebral artery (same case): small aneurysm of the left posterior cerebral artery, near to the start of the temporooccipital artery (arrow). **c**) selective catheterism of the left internal carotid artery: small sac-shaped aneurysm of the anterior communicating artery (arrow). **d**) selective catheterism of the left internal carotid artery: aneurysm of the anterior communicating artery (arrowhead); spasm of the anterior cerebral artery (arrow).

perfection of medical support have made it possible to extend PTA to the supraaortic vessels, albeit with application and selection criteria that are yet to be universally accepted. It may be that PTA is not absolutely required in hyperacute emergency situations, however, it may be useful to perform this therapeutic procedure in a timely manner subacutely in patients with rapidly worsening transient ischaemic syndromes, when preceding angiography demonstrates the presence of a severe stenosis that is felt to be responsible for the

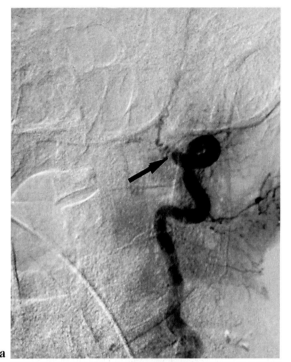

a

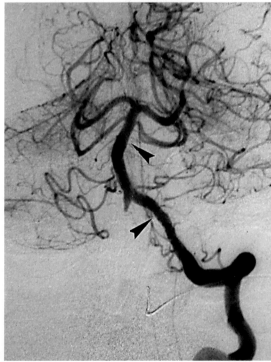

b

Fig. 1.104 - (**a, b**) Intraarterial fibrinolysis. **a**) selective catheterism of the left vertebral artery: acute thromboembolic occlusion of stretch V3, with impossibility of viewing the basilar stem and the posterior circulation (arrow tips). **b**) check-up after fibrinolytic treatment: complete recanalization of the vertebral artery with opacification of the basilar stem and posterior circle (arrowheads)

clinical picture; in such cases one may logically predict the vessel's rapid evolution to complete occlusion and perhaps resulting frank cerebral infarction. In some specialized centres, PTA of the supraaortic vascular branches is performed at the origins of the supraaortic vessels (Fig. 1.105) and within the vertebral arteries, the extracranial and sometimes even the intracranial segments of the internal carotid arteries (Fig. 1.106), and the first order branches of the major cerebral arteries. Although experience in this field is still somewhat limited, it is widely held that PTA represents a valid alternative to thromboendarterectomy, at least in patients who are at high surgical risk or who present with stenoses that are difficult to access surgically; however, it may well become more widely used as more sophisticated materials and instruments are made available.

Recent statistics have shown that PTA enables the recovery of vascular patency in more than 90% of cases; in the remaining 10% a modest residual stenosis remains. The frequency of intra- or postangiographic complications is relatively low (minor infarction: 1.6%, major infarction: 0.9%), as is the procedural death rate (0.4%) (1, 5, 6, 10-12, 19).

It should also be pointed out that emergency PTA can sometimes be performed on patients with subarachnoid haemorrhage caused by cerebral aneurysm rupture, where the clinical picture is dominated by the ischaemia caused by the vasospasm. It has been found that the arterial spasm responds well to dilation. Such patients are first treated with intraarterial papaverine (150-300 mg in 100 cm³ of physiological solution injected over 30 minutes) using a microcatheter that is introduced into the cerebral artery as far as the vascular spasm to be treated. In cases where papaverine treatment is unsuccessful, PTA is used first (Fig. 1.107) (4, 13, 14, 17).

In cases of subarachnoid haemorrhage, PTA's largest contribution to interventional radiology is in the percutaneous treatment of cerebral aneurysms using Guglielmi detachable coils (GDC). This widely used treatment is the most recent and perhaps the most fascinating and

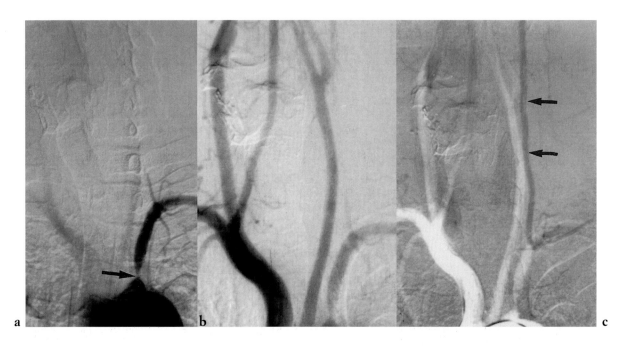

a   b   c

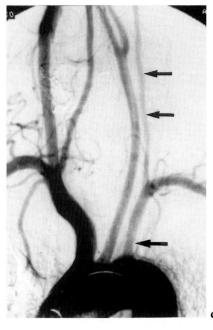

d

Fig. 1.105 - (**a-d**) Angioplasty of the left subclavian artery. (**a-c**) Aortography in early and late stages: suboccluding stenoses at the start of the left subclavian artery (arrow); in **a** and **b**, non-opaque homolateral vertebral artery; **c**) late opacification, against the stream of the homolateral vertebral artery (theft) (arrows). **d**) Check-up after angioplasty (same case): complete dilation of the stenotic tract (arrow); swift opacification of the homolateral vertebral artery (arrows).

promising interventional radiological technique in the neurological field. Through femoral arterial access, selective vascular catheterization into the specific vessel off of which the aneurysm originates is performed; using a microcatheter to selectively enter the lumen of the aneurysm, GDC's are introduced into the sack until a preferably complete occlusion is obtained. The technique's degree of invasiveness, if compared to surgical clipping, is far lower and the procedure is far easier for patients in any condition to tolerate. However, patients to be subjected to this treatment must be carefully chosen. The best results are obtained for small diameter aneurysms with narrow necks (90% success rate with low mortality and morbidity rates) (Fig. 1.108).

Obviously, this kind of procedure achieves the best results when practiced under ideal

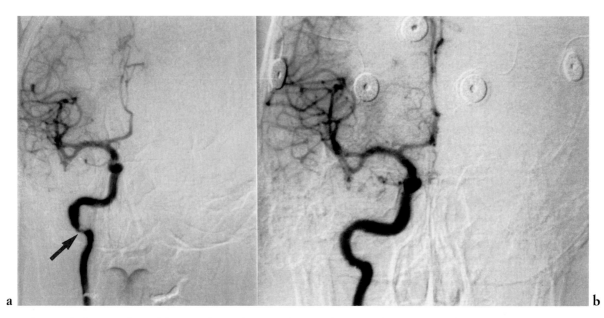

a   b

Fig. 1.106 - (**a, b**) Angioplasty of the internal carotid artery. Selective catheterism of the right internal carotid artery. 33 year-old patient with history of cerebral ischaemia. **a**) Segmentary stenosis at the passage between the extra- and intracranial tract, probably of a fibrodysplasic nature (arrow). **b**) Check-up after angioplasty (same case): complete resolution of stenosis.

conditions; however, it can still be used in emergency situations. According to Moret, of 124 cases presenting with subarachnoid haemorrhage related to ruptured aneurysms, 21 were treated in emergency conditions (17%), with a global success rate of coil embolization of 79% (9, 15, 16, 21).

CONCLUSIONS

In short, cerebral angiography offers a wide range of practical opportunities for use in the field of neurological emergency, and the role of this technique applied to various clinical situations is extremely varied. However, it should be pointed out how the role of angiography has changed in recent years both with regard to use in emergency and routine clinical conditions, thanks mainly to the invention of new imaging techniques. Angiographic semeiotics itself has also changed, and unfortunately a portion of its refined semeiological knowledge has gradually been forgotten. At the same time, the angiographic radiologist's role has also changed. From a certain point of view his or her task has become increasingly straightforward due to the technical advances made in angiographic appliances, and the sophistication of the instruments used have made angiographic examinations safer and more patient tolerable. In addition, newer imaging techniques have greatly simplified angiography's diagnostic role.

However, from other points of view, the radiologist's task has become more complex, due in part to the vast range of imaging techniques currently available. The imaging specialist's approach to any type of pathology has now become multidisciplinary, which makes obtaining sufficient expertise and experience with all the various diagnostic techniques and then choosing the optimal diagnostic-therapeutic pathway somewhat taxing.

However, the powerful development of interventional radiology has also made the radiologist's task more delicate by requiring a thorough knowledge of both routine and emergency clinical problems, a continuous upgrading of his knowledge of appliances and instruments that are themselves undergoing constant evolution, and familiarity with the use of a vast number of pharmacological preparations.

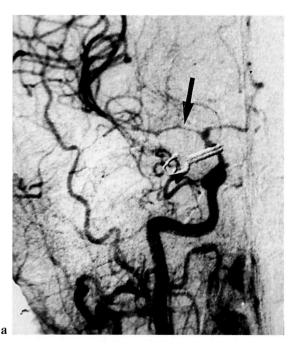
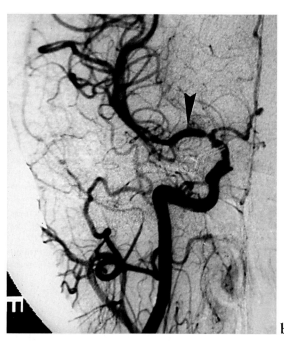

a
b

Fig. 1.107 - (**a, b**) Angioplasty of the middle cerebral artery. **a**) Selective angiography of the right internal carotid artery: serrated spasm post SAH of the M1 stretch of the middle cerebral artery (arrow) in patient operated for an aneurysm on the posterior communicating artery. **b**) Check-up after papaverine + PTA: complete resolution of the spasm with patent vessel of a good calibre (arrow tip).

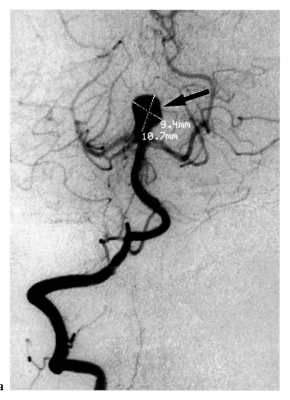
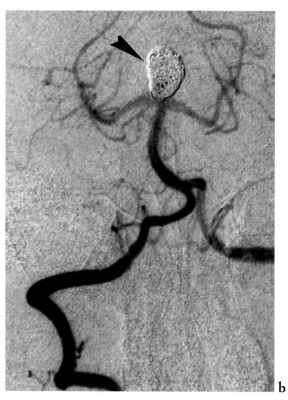

a
b

Fig. 1.108 - (**a, b**) Aneurysm embolization with Gugliemi's detachable coils. **a**) Selective angiography of the left vertebral artery: 1 cm aneurysm of the apex of the basilar artery (arrow). **b**) Check-up after embolization: complete occlusion of the aneurysmatic sack with well-compacted spirals (arrow tips).

REFERENCES

1. Borgey WM, Demasi RJ, Tripp MD, et al: Percutaneous transluminal angioplasty for subclavian artery stenosis. The American Surgeon 60: 103-106, 1994.

2. Bozzao L, Fantozzi LM, Bastianello S et al: Ischaemic supratentorial stroke: angiographic findings in patients examined in the very early phase. J Neurol. 236: 340-342, 1989.

3. Edwards MT, Murphy MM, Geraghty JJ et al: Intra-arterial cerebral thrombolysis for acute ischemic stroke in a community hospital. AJNR 20: 1682-1687, 1999.

4. Elliot JP, Newell DW, Lam DJ et al: Comparison of balloon angioplasty and papaverine infusion for the treatment of vasospasm following aneurysmal subarachnoid haemorrhage. J Neurosurg 88: 277-284, 1998.

5. Florio F, Balzano S, Nardella M et al: Terapia transluminale delle lesioni stenosanti dei tronchi epiaortici. Radiol. Med 86, 302-307, 1993.

6. Florio F, D'Angelo V, Nardella M et al: Displasia fibromuscolare dell'arteria carotide interna: angioplastica percutanea. Radiol. Med 84, 796-801, 1992.

7. Gonner F, Remonda L, Mattle H et al: Local intra-arterial thrombolysis in acute ischemic stroke. Stroke 29: 1894-1900,1998.

8. Grzyska U, Freitag J, Zeumer H: Selective cerebral intraarterial DSA. Complication rate and control of risk factors. Neuroradiology 32: 296-299, 1990.

9. Guglielmi G, Vinuela F: Intracranial aneurysms Guglielmi electrothrombotic coils. Neurosurg. Clinics North America 3: 427-435, 1994.

10. Henry M, Amor M, Henrry I et al: Percutaneous transluminal angioplasty of the subclavian arteries. In: Tenth international course book of peripheral vascular intervention. Europa Edition. Paris, pp. 617-627, 1999.

11. Henry M, Amor M, Henry I et al: Angioplasty and Stenting of the Extracranial Carotid Arteries. In: Carotid angioplasty and stenting. ISCAT ed. Europea pp. 267-280, 1998.

12. Higashida RT, Tsai FY, Halbach VV et al: Transluminal angioplasty for atherosclerotic disease of the vertebral and basilar arteries. J Neurosurg 78: 192-198, 1993.

13. Livigstone K et al: Intraarterial papaverine as on adjunct to transluminal angioplasty for vasospasm induced by subarachnoid haemorrage. AJNR 14: 346-347,1993.

14. Milburn JM, Moran CJ, Cross DT et al: Effect of intraarterial papaverine on cerebral circulation time. AJNR 18: 1081-1085, 1997.

15. Moret J, Boulin A, Castaings L: Endovascular treatment of berry aneurysms by endosaccular occlusion. In: Nacci G, Scialfa G: Atti 3° meeting neuroradiologico potentino: Neuroradiologia terapeutica, pp. 10-14, Ed. C.S.E. Potenza 1991.

16. Murayama Y, Vinuela F, Duckwiler GR: Embolization of incidental cerebral aneurysms by using the Guglielmi detachable coil system. J Neurosurg 90: 207-214, 1999.

17. Polin RS, Coenen VA, Hansen CA: Efficacy of transluminal angioplasty for the management of symptomatic cerebral vasospasm following aneurysmal subarachnoid hemorrhage. J Neurosurg 92: 284-290, 2000.

18. Redfern RM, Zygmunt S, Pickard JD et al: The natural history of subarachnoid haemorrhage with negative angiography: a prospectie study and 3 year follow-up. Br J Neurosurg 2: 33-41, 1998.

19. Sivaguru A, Venables GS, Beard JD et al: European carotid angioplasty trial. J Endovasc Surg 3: 16-20, 1996.

20. Smith TP: Radiologic intervention in the acute stroke patient. J Vasc Intervent Radiol 7: 627-40, 1996.

21. Vinuela F, Duckwiler G, Mawad M: Guglielmi detachable coil embolization of acute intracranial aneurysm: perioperative anatomical and clinical outcome in 403 patients. J Neurosurg 86:475-482, 1997.

22. Zeumer H, Freitag HJ, Grzyska U et al: Local intraarterial fibrinolysis in acute vertebrobasilar occlusion. Neuroradiology 31: 336-340, 1989

II

HEAD INJURIES

2.1

CLINICAL AND DIAGNOSTIC SUMMARY

G. M. Giannatempo, T. Scarabino, M. Armillotta

Overall, trauma represents the most frequent cause of death and permanent disability, with an annual incidence of 0.2-0.3% and with peak incidence in the 15-24 year age band (1). In the United States alone, approximately 2 million head injuries occur annually, of which some 10% are fatal. Approximately 5-10% of survivors experience neurological deficits of varying degrees (1, 4, 5). The most common causes of trauma are road accidents, firearm injuries, falls and assaults.

The brain lesions resulting from cranial trauma are usually classified as being either primary or secondary, according to how directly they correlate to the traumatic event (4, 20, 22, 29). Primary lesions include fractures of the skull, extraaxial haemorrhages (e.g., epidural haematoma, subdural haematoma and subarachnoid haemorrhage) and intraaxial lesions (e.g., diffuse axonal injury [DAI], cortical contusion, deep grey matter injury and intraventricular haemorrhage). Secondary lesions are constituted by pathological processes that occur due to the brain's response to the primary trauma and are generally more clinically devastating than primary ones. Secondary brain lesions include internal cerebral herniation, diffuse cerebral oedema, infarction and secondary haemorrhage (4, 20, 22, 29). Yet other lesions are the result of sequelae of severe cranial trauma; these changes are represented by pneumocephalus, CSF fistulae, leptomeningeal cysts, lesions of the cranial nerves, diabetes insipidus secondary to pituitary axis injury, cortical atrophy and encephalomalacia (9).

In recent decades, considerable progress has been made in the diagnosis and management of cranial trauma patients. The application of Computed Tomography (CT) has resulted in a revolution in head injury diagnosis, making it possible to detect cases suitable for surgical treatment in a rapid, non-invasive manner (6, 7, 11, 12, 14). Its near-universal availability in hospitals, the speed with which examinations can be conducted, the general absence of contraindications to emergency patient scanning, and its sensitivity in diagnosing haemorrhagic collections make CT the imaging technique of choice for the initial assessment of patients with acute head injuries (4, 22, 32, 33). Further advantages offered by this technique are found in its high spatial resolution allowing the possibility of documenting even the thinnest fractures and those located in critical positions such as the base of the skull or the temporal bone, and in identifying small splinters of metal or tiny fragments of bone displaced into the cranial cavity (24, 31). The drawbacks of CT include its limited sensitivity in studying small traumatic lesions in the inferior posterior fossa or elsewhere adjacent to the base of the skull, these limitations being principally due to bone artefacts generated by the technique. CT also has a relatively low sensitivity in the identification of small non-haemorrhagic lesions of the cerebral cortex, white matter and brainstem (4, 10, 20, 21, 23). However, these limitations do not prevent CT from identifying the nature, size and site of the most clinically significant acute phase traumatic brain lesions and from deciding whether or not surgical intervention is required (4, 22, 32, 33).

Magnetic Resonance Imaging (MRI) plays a limited role in the acute phase of cranial trauma, given its higher cost, relatively limited availability, longer examination times, lower sensitivity in recognising fractures, patient contraindications (internal electronic pacemakers, etc.) and the practical difficulty of effectively monitoring patients with severe clinical conditions requiring external support devices (4, 8). MR is also limited by problems encountered in recognising acute phase haemorrhages (e.g., oxy- and deoxyhaemoglobin within hyperacute haemorrhages) and small bone fragments dislocated into the skull. The use of MR in emergency situations also entails certain intrinsic risks, for example those linked to the difficulty in ascertaining the presence of electronic pacemakers in unconscious trauma patients.

Technological progress has to some extent reduced the drawbacks associated with long examination times and the difficulties in using instruments to monitor the patient's vital parameters during the MR examination. The use of fast scanning sequences (e.g., fast spin-echo, gradient-echo, echo-planar) has considerably reduced the amount of time required to perform MR studies, to the point where it is now possible to perform a basic MR scan in less than ten minutes. This scan protocol may include a T1-weighted spin-echo sequence, a T2-weighted fast spin-echo sequence and a T2*-weighted gradient-echo sequence, the latter being particularly sensitive to haemorrhagic extravasations. It must also be pointed out that considerable progress has been made in the development of new non-ferromagnetic alloys employed in the manufacture of electronic medical instruments used for vital parameter monitoring and life support, so that they are now compatible with MRI (4, 8).

MRI has greatest diagnostic sensitivity in many of the very cases in which CT encounters some of its greatest limitations. Given its greater sensitivity in the diagnosis of diffuse axonal injury (DAI), small cortical contusions and primary and secondary traumatic brainstem lesions, MRI is also used as a complement to other imaging methods in the acute phase of trauma, especially in patients with clinical signs and symptoms but with minor or absent CT findings (4, 20, 21). MR examinations are also suitable in subacute and chronic phase cranial trauma for the purpose of evaluating secondary lesions and other sequelae.

In the area of cranial trauma diagnosis, digital angiography currently plays only a marginal role and is principally utilized for cases in which traumatic vascular lesions are suspected (e.g., vascular dissections, lacerations, occlusions, pseudo-aneurysms and arteriovenous fistulae).

NEURORADIOLOGICAL PROTOCOLS

Although any diagnostic approach must be tailored to suit the requirements of each patient, some general guidelines can be identified to aid in the establishment of which technique is most suitable. Defining an efficient and efficacious diagnostic protocol requires compromising between the choice of a technique guaranteeing high diagnostic sensitivity and the limitations imposed on the number and complexity of the diagnostic examinations that can be performed.

Although CT is the examination technique of choice in cranial trauma, not all authors agree on the necessity of performing CT in asymptomatic patients with previous minor cranial traumatic incidents, the need for complementing CT examinations with MR scans in patients with intermediate or serious head injuries and the real contribution of traditional skull x-rays in patients with head injuries of any degree.

The choice of a specific imaging technique to be employed must be preceded by a definitive clinical evaluation of the patient. The most commonly used method for evaluating head injury patients is the Glasgow Coma Scale (GCS), based on a progressive score attributed to the patient's ability to open his/her eyes, perform movements and verbally respond to external stimuli (13, 22, 28) (Tab. 2.1). The degree of severity of the trauma is classified in three categories according to the GCS score: mild trauma for a GCS score of 13-15; moderate trauma for a GCS score of 12-8 and severe trauma for GCS scores lower than 8.

Patients with mild head trauma (GCS 13-15) usually complain of headaches and transient mental confusion or disorientation (30) and, by definition, they do not exhibit persistent problems with consciousness (30). Some authors hold that it is sufficient to keep patients with such mild degrees of cranial trauma under observation, and furthermore that they do not require imaging studies (18). On the contrary, others believe that mild head injuries warrant at a minimum a CT examination, because despite the paucity of symptoms, traumatic brain lesions may be observed (19, 27). In a recent survey conducted on 1,170 mild cranial trauma patients (GCS = 15), CT demonstrated the presence of brain lesions in 3.3% of cases, of which 18 in number were intracranial bleeds; in 1.8% the CT examination altered the treatment programme, and in four cases surgery was performed (19). The same authors also stressed the prognostic value of a negative CT examination: in the same patient sample, none of the patients with negative CT scans experienced clinical deterioration. The authors therefore believe that it is not necessary to keep asymptomatic mild head trauma patients under observation in the setting of negative CT findings (19). Patients with mild trauma can reveal skull fractures, as well as extraaxial and intraparenchymal haematomas, lesions that are usually clearly documented on CT images. Although MR is slightly more sensitive than CT in demonstrating extraaxial haematomas, those that are not detected by CT are small and generally do not require surgery (4). The diagnostic sensitivity of

Tab. 2.1 - Glasgow Coma Scale (GSGS)

Best Eye Response
- Eyes open spontaneously
- Eye opening to verbal command
- Eye opening to pain
- No opening of eyes

Best Motor Response
- Obeys commands
- Localising pain
- Withdrawal from pain
- Flexion to pain
- Extension to pain
- No motor response

Best verbal Response
- Oriented
- Confused
- In appropriate words
- Incomprehensible sounds
- No verbal response

Mild cranial trauma	GCS = 13 - 15
Moderate cranial trauma	GCS = 9 - 12
Severe cranial Trauma	GCS = 1 - 8

MR is clearly superior to that of CT in cases of small, non-haemorrhagic lesions (e.g., DAI, bland cortical contusions), but the recognition of this type of lesion in minor head trauma patients does not alter the therapeutic management nor the clinical outcome (18, 30).

Patients with moderate (GCS = 8-12) and severe (GCS< 8) head trauma share a number of clinical and therapeutic characteristics, and for the sake of simplicity they will be considered as a single group (4). It should be pointed out that before commencing any diagnostic examination, the stabilization of the patient's respiratory and circulatory systems must be ascertained, ensuring the freedom of the airways (with intubation, if necessary), cervical spine stabilization (in case of underlying fracture/subluxation), respiratory function (face mask with high flow O^2; controlled ventilation if the patient is intubated) as well as their haemodynamic condition (e.g., identification and treatment of serious internal and external haemorrhaging; volemic restoration with isotonic solutions or plasma expanders).

Once the patient's clinical stability has been ascertained, the neurological examination may commence with the evaluation of the GCS, pupillary analysis and the evaluation of lateralizing signs, as well as with a general clinical examination for the identification of any other non-cranial traumatic lesions. Patients with moderate and severe head injuries usually suffer from disorders of consciousness, often associated with focal neurological deficits. In such cases, the fundamental question to be answered is whether the patient has an intracranial haematoma that requires surgery; at present CT is the only technique that is able to exclude this type of lesion rapidly and with sufficient reliability.

Once the need for emergency surgery has been eliminated, certain authors recommend performing an MR examination during the first two weeks of the traumatic event in patients with moderate to severe head injuries. MR has a far greater sensitivity than CT in diagnosing DAI, small cortical contusions (especially when non-haemorrhagic) and brainstem lesions, conditions that usually demonstrate minor or completely negative CT findings that may contrast considerably with the impaired clinical picture. In such cases, MR permits a more accurate evaluation than does CT with regard to the extent of the involvement of the encephalon and the brainstem, thus offering important information on possible clinical evolution and outcome (3, 5).

It should be remembered that although clinical indicators such as the GCS are useful instruments in establishing the patient's clinical condition, they do not provide significant information on the actual lesion(s) underlying the signs and symptoms, the prognosis or the patient's clinical evolution. Low GCS scores can be obtained from a number of different brain injuries that ultimately are responsible for vastly different clinical evolutions. Prior to the advent of MRI, diagnostic studies had little impact on prognosis; for example, many authors have highlighted the poor prognostic value of CT findings (2, 3, 12). CT's poor sensitivity in documenting non-haemorrhagic lesions of the brain is believed to be partly responsible for the poor correlation between CT findings and clinical evolution, which appear to be much better correlated with MRI findings (3).

In particular, the number of DAI lesions would appear to be inversely correlated with the GCS score in the long term; whereas 80% of patients without DAI recover well, only 27% of those with more than 10 lesions have a good prognosis (3). Conversely, the number of cortical contusions and the presence of isolated subdural or epidural haematomas do not appear to be statistically correlated with clinical evolution, unless associated with significant mass effect (e.g., transtentorial cerebral herniation and brainstem compression) (3). Signs of brainstem compression and intrinsic brainstem lesions typically suggest a very severe prognosis, especially when observed in combination.

It should be pointed out that most authors agree that it is not necessary to perform skull x-rays for the purpose of diagnosing fractures (15, 17, 20, 25, 26). The presence or absence of fractures is often not indicative of the gravity of the underlying injury of the brain. Skull fractures can in fact be isolated and are not necessarily associated with intracranial haematomas; conversely, the absence of fractures does not exclude the possibility of serious brain damage: in 25-30% of patients with moderate and severe trauma and brain lesions, the skull is not fractured (16). Fractures shown on x-rays do not therefore necessarily indicate brain damage, nor is the absence of such fractures reassuring with regard to the patient's normality (15, 17). In short, the diagnosis of fractures is not as important as is the identification of depressed fractures, intracranial dislocation of bone fragments, fractures in critical positions such as the temporal bone and base of the skull (which can be associated with fluid fistulae and vascular lacerations or fistulae) and associated intracranial lesions (especially intra- and extraaxial haematomas). In all such cases, CT offers diagnostic potential that is far superior to conventional x-ray examinations.

REFERENCES

1. Frankowski RF, Annegers JF, Whitman S. Epidemiological and descriptive studies. Part I: The descriptive epidemiology of head trauma in the United States. In: Becker DP, Polishock J, eds. Central Nervous System Trauma Status Report. Bethesda, MD National Institute of Health, 33-51, 1985.

2. French BN, Dublin AB: The value of computerized tomography in the management of 1000 consecutive head injuries. Surg Neurol 7:171-183, 1977.

3. Gentry LR, Godersky JC, Thompson BH: Prognosis after severe head injury: MRI correlation with Glasgow outcome scale. (Submitted).

4. Gentry LR: Head trauma. In: Atlas SW:Magnetic resonance of the brain and spine.(2nd ed.), Lippincott-Raven, Philadelphia, pp. 611-647, 1996.

5. Gentry LR: Imaging of closed head injury. Radiology 191:1-17, 1994.

6. Grumme T, Kluge W, Kretzschmar K et al: Head Trauma. In: Cerebral and spinal computed tomography. Blackwell Science, Berlin pp. 49-69, 1998.

7. Johnson MH, Lee SH: Computed tomography of acute cerebral trauma. Radiol Clin N Am 30:325-352, 1992.

8. Kanal E, Shellock FG: Patient monitoring during clinical MR imaging. Radiology; 185:623-629, 1992.

9. Keskil S, Baykaner K, Ceviker N et al: Clinical significance of acute traumatic intracranial pneumocephalus. Neurosurg Rev. 21(1):10-3, 1998.

10. Klufas RA, Hsu L, Patel MR: Unusual manifestations of head trauma. AJR 166:675-681, 1996.

11. Kuntz R, Skalej M, Stefanou A: Image quality of spiral CT versus conventional CT in routine brain imaging. Eur J Radiol. 26(3):235-40, 1998.

12. Lanksch W, Grumme T, Kazner E: Computed tomography in head injuries Springer, Berlin, 1979.

13. Lee TT, Aldana PR, Kirton OC et al: Follow-up computerized tomography (CT) scans in moderate and severe head injuries: correlation with Glasgow Coma Scores (GCS), and complication rate. Acta Neurochir Wien. 139(11):1042-7; discussion 1047-8, 1997.

14. Leidner B, Adiels M, Aspelin P et al: Standardized CT examination of the multitraumatized patient. Eur Radiol. 8(9):1630-8, 1998.

15. Lloyd DA, Carty H, Patterson M et al: Predictive value of skull radiography for intracranial injury in children with blunt head injury. Lancet. 22; 349(9055):821-4, 1997

16. Macpherson BCM, Macpherson P, Jennett B: CT incidence of intracranial contusion and hematoma in relation to the presence, site and type of skull fracture. Clin Radiology 42:321-326, 1990.

17. Mogbo KI, Slovis TL, Canady AI et al: Appropriate imaging in children with skull fractures and suspicion of abuse. Radiology. 208(2):521-4, 1998.

18. Mohanty SK, Thompson W, Rakower S: Are CT scan for head injury patients always necessary? J Trauma 31:801-805, 1991.

19. Nagy KK, Joseph KT, Krosner SM et al: The utility of head computed tomography after minimal head injury. J Trauma. 46(2):268-70, 1999.

20. Osborn A: Craniocerebral trauma. In Osborn A: Diagnostic neuroradiology. St Louis, pp 199-247, 1994.

21. Parizel PM, Ozsarlak P, Van-Goethem JW et al: Imaging findings in diffuse axonal injury after closed head trauma. Eur Radiol. 8(6):960-5, 1998.

22. Pellicanò G, Bartolozzi A: La TC nei traumi cranioencefalici. Edizioni del Centauro, Udine,1996.

23. Petitti N, Williams DW 3rd: CT and MR imaging of nonaccidental pediatric head trauma. Acad Radiol. 5(3):215-23, 1998.

24. Rhea JT, Rao PM, Novelline RA: Helical CT and three-dimensional CT of facial and orbital injury. Radiol Clin North Am 37:489-513, 1999.

25. Shane SA, Fuchs SM: Skull fractures in infants and predictors of associated intracranial injury. Pediatr Emerg Care. 13(3):198-203, 1997.

26. Snoek J, Jennet B, Adams JH: Computerized tomography after recent severe head injury in patients without acute intracranial hematoma. J Neurol Neurosurg Psychiat 42:215-225, 1979.

27. Stein SC, Ross SE: The value of computed tomographic scans in patients with low-risk head injuries. Neurosurgery 26:638-640, 1990.

28. Teasdale G, JennettB: Assessment of coma and impaired consciousness: a practical scale. Lancet 2:81-84, 1974.

29. Weisberg L., Nice C.: Cerebral computed tomography. W.B. Saunders, Philadelphia, pp 321-343, 1989.

30. Williams DH, Levin HS, Eisenberg HM: Mild head injury classification. Neurosurgery, 27:422-428, 1990.

31. Wilson AJ: Gunshot injuries: what does a radiologist need to know? Radiographics 19:1358-1368, 1999.

32. Wysoki MG, Nassar CJ, Koenigsberg RA et al: Head trauma: CT scan interpretation by radiology residents versus staff radiologists. Radiology. 208(1): 125-8, 1998.

33. Zee CS, Go JL: CT of head trauma. Neuroimaging Clin N Am. 8(3): 525-39, 1998.

2.2

CT IN HEAD INJURIES

G.M. Giannatempo, T. Scarabino, A. Simeone, A. Casillo, A. Maggialetti, M. Armillotta

INTRODUCTION

Trauma constitutes the most frequent cause of death and permanent disability in the western world (3, 20). For example, each year in the United States of America alone, some 2 million incidents of head injury occur (9), representing the most frequent cause of death among children and young adults (3, 20). Annual mortality from head injuries is estimated to be 25 per 100,000 population and is four times higher in males than females (2, 4). In the United States, 20-50% of head injuries are the result of road traffic accidents, 20-40% of firearm injuries, and assault or falls in the remainder (2, 4). Falls are particularly dangerous in children under ten years of age and the elderly, representing approximately 75% of all head injuries in the preschool population (2, 4).

Head injuries can be classified as open or closed, depending on whether or not the dura mater is intact (11, 12, 26). Closed cranial traumas are the more frequent of the two types and produce violent accelerations of the brain tissue, which are responsible for tissue contusion and vascular laceration at both the site of the direct trauma as well as on the opposite side. Among other injuries, skull fractures, extracerebral intracranial haemorrhages and parenchymal lesions are typically observed alone or in varying combinations. Open head trauma includes lesions of the skull such as depressed fractures associated with interruptions of the dura mater, and intracranial lesions secondary to the action of penetrating foreign bodies or dislocated calvarial fracture fragments.

Brain lesions can also be divided into primary and secondary categories according to how closely they are linked to the traumatic event (3, 20, 22, 26). Primary lesions include skull fractures, extraaxial haemorrhages (e.g., epidural and subdural haematomas and subarachnoid haemorrhages) and intraaxial lesions (e.g., diffuse axonal injury [DAI]), cortical and deep grey matter contusion [bland or haemorrhagic], and intraventricular haemorrhage) (Tab. 2.2). Secondary lesions are caused by pathological processes that arise from the brain's response to the trauma, as a complication of the primary traumatic brain lesions or as neurological involvement associated with systemic extracranial trauma (Tab. 2.3). In general, the secondary types of trauma are more clinically devastating than are the primary brain injuries. They are generally caused by compression of the brain, cranial nerves and blood vessels against the bony cranial structures and the non-expandable dural margins. Secondary brain injuries include cerebral herniations, diffuse cerebral oedema, infarction and secondary haemorrhages (3, 20, 22, 26).

Tab. 2.2 - Primary traumatic cranioencephalic lesions.

1) Fractures

2) Intraaxial lesions
   a) diffuse axonal injury (damage)
   b) cortical contusion
   c) intraparenchymal haematoma
   d) intraventricular haemorrhage
   e) lesions of the deep grey matter
   f) brainstem lesions

3) Extraaxial lesions
   a) epidural haematoma
   b) subdural haematoma
   c) subarachnoid haematoma
   d) subdural hygroma
   e) vascular lesions

Tab. 2.3 - Secondary traumatic cranioencephalic lesions

1) Cerebral herniation
2) Diffuse cerebral oedema
3) Posttraumatic ischaemia
4) Posttraumatic infarction

In the study of acute head injuries, CT currently represents the diagnostic methodology of choice (3, 7, 20, 22, 28). Its ability in distinguishing between minor differences in tissue density, its high spatial definition, capacity to demonstrate even very subtle or critically positioned (e.g., base of the skull, temporal bone) fractures, fast scanning times and compatibility with life support devices all contribute to making CT the most suitable technique in acute phase head injury evaluation (3, 7, 20, 22, 29).

TECHNIQUES

Despite the speed with which CT must be performed in emergency conditions, head injuries warrant the observance of certain technical and methodological parameters that ensure diagnostic efficiency and the reproducibility of the results in the event of serial evaluations (14, 22, 29).

Caution is required when positioning the patient on the CT bed, taking care that any tubes and electrode cables are sufficiently long to enable suitable scan table indexing during the scan. Particular care must be observed in positioning the patient's head in the supine position: the chin must be extended in order to prevent breathing difficulties. And, to prevent a potential cervical spinal cord injury resulting from a suspected or occult unstable spinal column fracture-dislocation, immobilization of the head and cervical spine should be undertaken.

The CT examination begins with a projection digital scanogram that includes the cervical spine. This serves to define the scanning limits for an evaluation of skull vertex fractures, gross subluxations and fractures of the cervical spinal column, gross soft tissue alterations and for the recognition of any radioopaque foreign bodies. The CT scan gantry should be oriented along the orbitomeatal plane, or alternatively along the so-called horizontal "German plane" parallel to the hard palate, and should be directed in such a way as to avoid if possible sectioning through any metal foreign bodies (e.g., dental fillings, etc.) that might be likely to cause beam-hardening artefacts (5, 7, 22, 29). The examination continues with contiguous 5 mm-thick axial slices through the structures of the posterior fossa and then concludes with a stacked series of 10 mm-thick axial slices through the cranial vertex to cover the supratentorial structures (5, 7, 22, 29).

For small lesions or in order to visualize fractures at the base of the skull, the acquisition of 2-3 mm sections is recommended. Coronal scans may be required at a later point beyond the emergency period in order to identify or exclude fractures at the base of the skull, the bony orbit and the petrous bone, and for visualization of parenchymal or bony lesions adjacent to the vertex. It should also be pointed out that coronal scans require optimal patient cooperation and should only be performed when it is absolutely certain that there are no fractures/instability of the cervical spine or at the atlanto-occipital junction.

When an otorrhagia or acute paralysis of the facial nerve suggests a fracture of the temporal bone, the examination must be completed with a detailed study of the petrous bone using thin slices (1-2 mm), a reduced field of view (FOV) and utilizing bone reconstruction algorithms (14, 24, 29).

Generally speaking the examination should be filmed/reviewed using window and level values that permit an optimal viewing of the cerebral parenchyma (e.g., 100 H.U. window and 40-50 H.U. level), and those that also enable visualization of the bony structures (e.g., 2000-3000 H.U. window and 500-700 H.U. level). In certain cases, especially for the visualization of thin epidural or subdural haemorrhages, it is advisable to film the examination with window values equal to 200-350 H.U. and level values equal to 40-80 H.U. in order to distinguish the mildly hyperdense blood collection from the adjacent bony hyperdensity (9, 15, 22, 28).

The intravenous administration of iodine contrast medium does not significantly improve the diagnostic sensitivity of the examination in cases of cranial trauma; in fact, it can conceal intracranial haemorrhage, causing minor blood collections to be overlooked. The administration of contrast agents is also usually avoided as it can produce renal injury or even potentially worsen brain function in patients with traumatic cerebral lesions. However, the utilization of contrast media can be useful in certain limited cases when better definition of the dural venous sinuses is desired, better visualization of chronic isodense subdural haematomas is necessary, and above all, in order to document simultaneous underlying pathology such as neoplasia or AVM's. Of course, intravascular contrast media are required for performing CT angiography in cases where there is a suspicion of posttraumatic intracranial vascular pathology (e.g., vascular lacerations, arteriovenous fistulae and posttraumatic pseudo-aneurysms). In all of these cases, MR may be more sensitive and is sometimes preferable to CT.

Modern CT appliances with spiral (helical) scanning capability greatly reduce the time required for scanning, these units acquiring the entire scan volume in just a few seconds; when acquired in sufficiently thin sections (e.g., 1-2 mm) these scans can then subsequently be reconstructed in different spatial planes (1, 10, 22, 24). Helical scans are most useful in cases where scanning time must be reduced to a minimum, such as in children or in non-cooperative patients. It can also be very helpful when there is a suspicion of lesions of the orbit or the facial skeleton in which it is possible to quickly obtain high resolution two- or three-dimensional reconstructions (1, 10, 24).

It is useful, however, to stress that spiral CT examinations can sometimes produce images that simulate non-existent pathology, such as minor subdural haematomas, in part due to the partial volume averaging effects along the z-axis of scanning. This kind of artefact appears principally along sloping surfaces such as the skull-brain interface over the frontoparietal convexity (1, 10, 22).

Another type of artefact associated with spiral CT that can simulate a chronic subdural haematoma is the so-called "stairstep" artefact that produces images with hypodense peripheral areas, especially at the skull vertex (1, 10, 22). Such problems can be partly or completely resolved by reducing the collimation, the reconstruction interval, the scan bed's index speed and/or the tube rotation speed (22). Recent research shows that traditional, non-helical CT is superior to spiral CT with regard to the signal/noise ratio, in visualizing the interface between white and grey matter and in observing low contrast, small, complex structures (e.g., the internal capsule) (1).

In summary, the use of spiral CT in cases of cranial trauma should be restricted to those cases in which scanning time must be as brief as possible, instances in which a three-dimensional study of the bony structures is required or when CT angiography of intracranial circulation is necessary.

SEMEIOTICS

PRIMARY TRAUMATIC LESIONS

Skull fractures

Skull fractures associated with cranial trauma are common and are discovered in approximately 60% of all cases (20). The presence of a fracture is not necessarily significant with regard to the clinical severity of the trauma, nor does the absence of a fracture exclude the possibility of severe brain damage; records show that in 25-35% of patients with severe trauma and underlying brain injury, no fracture is present. For this reason, many practitioners feel that x-rays aimed at diagnosing skull fractures are superfluous with reference to patient care (16, 20, 25). In addition to the parietal, frontal and occipital areas, skull fractures can affect the vertex or base of the skull. And, depending on the intensity of the force applied, they can be classified as linear fractures usually caused by lesser forces (Fig. 2.1), and comminuted and depressed fractures typically caused by greater forces (Fig. 2.2) (16, 17, 22, 25, 29). Fractures of the skull base can be caused by superficial or penetrating trauma, the caudal extension of a fracture of the calvaria, or alternatively, the upward transmission of traumatic forces along the vertebral column. Although CT is sensitive in detecting these types of lesions, thin, linear fractures and those oblique/parallel to the plane of section can go unnoticed (16, 17, 25). However, the practical importance of fracture recognition is secondary, as efforts are principally concentrated on the search for associated intracranial lesions. Linear fractures are often associated with epidural and subdural haematomas, whereas depressed fractures are more frequently associated with focal parenchymal lesions adjacent to the bony lesions (20).

In more severe cases, such as in open head injuries that are often consequences of knife or firearm wounds, fractures may be associated with a laceration of the dura mater and a penetration of bone fragments, air or foreign bodies into the cranial cavity (3, 20, 27). In the study of such open head injuries, CT permits the accurate localization of foreign bodies or bone fragments in large part due to their relative high density (Fig. 2.3). CT also provides a detailed picture of the spatial characteristics of depressed fractures (Fig. 2.4) and at the same time, documents any related cerebral lesions.

Lesions of the dura mater at the base of the skull, associated with fractures of the adjacent bone, can be complicated by a CSF fistula formation, with consequent oto- and/or rhinorrhea (Fig. 2.5). In such cases, the site of the fistula can be suggested by means of a detailed study of the bone using high resolution CT. This study should be performed employing axial slices to study fractures of the posterior wall of the frontal sinuses and the petrous bone, and coronal acquisitions to study ethmoid fractures and also to supplement the evaluation of petrous fractures.

In addition, fractures of the paranasal sinuses, the mastoid cells or the middle ear may result in the introduction of air into the subarachnoid spaces or the cerebral ventricles (pneumocephalus) (8, 27). These conditions can occasionally behave as space-occupying lesions (e.g., pneumatocele formation) when a valve mechanism is formed at the dural laceration resulting in a considerable increase in the volume of intracranial air, and therefore will require treatment (Fig. 2.6).

Intraaxial lesions

Diffuse axonal injury

Diffuse axonal injury (DAI) is one of the most common primary brain lesions associated with severe trauma and accounts for approximately 48% of all traumatic intraaxial injuries (3). DAI typically results from abrupt accelerations or decelerations or when violent rotational forces obtain causing a differential inertia between grey and white matter, between the cerebral hemispheric connecting structures or within the diencephalon and brainstem with consequential axonal stretching, twisting and tearing (3, 20). Clinically, DAI is characterized by a loss of consciousness beginning immediately at the time of the trauma which can evolve into a coma that is often irreversible (3, 13, 22). DAI is the most severe of all primary brain lesions, being ahead in degree of severity of that of cortical contusions, intraparenchymal haematomas and extraaxial haemorrhages. Pathoanatomically,

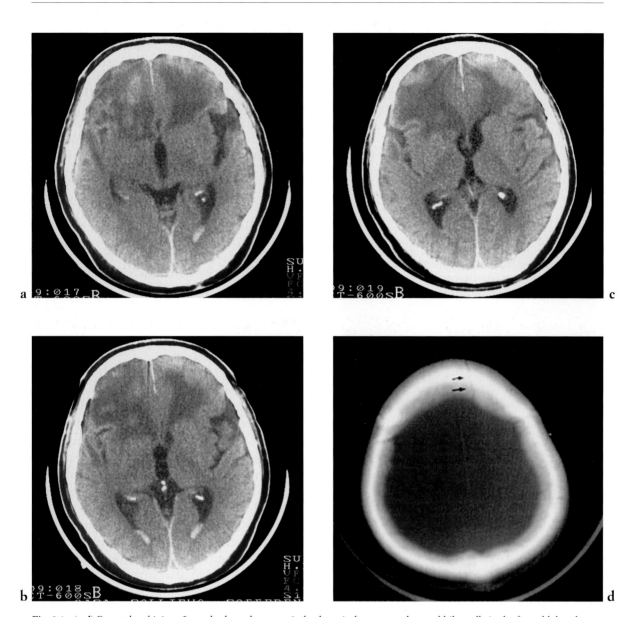

Fig. 2.1 - (**a-d**) Recent head injury. Irregular hypodense cortical-subcortical areas are observed bilaterally in the frontal lobes; hyperdense haemorrhagic material is noted in the occipital horns of the lateral ventricles (**a-b**). Also seen is a frontal bone fracture line (**c**).

ball-shaped deformations of the damaged axons can be observed; the lesions are not usually haemorrhagic, although in 20% of cases they can be associated with small haemorrhages resulting from the rupture of penetrating arterial vessels (3). DAI usually occurs in one of three typical positions: the cerebral hemispheric white matter, the corpus callosum and the dorsolateral aspect of the midbrain. More precisely, in approximately two thirds of cases the lesions are located at the subcortical grey-white matter junction in the frontotemporal region, 20% are located in the corpus callosum (especially the body and the splenium), and less frequently the alterations affect the dorsolateral side of the brainstem tegmen, the internal capsule, the thalamus and the caudate nucleus (20). During the early phases of a traumatic injury, the CT picture is often normal despite the fact that the clinical status is that of a seriously compromised

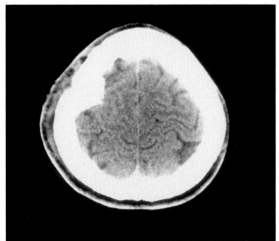

a

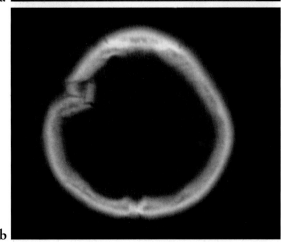

b

Fig. 2.2 - (**a**, **b**) Demonstrated is a depressed fracture of the right parietal bone.

patient; research indicates that alterations can only be documented by imaging in 20-50% of patients with DAI (3, 20, 24). The alterations that can be documented by CT consist of small haemorrhages and hypodense lesions that affect the corpus callosum and the grey-white matter junction of the cerebral hemispheres (Fig. 2.7). Small haemorrhages also occur in the internal capsule, in the periventricular grey matter and in the dorsolateral quadrants of the brainstem, the latter being a somewhat vulnerable area in patients subjected to angular accelerations-decelerations. Although MRI also underestimates the real extent of axonal damage in DAI relative to the pathoanatomical findings, it is currently the most sensitive imaging technique available (3, 20, 21).

Cortical contusion

Cortical contusion is the second most frequent form of parenchymal lesion following DAI and represents approximately 45% of all intraaxial primary traumatic injuries (3, 20). Unlike DAI, cortical contusion is less frequently associated with loss of consciousness and occurs following a violent traumatic shaking injury of the cerebral tissue (3, 13). It can occur secondary to linear accelerations of the cerebrum that produce the typical coup and countercoup parenchymal contusions, or alternatively after angular accelerations that produce cortical contusions resulting from collisions of the brain against the inner surface of the skull. As the grey matter is far more vascularized than the white matter, cortical contusions tend to be more frequently haemorrhagic than do those lesions associated with DAI (7, 29). Pathoanatomically, these contusions are characterized by isolated or multiple foci of focal or linear microhaemorrhages of the cortical gyri. The lesions may be associated with focal oedema resulting from alterations of the permeability of the regional capillaries and the walls of involved glial cells. Petechial lesions, which are often combined with overlying bony skull fractures, tend to expand into more widespread haemorrhagic foci that often manifest 24-48 hours after the trauma (3, 20, 29). Because the lesions are caused by the impact of the cerebral parenchyma against the surrounding bony structures, most contusions are located in characteristic locations. In approximately half of all cases, the lesions are situated within the temporal lobes (especially in the poles), over the lower surface of the frontal lobes and in the cortex surrounding the Sylvian fissure (Fig. 2.8).

The CT appearance of cortical contusions varies in part with the manner in which the lesions evolve over time. At the onset, the CT picture can be negative because the lesions are initially isodense, and therefore are impossible to distinguish from the surrounding healthy parenchyma. In other cases, early stage contusions appear as small hypodense areas often in-

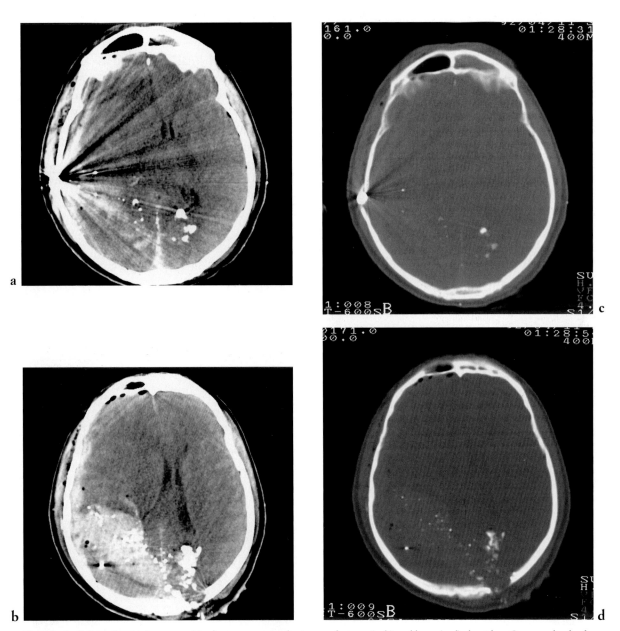

Fig. 2.3 - (**a-d**) Open head injury caused by firearm, examined using a soft tissue (**a, b**) and bone (**c, d**) algorithm. One can clearly observe the bullet entrance hole (**b, d**) in a left paramedian parieto-occipital location, the bullet's pathway that ends against the fractured parietal bone (**a-c**), various metal and bone fragments which appear hyperdense a right parietal subdural haematoma, midline shift to the left and obliteration of the cortical sulci (**a, b**).

termingled with small hyperdense haemorrhagic foci.

In serial CT scans performed 24-48 hours following the trauma, the lesions become more obvious due to the increase in oedema and the resulting enlarging mass effect. The trauma may also be responsible for frank damage to the intracerebral vessels with consequent progres-

sive haemorrhagic extravasation (7, 29). Therefore, it is important that repeat CT scans be performed within the first 24 hours of the initial trauma to reassess the condition of the brain for possible intervention.

In such cases the CT shows areas of mixed density due to a combination of hyperdense haemorrhagic foci often in combination with

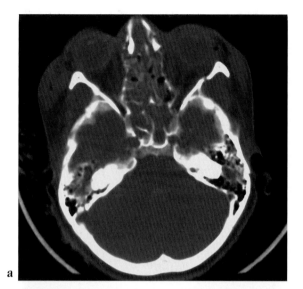

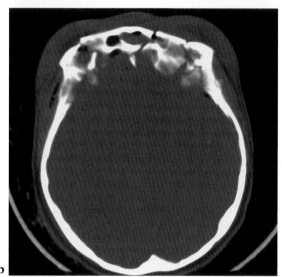

Fig. 2.4 - (**a**, **b**) Open head-facial injury caused by road traffic accident. Multiple fractures of the left orbital, ethmoidal and frontal bones are noted, with fluid within the ethmoid air cells and frontal sinus (**a**, **b**).

Traumatic intraparenchymal haematoma

Intraparenchymal haematomas are usually caused by combined torsion and compression forces applied to the intraparenchymal vessels, causing them to rupture; less frequently they are a consequence of direct vascular damage in-

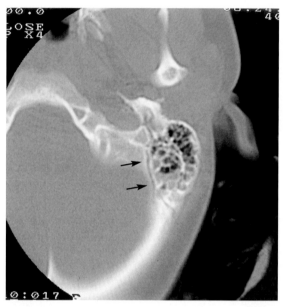

Fig. 2.5 - Fracture of the left petrous bone, with fluid within the mastoid air cells (arrows).

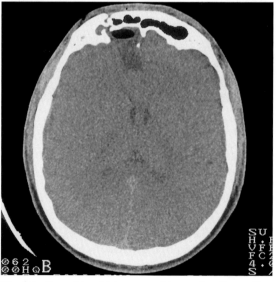

Fig. 2.6 - Frontal head injury caused by road traffic accident with fractures of the walls of the right frontal sinus and the formation of an air-fluid level.

confluent hypodense non-haemorrhagic areas (Fig. 2.8 a, b). The haemorrhagic component gradually resolves and disappears completely within 2-4 weeks (Fig. 2.8 c, d), whereas the oedematous areas may persist for longer periods before complete recovery; alternatively, irregular areas of hypodensity may remain indicating residual encephalomalacia (Fig. 2.8 e, f), and in some cases parenchymal cavitation occurs (3, 20).

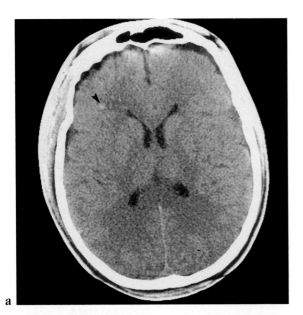

a

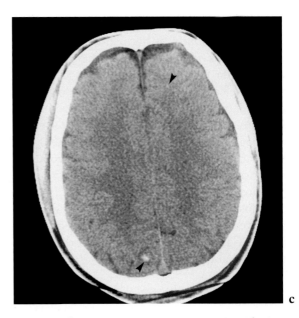

c

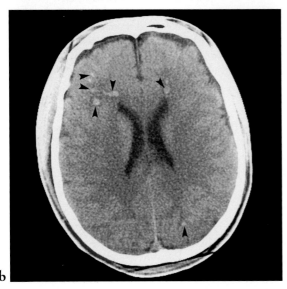

b

Fig. 2.7 - (**a-c**) Diffuse axonal injury (damage). Multiple hyperdense foci are observed with haemorrhage and compression of the white-grey matter junction bilaterally (arrow heads).

curred from penetrating injuries. These haemorrhages vary in dimension from a few mm to several cm and occur in 2-16% of all head injury patients (3). Haematomas can occur acutely, typically due to primary vessel rupture, or may appear sometime after the trauma, as a result of the confluence of multiple small laceration-contusion foci; CT scans performed in such cases immediately after the traumatic incident may be completely negative. Unlike patients with DAI

or cortical contusion, trauma patients with single intraparenchymal haematomas may not lose consciousness; in 30-50% of cases these patients remain lucid for the entire duration of the clinical outcome (3, 15). Signs and symptoms in parenchymal haematomas and their clinical evolution are similar to those observed in extraaxial haematoma patients, with the exception of large or temporal lobe haemorrhages that have an unpredictable outcome; even when small, these haematomas can cause brainstem damage due to associated transtentorial herniation (3, 7, 29).

Intraparenchymal haematomas usually occur in the same or nearly the same position in which the primary trauma was applied to the cranium as a typically well-circumscribed hyperdensity with or without a rim of perilesional oedema, depending upon the time of the CT acquisition relative to the traumatic incident (acute: no perilesional oedema; subacute: perilesional oedema; Fig. 2.9). These haematomas are frequently observed within the frontal and temporal lobes. Up to 60% of cases are associated with extradural haematomas, either epi- or subdural in location. If the haematoma develops in a periventricular position, it can rupture into the cerebral ventricles. Larger haemorrhages result in considerable mass effect and have the added risk of downward transtentorial internal herniation of cerebral and brainstem tissue through the tentorial incisura, or even the possibility of herniation of the cerebellar tonsils through the foramen magnum later in the process of haemorrhagic expansion. Clinically it is not always easy to distinguish intraparenchymal haemorrhage from DAI or parenchymal contusion; this differential diagnostic difficulty probably accounts for the marked variability in the clinical evolution statistics as reported in the literature (3). The prognosis for isolated intraparenchymal haematomas is fairly good, but worsens considerably with increasing degrees of mass effect or when it is associated with DAI or haemorrhages into the basal ganglia.

rhages are occasionally seen in combination with choroid plexus haematomas, haematomas of the deep grey or white matter and subarachnoid haemorrhage (Fig. 2.22c).

Traumatic lesions of the deep grey structures and the brainstem

This type of lesion is caused by stretching and torsional forces that cause the rupture of small perforating vessels, or by the direct impact of the dorsolateral surface of the brainstem against the tentorial incisura. These lesions are less frequently observed than those

Tab. 2.4 - Comparison between subdural and epidural haematomas

	EPIDURAL HAEMATOMA	SUBDURAL HAEMATOMA
Incidence	1-4% of trauma cases; 10% of fatal trauma cases	10-20% of all trauma cases; 30% of fatal trauma cases
Aetiology	Associated fractures in 85-95% of cases; Laceration of middle meningeal artery/dural venous sinus in 70-80% of cases.	Tearing of the cortical veins of the pons
Site	Between skull and dura mater; Crosses the dura mater but not the cranial sutures; 95% are supratentorial 5% are subtentorial; 5% bilateral	Between dura mater and arachnoid mater; Crosses the cranial sutures but not the dura mater; 95% are supratentorial; 5% are bilateral
CT findings	Biconvex (lens) shape; Shifts the white-grey matter interface; 66% are hyperdense; 33% are mixed (hyper-/hypodense) Crescent shape;	*Acute*: 60% hyperdense; 40% mixed (hyper-/hypodense) *Subacute*: isodense; *Chronic*: hypodense

Intraventricular haemorrhage

Traumatic intraventricular haemorrhage is somewhat uncommon and is only present in 1-5% of closed head injuries; it is usually a consequence of particularly severe trauma and tends to be associated with DAI and traumatic lesions of the deep grey matter and brainstem. The clinical prognosis is generally poor (3, 13, 20, 22). CT shows hyperdense intraventricular collections, which may or may not have associated fluid-fluid levels. Intraventricular haemor-

mentioned in the preceding sections and represent approximately 5-10% of primary traumatic pathology (3, 20, 22). They are associated with severe clinical states, and usually have unfavourable prognoses. Depending upon the clinical severity, CT can be entirely negative or may show relatively minor findings, including small haemorrhages in the areas of the brainstem surrounding the cerebral aqueduct and in the basal grey nuclei. As compared to CT, on MRI these types of lesions appear relatively more clearly.

Extraaxial traumatic lesions

Epidural haematomas

Overall, epidural haematomas are present in 1-4% of head injury cases, and in 10% of fatal cranial head injuries. These injuries are quite rare in patients over 60 years of age, because of the increased adherence of the parietal dura mater to the overlying inner table of the skull (Tab. 2.4).

Epidural haematoma patients may present with few or minor signs and symptoms. In almost 50% of all cases there is a typical interval of mental lucidity between the traumatic event and the onset of severe neurological deterioration or coma (3, 13). In 10-30% of cases, the imaging findings may first appear and even progress over the first 24-48 hours following the traumatic incident (20, 22).

Epidural haematomas are situated between the dura mater and the internal bony table of the skull, and they are almost always associated with skull fractures (Fig. 2.10). On occasion, parenchymal countercoup lesions may be observed on the side of the cranium opposite to the primary traumatic blow (3, 20, 22). These haematomas are often secondary to lacerations of the middle meningeal artery (when in the temporoparietal region), or more rarely, tears of the cranial veins such as the diploic and meningeal veins, and the dural venous sinuses. In this latter case, the epidural haematoma straddles the midline when the sagittal venous sinus is involved (direct coronal acquisitions or scans reconstructed in the coronal plane may be required for precise demonstration); alternatively, the epidural haemorrhage may extend between the supra- and infratentorial compartments, if the lateral dural venous sinuses are involved. Arterially fed epidural haematomas are typically observed in the acute phase because they grow under arterial blood pressure, thus compressing the brain and resulting in early downward internal cerebral herniation coupled with rapid clinical deterioration and eventual coma (7, 29). Venous epidural haematomas are usually small by comparison as the accumulation of blood takes place under relatively low venous pressure. Larger ve-

nous epidural haematomas are typically seen when resulting from the rupture of one of the larger dural venous sinuses. The CT density of the extraaxial blood collection depends in part upon the phase in which the haematoma is imaged. In the acute phase, epidural haematomas appear as homogeneously hyperdense lesions, with a biconvex or lens shape; the varying mass effect can be observed in the contralaterally displaced ventricular and extraventricular CSF

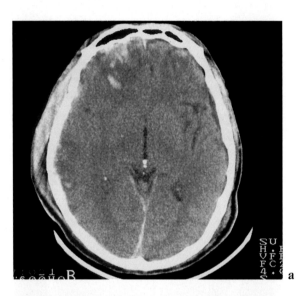

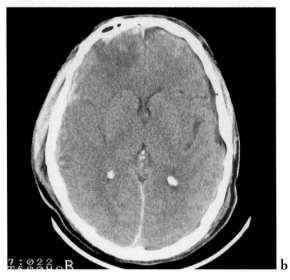

Fig. 2.8 - (**a-f**) Temporal evolution of contusive haemorrhagic focus. (**a-b**) CT examination a few hours following trauma: irregular haemorrhagic foci are seen in both frontal lobes and in right temporal-parietal region with the obliteration of the ipsilateral Sylvian fissure cistern.

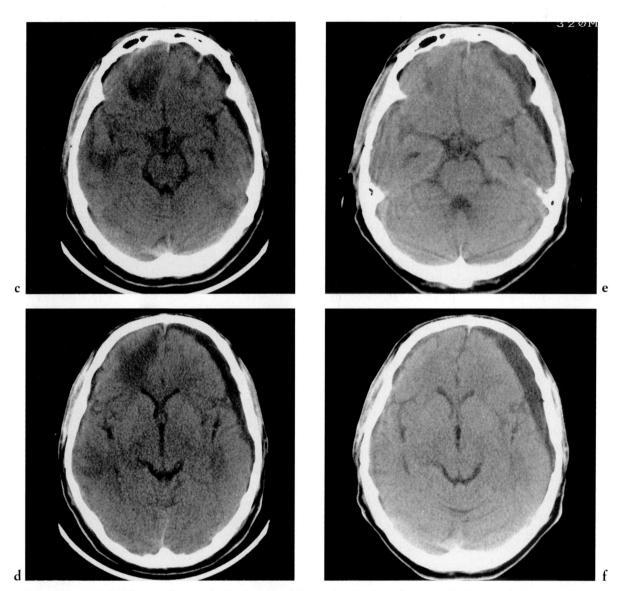

Fig. 2.8 (*cont.*) - (**c-d**) Follow up after 3 weeks: The hyperdense haemorrhage has been almost completely resolved, whereas the hypodense component is still clearly visible; a subdural hygroma has accumulated on the left side. (**e-f**) Follow up after 6 weeks: There is partial resolution of the hypodense component, a residual of which persists in a right frontal region; the hygroma on the left side remains.

spaces (Figs. 2.10 and 2.11). Rarely epidural haematomas can have an isodense appearance immediately subsequent to the traumatic incident, if imaging is undertaken before the fresh blood clots (another cause may be a very anaemic patient).

In certain cases of venous epidural haematoma, CT examinations conducted immediately after the trauma may reveal little, whereas the haematoma appears only 2-3 days later. This delay in the appearance of the haemorrhage is due to the fact that in venous epidural haematomas the injured veins bleed relatively slowly; alternatively, a delay in epidural haemorrhage from a traumatized arterial source may occur because blood can only flow into the epidural space after resolution of the trauma-induced arterial spasm. The haematoma can also be dampened by the mass effect of overlying brain contusion. In the case of persistent bleeding within an extraaxial blood collection, the haematoma can appear of mixed den-

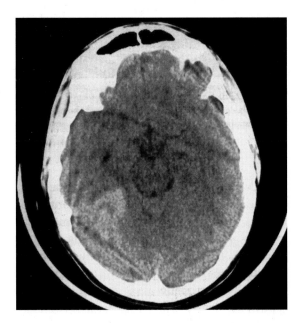

Fig. 2.9 - An acute post-traumatic intraparenchymal haematoma in observed in the right temporal-occipital area.

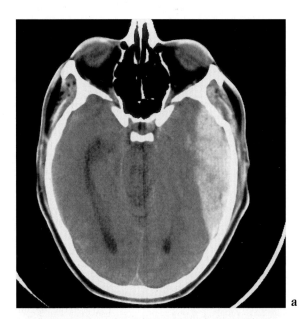

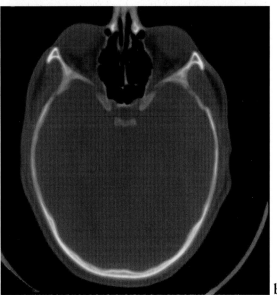

Fig. 2.10 - (**a-b**) A large epidural haematoma is seen in left temporal-parietal region (**a**) associated with an overlying skull fracture (**b**).

sity due to the presence of non-clotted new blood alternating with older clotted haemorrhage (7, 29). In subacute forms, as in the case of bleeding caused by the rupture of the dural venous sinuses, the density of the clotted haemorrhage varies in part according to the resorption of the solid blood constituents (Fig. 2.12).

Acute epidural haematomas represent the most urgent of all cases of cranial trauma. They require swift treatment before irreversible parenchymal damage occurs, caused by the compression of brain structures, especially the brainstem. Although rare (5% of extraaxial haematomas), extradural haematomas in the posterior fossa are potentially the most worrisome and tend to demonstrate the most rapid compromise of patient vital functions. As an additional factor, the compression of the aqueduct of Sylvius may cause acute obstructive hydrocephalus resulting in progressive supratentorial mass effect and accelerated downward transtentorial internal cerebral herniation.

Subdural haematoma

Subdural haematomas (SDH's) are one of the most life threatening events that can occur

Tab. 2.5 - Post-traumatic sequelae of head injuries

---

1) - Cortical atrophy
2) - Encephalomalacia
3) - Pneumocephalus
4) - Leptomeningeal cyst formation
5) - Cranial nerve lesions
6) - Diabetes insipidus (pituitary injury)
7) - Hydrocephalus (communicating or obstructive)

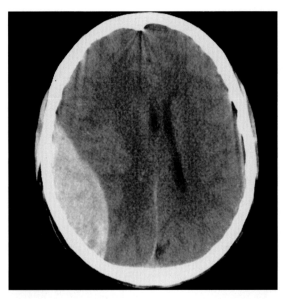

Fig. 2.11 - Axial CT shows an epidural haematoma with biconvex lens shape, in right parietal region with compression of the cerebral parenchyma and midline shift.

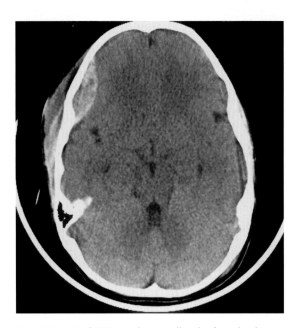

Fig. 2.12 - Axial CT reveals a small right frontal subacute epidural haematoma with mixed hypodense and hyperdense component, concomitant extracranial haematoma.

following head injuries, having a 50-85% mortality rate (20) (Tab. 2.5). They occur in 10-20% of all cases of cranial trauma and are frequent in the elderly with underlying brain atrophy and large intracranial subarachnoid spaces, and in physically abused children who have

been subjected to strong shaking (i.e., "shaken baby syndrome") (3, 6, 20, 23). In elderly patients they may arise in the absence of a traumatic episode (18, 19). If the haematoma is isolated and small, symptomatology may be absent or minor (e.g., headache). However, the SDH is often associated with DAI and/or severe mass effect, and patients therefore tend to be clinically compromised, with low Glasgow Coma Scores; in up to 50% of cases, patients appear flaccid or even decerebrate (13).

SDH is a collection of blood in the subdural space between the external surface of the leptomeninges and the dura mater secondary to the laceration of veins (in particular the veins involved are those that join the cerebral cortical veins and veins of the pons with the dural sinuses), or in the more severe forms, secondary to or associated with underlying cortical laceration. SDH's can occur at any age, but are most frequently observed in patients aged 60-80 years because of the greater mobility of the brain within the skull secondary to senile atrophy and therefore the greater ease with which veins rupture upon acute traumatic stretching of the attached cortical venous structures (18, 19). SDH's are more frequent than are epidural haematomas and are relatively more often associated with contusion-type injuries rather than skull fractures. This relationship is useful in predicting patient prognosis and in part explains why the overall intracranial mass effect is larger than are the actual dimensions of the SDH. Distinctions are made between the acute (i.e., within 3 days from the trauma), subacute (i.e., within 3 months) and chronic (i.e., more than 3 months) forms of SDH. In the acute phase, subdural haematoma appears as a hyperdense, sickle-shaped extraaxial lesion (Fig. 2.13); in some cases there may be a medial beak at the level of the pterion, where it penetrates the anterior and lateral aspects of the Sylvian fissure between the opercula of the frontal and the temporal lobes. Atypical configurations may be encountered in very large SDH's (Fig. 2.14a) or in the presence of fibrous bands traversing the subdural space resulting from previous trauma or inflammation; these cases of SDH can take the form of a biconvex lens or a multilocular appearance.

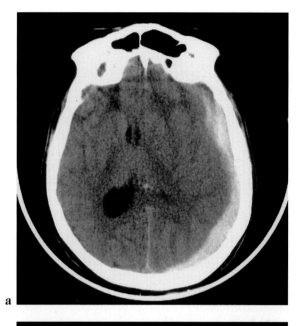

a

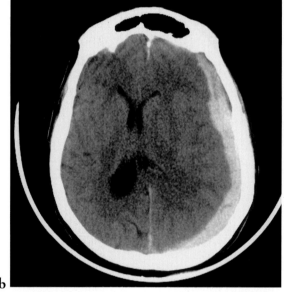

b

Fig. 2.13 - Axial CT demonstrates an acute subdural haematoma along the left hemisphere convexity with right shift of the midline structures and compression of the left lateral ventricle. [**a**), **b**) axial CT].

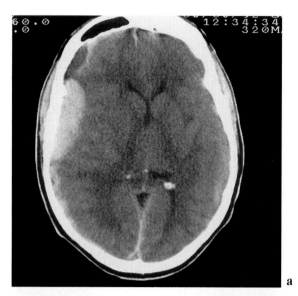

a

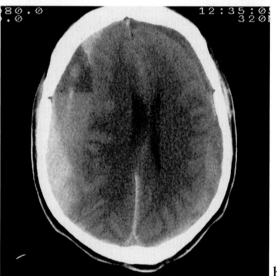

b

Fig. 2.14 - Bilateral subdural haematomas. There is a biloculated acute-subacute subdural haematoma on the right side (**a**), a heterogeneous appearance of the two haematomas with fluid-fluid levels (**b**), and presence of haemorrhagic components of different ages. The left sided subacute subdural haematoma is almost isodense as compared to the underlying brain and is therefore somewhat difficult to visualise. [**a**), **b**) axial CT].

Subsequently, due to the effect of the metabolism of the protein content of haemoglobin, SDH's initially become isodense (e.g., between the 7th and 21st day following the traumatic incident) (Fig. 2.15), and then evolve into a generally hypodense lesion (Figs. 2.16, 2.17) relative to the density of the underlying brain tissue. In practice, an SDH can also be isodense or hypodense outside of this predicted phase density pattern if the patient is anaemic, or if the systemic blood is diluted with iatrogenically administered fluid; conversely, chronic SDH's can show progressive hyperdensity due to interim haemorrhage(s) which can be asymptomatic and unprovoked by recurrent trauma (i.e., spontaneous) (Fig. 2.16). In cer-

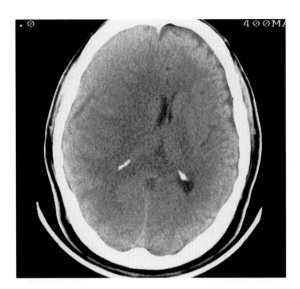

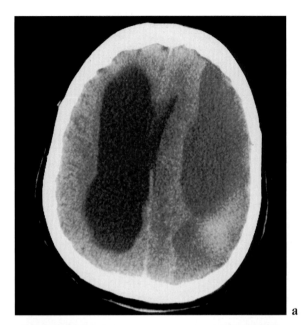

a

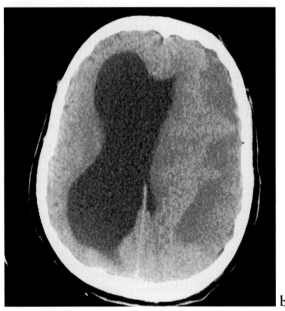

b

Fig. 2.15 - Subdural haematoma. Axial CT shows a subacute right frontal subdural haematoma is noted that is isodense and associated with obliteration of the cortical sulci, displacement of the corticomedullary junction away from the overlying skull, leftward shift of the midline structures and compression of the adjacent lateral ventricle.

tain cases in the subacute or chronic phases, a blood-fluid level can be observed following blood clot liquefaction, perhaps contributed to by haemorrhagic sedimentation (hypodensity superiorly and iso- or hyperdensity inferiorly) (Fig. 2.14b). In some cases, haemorrhagic events are followed by blood clot organization, which gives the crescent image a layered curvilinear appearance, with the older, hypodense collections on the medial and lateral margins and the more recent haematomas showing a relatively denser core; complex, crescent-shaped layers of varying density, representing haematomas and membranes of different ages, may subsequently occur.

In rare cases SDH's can reabsorb spontaneously, although some increase in volume and become chronic in duration. The eventual evolution depends in part upon the hyperosmolarity of liquefied blood products, as well as on whether or not new bleeds have occurred over the interim. The sites of SDH's are usually supratentorial and especially over the convexity; due to the lack of barrier to progression at this level, the extravasated blood easily extends along the entire hemicranium. If the SDH is situated at the vertex, it can go unnoticed on axial slices, and there-

Fig. 2.16 - Subdural haematoma. Axial CT reveals and unusual appearing left frontoparietal subdural haematoma with a hyperdense acute haemorrhagic component layering posteriorly. The left lateral ventricle is compressed by the haematoma and the contralateral lateral ventricle is dilated. [**a**), **b**) axial CT].

fore coronal scans are required in appropriate cases (Fig. 2.18). If unilateral, SDH's are accompanied by a contralateral shift of the midline structures and the lateral cerebral ventricles (Fig. 2.19); if bilateral, these extraaxial haemorrhages cause compression of the ventricles that assume a

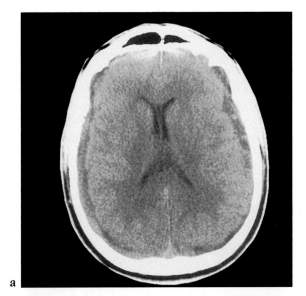

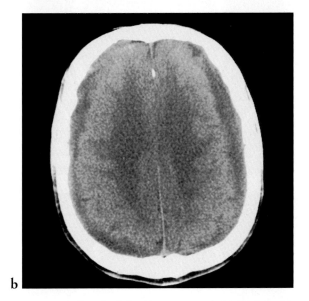

Fig. 2.17 - Bilateral subdural haematomas. Axial CT shows bilateral hypodense subdural haematomas. [**a**), **b**) axial CT].

thinner, elongated and parallel appearance (Fig. 2.20). In both instances, the characteristic finding is the disappearance of the underlying cortical sulci and the displacement of the superficial brain parenchyma away from the bony inner table of the skull. For the demonstration of these SDH's, especially when the haemorrhage is isodense, it is important to identify the corresponding cortico-medullary junction and the digitations of the white matter that penetrate into the gyral folds. The centrum semiovale usually has a

convex lateral margin; however, in the presence of an SDH this margin becomes flattened, concave or irregularly distorted. If the cortico-medullary junction is not visible, a bolus injection of contrast medium administered during the scan may be useful in identifying the cortical surface and delineating the border of an isodense SDH. This image enhancement method can document

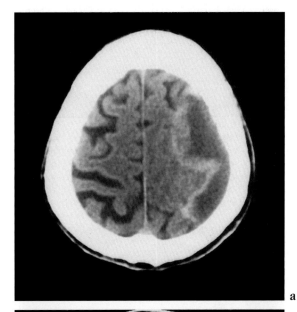

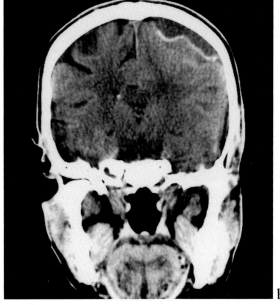

Fig. 2.18 - Subdural haematomas. Axial and coronal CT shows small, chronic subdural haematoma over the convexity of the brain is observed which is better seen on coronal scans. [**a**) axial CT; **b**) coronal CT].

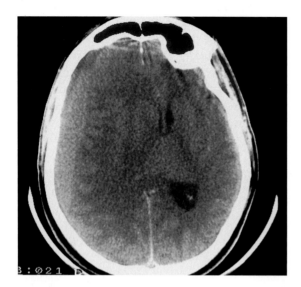

Fig. 2.19 - Subdural haematoma. The axial CT shows a right frontoparietal subdural haematoma with associated mass effect upon the adjacent cerebral parenchyma, which causes a subfalcian herniation of the cingulate gyrus and the compressed right lateral ventricle. The left lateral ventricle is dilated due to a CSF obstruction at the level of the left foramen of Monro.

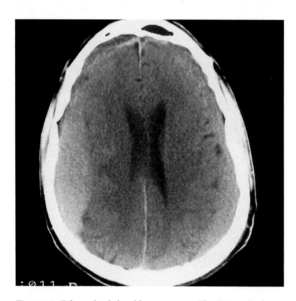

Fig. 2.20 - Bilateral subdural haematomas. The CT study shows lateral ventricles that are thinned, elongated and parallel to one another. The left sided subdural haematoma is almost isodense as compared to the underlying brain.

a thin line of enhancement at the brain surface (perhaps due to compression ischaemia), a focal traumatic rupture of the blood-brain barrier, visualization of a membrane related to the prior haemorrhage or prominent enhancement of dilated cortical veins.

SDH's do not cross the midline because the subdural spaces on the two sides of the cranium do not communicate. These haematomas are occasionally observed beneath the temporal lobe within the middle cranial fossa and under the occipital lobes extending along the tentorium cerebelli, and are often difficult to see with axial slices alone. In these instances, supplemental coronal slices are helpful for visualization.

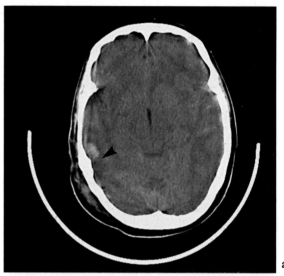

a

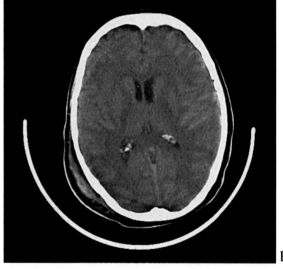

b

Fig. 2.21 - Subarachnoid haemorrhage. Hyperdensity is noted within the cortical sulci over the left cerebral hemisphere. Small haemorrhagic cortical contusions are also seen, the largest of which can be observed in the right temporal region (arrowhead). [**a**), **b**) axial CT].

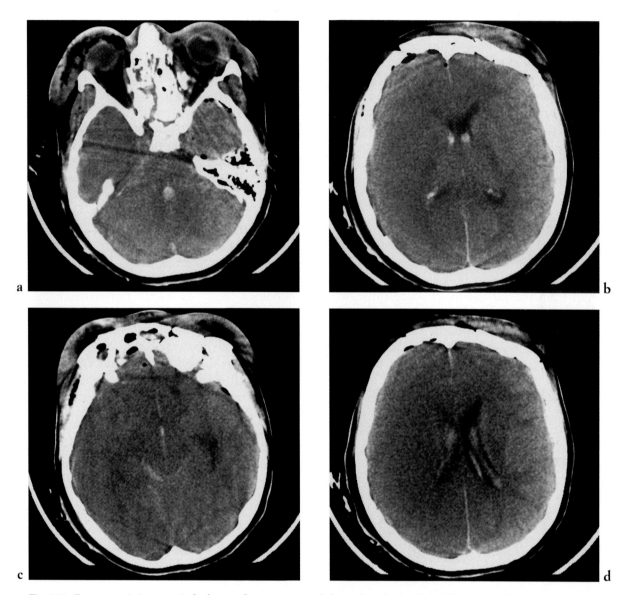

Fig. 2.22 - Posttraumatic intraventricular haemorrhage, pneumocephalus, and cerebral oedema. Bilateral eyelid haematomas are seen associated with subcutaneous emphysema (**a**). Intracranially are observed subarachnoid (**b**) and intraventricular haemorrhage (**a**), air bubbles in the CSF spaces (**c**) and the widespread oedema within the right cerebral hemisphere (**d**). [**a**]-**d**] axial CT].

Subarachnoid haemorrhage (SAH)

SAH's typically occur after severe cranial trauma and are usually associated with haemorrhagic parenchymal contusions (Figs. 2.21 and 2.22) (3, 29). Traumatic SAH's are usually somewhat insignificant from a clinical point of view, being linked pathologically to the rupture of small cortical vessels that traverse the subarachnoid space. These haemorrhages are seen as hyperdense collections of blood in the sulci, fissures and cisternal spaces, especially around the Sylvian fissure and the interpeduncular cistern (Figs. 2.21 and 2.22) (20, 22).

The site of the SAH is often somewhat distant from that of the trauma because the blood tends to diffuse within the subarachnoid spaces. In some cases the blood can reach the ventricular system, due to retrograde flow through the foramina of Luschka and Magendie. The ability of CT to detect SAH is directly related to the quantity of extravasated blood as well as to the time from the traumatic incident; the SAH can be negative if the CT scan is performed some days after the event. SAH's can sometimes be falsely simulated in certain particularly severe cases of diffuse cerebral oedema, in which the brain appears relatively hypodense in comparison to the underlying dura mater and neural tissue (20).

Subdural hygroma

A subdural hygroma is an extraaxial collection of CSF caused by the extravasation of this fluid from the subarachnoid space through a traumatic tear in the arachnoid mater (Fig. 2.23). The acute form is particularly frequent in children and less so in adults (6, 23). Subacute

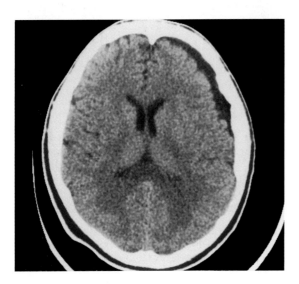

Fig. 2.23 - Posttraumatic subdural hygroma. The axial CT shows a left sided frontal posttraumatic subdural hygroma.

and chronic forms can be seen following surgery performed to treat severe head injuries. In such cases, the hypodense subdural collection is either located in the region of the operation or alternatively on the opposite side due to an *ex vacuo* mechanism following the evacuation of a contralateral haematoma. The differential diagnosis includes chronic, hypodense SDH.

Traumatic vascular lesions

Traumatic cerebrovascular lesions are somewhat rare, but are probably less infrequent than reported in the medical literature (3, 9, 20). In certain cases these lesions can be asymptomatic or have a clinical onset sometime after the initial traumatic incident and can therefore be overlooked on routine imaging studies in patients having undergone trauma. In other cases the presence of other craniocerebral lesions related to trauma can conceal the presence of related underlying vascular lesions, as both clinical symptoms and imaging findings may be attributed to other dominant traumatic parenchymal pathology such as DAI, intraparenchymal haematomas or extraaxial haematomas. CT is a most useful technique for identifying patients with an increased risk of vascular lesions such as those with fractures at the base of the skull extending into the bony internal carotid canal, the sphenoid bone, and the petrous pyramid of the temporal bone and the basiocciput. Of course, it should be pointed out that the presence of fractures in such sites does not necessarily indicate the presence of associated vascular lesions (7, 29).

The internal carotid artery, which is the most frequently affected vessel in cranial trauma, can undergo dissection due to the forced extension and torsion of the neck or due to the direct laceration of the arterial wall by a skull base fracture; this is especially true with trauma to the region directly adjacent to the anterior clinoid processes and the bony internal carotid canal (9). In certain cases the adventitia of the carotid artery wall can remain intact and thereby develop a pseudo-aneurysm (3, 9, 20). Other possible cerebrovascular lesions related to the trauma include dissections, lacerations and frank vessel occlusions, which may or may not be associated with perivascular haematomas.

Another pathological entity connected with brain trauma is the formation of arteriovenous fistulae. The most typical site is a fistula between the internal carotid artery siphon and the cavernous venous sinus, usually a consequence of the fracture of the central skull base. In such

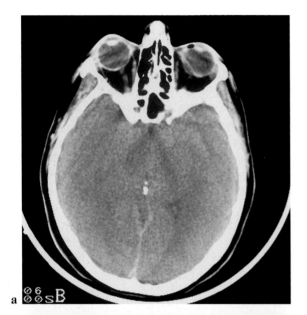

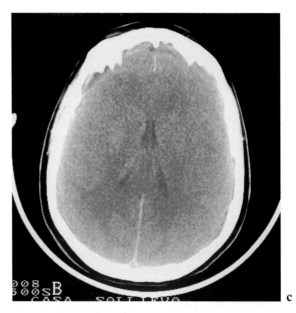

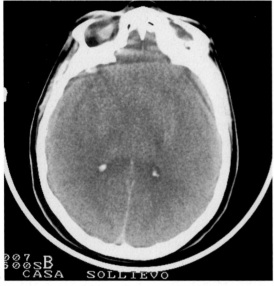

Fig. 2.24 - Posttraumatic cerebral swelling. The CT demonstrated diffuse posttraumatic cerebral swelling is seen with obliteration of the basal subarachnoid cisterns and superficial cortical sulci, compression of the 3rd ventricle and reduction in size of the lateral ventricles. The midline structures are not shifted, and there are no focal haemorrhages are present. [a), b), c) axial CT].

cases, one suggestive indirect sign on imaging is the CT finding of an enlarged, arterialized superior ophthalmic vein.

CT is very accurate in demonstrating fractures of the base of the skull, whereas greater diagnostic sensitivity in demonstrating traumatic vascular lesions can be obtained with MR or MR angiography examinations (3, 20). In selected cases where such traumatic cerebrovascular lesions are suspected on the basis of non-invasive imaging studies and clinical information, selective cerebral angiography is required to clearly define the diagnosis and to suggest optimal treatment options.

SECONDARY LESIONS

Internal cerebral herniation

Bony and dural structures grossly subdivide the cranial cavity into functional supra- and infratentorial compartments. Internal cerebral herniations are a mechanical shift of the cerebral parenchyma, cerebrospinal fluid and the attached blood vessels from one compartment to another. These alterations are the most common secondary effects of expanding intracranial processes. Based on the site and direction of the shift, they can be divided into subfalcian, transtentorial (ascending and descending), cerebellar tonsillar and transphenoid (ascending and descending) in type. Patients with internal cerebral herniations are usually in compromised clinical states that only permit the use of axial CT acquisitions, which are not the most suitable for viewing craniocaudal shifts of the cerebral parenchyma. Therefore, due attention must be paid to gleaning the indirect signs of internal cerebral herniation (3, 20).

Subfalcian and descending transtentorial herniations are the most common subtypes. A subfalcian herniation is defined by a shift of the cingulate gyrus across the midline, traversing below the free margin of the falx cerebri. As the shift progresses, the compressed ipsilateral cerebral ventricle becomes thinner, while the contralateral ventricle dilates as a consequence of CSF obstruction at the level of the foramen of Monro (Fig. 2.19). In addition, distal branches of the anterior cerebral artery are also shifted towards or across the midline, and, in the most severe cases these vessels can be compressed against the free edge of the falx cerebri; this in turn may result in secondary ischaemia or infarction due to pressure-occlusion of the pericallosal or callosomarginal arteries.

Descending transtentorial herniations consist of a medial and caudal shift of the uncus and the parahippocampal gyrus of the temporal lobe beyond the free margin of the tentorium cerebelli. This results in an asymmetric appearance of the peripontine cisterns and the cerebellopontine angle, which are widened on the side of the mass lesion due to a contralateral shift of the brainstem; the contralateral cisterns are consonantly narrowed by both the lateral shift as well as the downward herniation of cerebral tissue. The anterior choroid, posterior communicating and posterior cerebral arteries are also displaced medially and downward and can be compressed against the free edge of the tentorium cerebelli with resulting ischaemia or infarction of the occipital lobe if severe. In rare cases, compression of the perforating vessels emerging from the arterial circle of Willis can cause ischaemia and infarction in the basal cerebral nuclei. Other possible complications of transtentorial herniations include periaqueductal brainstem necrosis, brainstem haemorrhage (i.e., Duret haemorrhages) and direct contusion of the cerebral peduncle(s) due to traumatic impact against the free edge of the tentorium cerebelli (i.e., Kernohan's notch) (20).

Ascending transtentorial herniations are more rare, and are defined by the cranial shift of the cerebellar vermis and parts of the superi-

or-medial aspects of the cerebellar hemispheres through the tentorium incisura. This in turn results in compression of the superior cerebellar and superior vermian cistern and the upper fourth ventricle. If severe, hydrocephalus may develop due to the compression of the aqueduct of Sylvius.

Tonsillar herniations are usually caused by an increase in mass effect within the posterior fossa, which causes a downward displacement of the cerebellar tonsils through the foramen magnum. It is estimated that up to half of all descending transtentorial herniations and approximately two-thirds of ascending transtentorial herniations are associated with tonsillar herniations at some point in the evolution of the herniative process.

Descending transphenoid herniations are produced by a posterior and downward (caudal) shift of the frontal lobe beyond the margin of the greater wing of the ipsilateral sphenoid bone, with backward displacement and compression of the Sylvian fissure, the middle cerebral artery and the temporal lobe on the same side. Conversely, in ascending transphenoid herniations, the frontal lobe is pushed upwards and anteriorly, to extend above the margin of the greater wing of the sphenoid.

Posttraumatic diffuse cerebral oedema

Diffuse cerebral oedema with generalized swelling of the brain occurs in up to 10-20% of all severe head injuries; this is encountered more commonly in children and can be either unilateral or bilateral (Figs. 2.24, 2.25). Unilateral diffuse cerebral oedema is associated with ipsilateral subdural haematoma formation in 85% of cases and with epidural haematoma in 9% of cases; it is an isolated finding in only 4-5% of cranial trauma patients (3, 20). Despite the fact that it can develop in just a few hours in the most serious cases, it usually evolves over a period of 24-48 hours. Posttraumatic diffuse cerebral oedema is caused by an increase in the water content of the brain and/or an increase in intravascular blood volume, both of which can

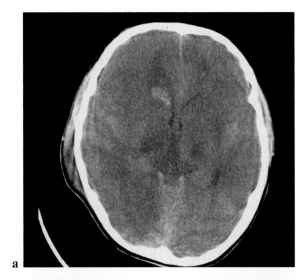

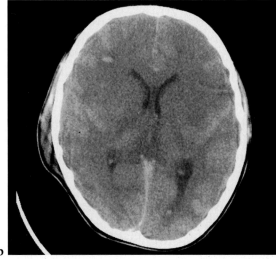

Fig. 2.25 - Posttraumatic cerebral oedema. The CT reveals posttraumatic cerebral oedema is observed associated with diffuse hypodensity of the white matter and obliteration of the Sylvian and perimesencephalic cisterns, a reduction in the size of the ventricular system and small intraparenchymal right haemorrhages in the right frontal region.

matter interface. The cerebellum is generally spared and can appear relatively hyperdense as compared to the cerebral parenchyma which is isodense. In the later stages of evolution in severe cases, diffuse cerebral oedema is often accompanied by transtentorial internal cerebral herniation (3, 20, 22).

Posttraumatic cerebral ischaemia and infarction

The herniation of brain parenchyma across the falx cerebri and through the tentorium cerebelli is the most common cause of posttraumatic infarction. The occipital lobe is the territory most frequently affected by ischaemic events, which are usually associated with herniation of the temporal lobe through the tentorial incisura, with consequent compression-occlusion of one or both of the posterior cerebral arteries (3, 20). The second most common area of infarction associated with cranial trauma is the vascular territory of the anterior cerebral branches contralateral to the traumatic mass lesion, to include the pericallosal and callosomarginal arteries, consequent to subfalcian herniation of the cingulate gyrus. More rarely, infarcts may occur in the basal ganglia due to the compression of the choroid, lenticulostriate and thalamoperforating arteries against the structures at the base of the skull (7, 29).

Another category of important secondary manifestations of brain injuries is that of posttraumatic haemorrhages related to direct injury of larger arteries and veins. The caudal shift of the upper portion of the stem in transtentorial herniations can cause a compression of the perforating vessels in the interpeduncular cistern. This in turn causes small haemorrhagic foci, which can be confluent, in the tegmen (i.e., Duret haemorrhage), which must not be confused with the rarer primary haemorrhagic contusion lesions in the dorsolateral portion(s) of the midbrain resulting from collision of the brainstem with the free edge of the tentorium cerebelli. As an additional factor in descending transtentorial herniations, the impact of the cerebral peduncle contralateral to the traumatic mass lesion(s) against the free edge of the

be precipitated by a number of factors. This is a severe clinical condition and is fatal in approximately 50% of cases (20). The CT picture is characterized by a generalized obliteration of the cerebral cortical sulci and the intracranial subarachnoid spaces of the suprasellar and perimesencephalic cisterns (e.g., ambiens and quadrigeminal), and the cerebral ventricles appear thinned and compressed.

The brain appears diffusely hypodense, with a loss of the distinction of the grey-white tentorium cerebelli may cause oedema, ischaemia and/or haemorrhagic necrosis of this structure which results in focal atrophy that may take the gross form of a notch (i.e., Kernohan's notch). Clinically this may result in hemiparesis ipsilateral to the side of the primary traumatic effects; this is known by the term "false localizing sign" because it occurs in the peduncle contralateral to the supratentorial traumatic mass effect (20).

POSTTRAUMATIC SEQUELAE

The most common sequelae of severe cranial trauma include cortical atrophy, encephalomalacia, pneumocephalus, CSF leaks (i.e., fistulae), leptomeningeal cysts, cranial nerve lesions and diabetes insipidus (Tab. 2.8).

Encephalomalacia is characterized by foci of cerebral parenchyma loss in the area of the contusion and by diffuse cortical atrophy (3, 20). Encephalomalacic foci appear on CT as hypodense areas, often associated with varying degrees of dilation of the adjacent cerebral ventricles and overlying cortical sulci.

Skull base fractures with interruption of the dura resulting in direct communication of the cranium with the paranasal sinuses, can lead to intracranial air collection(s) (i.e., pneumocephalus). This is easily detected using CT because of the extremely low attenuation coefficient of air (Figs. 2.3, 2.22) (8). Air limited to the epidural space tends to remain localized and does not vary in position with the placement of the head; conversely, air localized to the subdural space tends to move its principal focus with head movements (20). Subarachnoid air is typically multifocal, non-confluent, has a "bubble-like" appearance and is often localized within the cerebral sulci. Posttraumatic intraventricular air occurs in association with fractures at the base of the skull with lacerations of the dura mater. Intravascular air is only rarely observed and is usually detected only in cases of fatal trauma.

CSF leaks are a consequence of fractures of the base of the skull in 80% of cases (20). Typically they are frontally positioned with CSF draining via a fistula into the ethmoid or the sphenoid paranasal sinus, and in 20% of cases they are complicated by meningitis, which if untreated can in turn lead to the formation of cerebral abscess or extraaxial empyema (20). Clinical onset of a posttraumatic CSF leak usually occurs within a week of the initial trauma, but can develop as late as several years after the event. High resolution coronal acquisition CT is the examination of choice to identify the associated skull base fracture, although the visualization of the fistula is often difficult or impossible to achieve. Positive contrast CT or MR cisternography may be required to prove the presence and pinpoint the location of the fistula preoperatively.

Cranial fractures can later cause leptomeningeal cysts. These cysts are typically limited to children, occurring months to years after the cranial trauma. They are associated with underlying meningeal lacerations and theoretically result from an interposition of meningeal tissue within the space of the fracture line of the overlying calvaria at the time of the traumatic event. Sometimes known as an "expanding posttraumatic fracture", CSF pulsations have been hypothesized to be the mechanism of cyst accumulation as well as fracture expansion.

Diabetes insipidus is an infrequent sequela of cranial trauma, most commonly seen in infants as a result of birth trauma. Diabetes insipidus can be a direct result of either descending transtentorial herniation causing hypothalamic infarction or pituitary stalk transection occurring at the time of the traumatic event.

Posttraumatic paralysis of one or more of the cranial nerves, especially the second, third, fourth and sixth nerves and the second division of the fifth cranial nerve, are typically due to cranial base fractures that involve the cavernous venous sinus and the apex of the orbit. The third cranial nerve can also be affected individually by transtentorial herniation of the temporal lobe, whereas the fourth cranial nerve can be injured by compression against the free margin of the tentorium cerebelli during violent shaking movements of the head.

One final sequela to cranial trauma is hydrocephalus, usually secondary to intraventricular haemorrhage or traumatic adherence of the meninges over the cerebral convexity, the basal cisterns or the aqueduct of Sylvius. This is caused by an inflammatory meningeal reaction to the effects of the trauma and the presence of blood products with consequent defective CSF resorption.

CONCLUSIONS

The advent of CT and its progressive technological improvement have revolutionized the diagnosis and clinical management of acute cranial trauma patients, resulting in early accurate analysis and swift evidence-based treatment of potentially fatal head injuries. Unenhanced CT is the examination technique of choice in these cases as it is quickly accomplished, readily available and does not require ancillary studies using other imaging technologies in most cases.

The spiral (helical) CT technique is principally useful in those cases in which the examination must be performed within an extremely limited time frame and in cases in which three-dimensional acquisition is necessary for multiplanar reconstruction of fractures of the orbit and the facial skeleton or CT angiographic studies of the intracranial vessels. Otherwise, standard CT acquisitions are preferred for their accuracy and absence of artefacts.

The use of IV contrast media is restricted to those rare cases in which a CT angiographic examination is needed when posttraumatic vascular pathology is suspected. Intrathecal positive contrast cisternography coupled with either CT or MRI may be required to analyse the presence and focus of a CSF fistula preoperatively.

One important limitation of the use of CT is the difficulty in detecting small parenchymal lesions located in the posterior fossa or at base of the skull, principally because of beam hardening artefacts typically present. However, this problem is of little practical significance clinically in the acute stage of trauma, as such pathology seldom requires surgical intervention.

It should be noted that MRI is more sensitive than is CT in detecting small cortical contusion lesions at the grey-white matter interface, DAI, extracerebral haematomas (especially when hypodense) and primary and secondary brainstem lesions. However, these changes are relatively minor and do not usually demand operative therapy in the emergency time frame. On the other hand, MRI can be a useful complement in the acute phase of cranial trauma in patients with significant clinical findings but no or few CT observations. And finally, MRI is the technique of choice in the evaluation of the subacute and chronic phases of symptomatic head injury.

REFERENCES

1. Bahner ML, Reith W, Zuna I et al: Spiral CT vs incremental CT: is spiral CT superior in imaging of the brain? Eur Radiol. 8(3): 416-20, 1998.
2. Frankowski RF, Annegers JF, Whitman S: Epidemiological and descriptive studies. Part I: The descriptive epidemiology of head trauma in the United States. In: Becker DP, Polishock J, eds. Central Nervous System Trauma Status Report. Bethesda, MD National Institute of Health, 33-51, 1985.
3. Gentry LR: Head trauma. In: Atlas SW:Magnetic resonance of the brain and spine.(2nd ed.), Lippincott-Raven, Philadelphia, pp 611-647, 1996.
4. Gentry LR: Imaging of closed head injury. Radiology 191:1-17, 1994.
5. Grumme T, Kluge W, Kretzschmar K et al: Head trauma. In: Cerebral and spinal computed tomography. Blackwell Science, Berlin pp 49-69, 1998.
6. Hymel KP, Rumack CM, Hay TC et al: Comparison of intracranial computed tomographic (CT) findings in pediatric abusive and accidental head trauma. Pediatr Radiol. 27(9):743-7, 1997.
7. Johnson MH, Lee SH: Computed tomography of acute cerebral trauma. Radiol Clin N Am 30:325-352, 1992.
8. Keskil S, Baykaner K, Ceviker N et al: Clinical significance of acute traumatic intracranial pneumocephalus. Neurosurg Rev. 21(1):10-3, 1998.
9. Klufas RA, Hsu L, Patel MR: Unusual manifestations of head trauma. AJR 166:675-681, 1996.
10. Kuntz R, Skalej M, Stefanou A: Image quality of spiral CT versus conventional CT in routine brain imaging. Eur J Radiol. 26(3): 235-40, 1998.
11. Lanksch W, Grumme T, Kazner E: Computed tomography in head injuries Springer, Berlin, 1979.
12. Lee SH, Rao KL: Cranial computed tomography. MC Graw-Hill, New York, 1983.
13. Lee TT, Aldana PR, Kirton OC et al: Follow-up computerized tomography (CT) scans in moderate and severe head injuries: correlation with Glasgow Coma Scores (GCS) and complication rate. Acta Neurochir Wien. 139(11): 1042-7; discussion 1047-8, 1997.
14. Leidner B, Adiels M, Aspelin P et al: Standardized CT examination of the multitraumatized patient. Eur Radiol. 8(9):1630-8, 1998.

15. Lerner C: Detecting acute extraaxial blood with bone algorithm CT images. AJR 17:1707, 1998.

16. Lloyd DA, Carty H, Patterson M et al: Predictive value of skull radiography for intracranial injury in children with blunt head injury. Lancet. 22; 349(9055): 821-4, 1997.

17. Mogbo KI, Slovis TL, Canady AI et al: Appropriate imaging in children with skull fractures and suspicion of abuse. Radiology. 208(2): 521-4, 1998.

18. Nagurney JT, Borczuk P, Thomas SH: Elderly patients with closed head trauma after a fall: mechanisms and outcomes. J Emerg Med. 16(5): 709-13, 1998.

19. Nagy KK, Joseph KT, Krosner SM et al: The utility of head computed tomography after minimal head injury. J Trauma. 46(2): 268-70, 1999.

20. Osborn A: Craniocerebral trauma. In Osborn A: Diagnostic neuroradiology. St Louis, pp 199-247, 1994.

21. Parizel PM, Ozsarlak P, Van-Goethem JW et al: Imaging findings in diffuse axonal injury after closed head trauma. Eur Radiol. 8(6): 960-5, 1998.

22. Pellicanò G, Bartolozzi A: La TC nei traumi cranioencefalici. Edizioni del Centauro, Udine ,1996.

23. Petitti N, Williams DW 3rd: CT and MR imaging of nonaccidental pediatric head trauma. Acad Radiol. 5(3): 215-23, 1998.

24. Rhea JT, Rao PM, Novelline RA: Helical CT and three-dimensional CT of facial and orbital injury. Radiol Clin North Am 37:489-513, 1999.

25. Shane SA, Fuchs SM: Skull fractures in infants and predictors of associated intracranial injury. Pediatr Emerg Care. 13(3):198-203, 1997.

26. Weisberg L., Nice C: Cerebral computed tomography. W.B. Saunders, Philadelphia, pp 321-343, 1989.

27. Wilson AJ: Gunshot injuries: what does a radiologist need to know? Radiographics 19:1358-1368, 1999.

28. Wysoki MG, Nassar CJ, Koenigsberg RA et al: Head trauma: CT scan interpretation by radiology residents versus staff radiologists. Radiology. 208(1):125-8, 1998.

29. Zee CS, Go JL: CT of head trauma. Neuroimaging Clin N Am. Aug; 8(3):525-39, 1998.

2.3

MRI IN HEAD INJURIES

M. Gallucci, G. Cerone, M. Caulo, A. Splendiani, R. De Amicis, C. Masciocchi

INTRODUCTION

Trauma is the most common cause of death among children and infants, of which head injuries account for some 60%. The mortality and morbidity rates concerning primary lesions and posttraumatic sequelae in patients with head injuries have been considerably reduced by the advent of computed tomography (CT), which is still the examination technique of choice in the acute phase, thanks to the rapidity with which it can be performed, the ready availability of the imaging equipment and the absence of contraindications (6, 25, 29). The drawback of this technique is the difficulty encountered in detecting smaller lesions, which are often located at the grey-white matter junction or in the vicinity of bone (e.g., temporal and frontal lobe poles, posterior fossa). In certain cases, the patient's clinical condition can be quite in contrast with the information yielded on their respective CT examinations (4, 7).

Due to its greater sensitivity in detecting these types of lesions, magnetic resonance imaging (MRI) can be used as a complement to or even a substitute for CT in some instances (5, 10, 14, 16, 18, 19, 24, 26). This said, performing an MR examination in the acute phase of trauma can prove somewhat difficult and entails a number of risks. These drawbacks, which will be discussed briefly below, make MR a technique of secondary importance in the overall imaging evaluation of head injuries (12).

DRAWBACKS

Intrinsic limits

The intrinsic limits of the MR technique consist in the absolute contraindication of examining subjects having ferromagnetic foreign bodies or electronic device implants (e.g., cardiac pacemakers). This problem becomes important in polytrauma patients, who may have acquired metal splinters from the traumatic event itself, and even more so in subjects with disorders of consciousness in whom it is not possible to reconstruct an accurate medical history with regard to previous surgical or prosthetic implant procedures (22, 9). It is therefore necessary if possible to determine the compatibility of any metallic foreign materials that are known or suspected to be present before exposure of the patient to the strong magnetic fields inherent in MRI.

Semeiological limits

The semeiological limits of MRI during the acute phase of cranial trauma include its lower

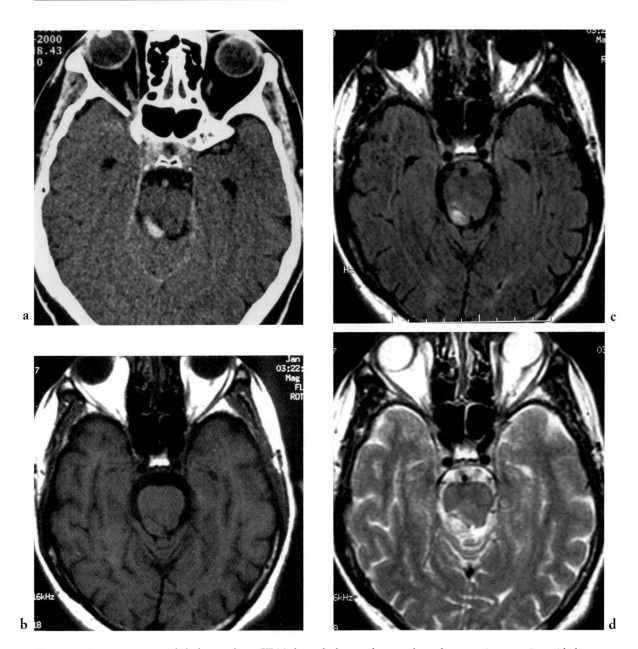

Fig. 2.26 - Hyperacute mesencephalic haemorrhage. CT (**a**) shows the haemorrhage as a hyperdense area in comparison with the surrounding brain tissue. The MRI examination conducted in the acute phase shows the haemorrhage to be isointense on T1-weighted sequences (**b**) and hyperintense on T2-dependent, FLAIR and turbo spin echo (TSE) (**c**, **d**) sequences because blood cannot be distinguished from oedema in this phase on the basis of MRI (i.e., oxyhaemoglobin).

sensitivity as compared to CT in identifying bony fractures of the skull, especially small ones, and acute intracranial bleeds (1, 30). Whereas in CT the densitometric value of the blood is due primarily to the quantity of the haemoglobin protein component, in MRI the intensity of the signal depends in large part on the magnetic properties of the iron contained in blood, or rather, on the electronic configuration that the hemoglobin iron assumes during evolution of the haemoglobin breakdown process (2). Therefore, although CT is clearly able to detect a hyperacute phase haemorrhage as an obvious area of hyperdensity due to the

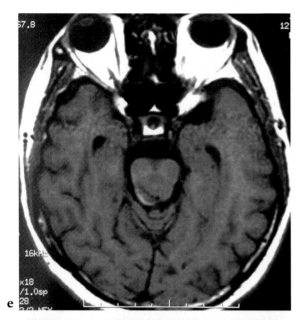

e

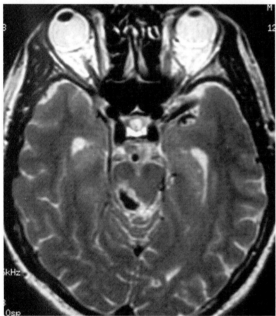

f

Fig. 2.26 (*cont.*) - An MRI examination conducted three days later shows an area of hyperintense signal on T1-weighted sequences (**e**) and hypointense signal on T2-weighted sequences as a result of haemoglobin breakdown products (i.e., deoxyhaemoglobin). [**a**), **b**), **c**) axial CT; **d**), **f**) axial T2-weighted MRI; **e**) axial T1-weighted MRI].

high concentration of haemoglobin, MRI in this same phase has characteristically poor sensitivity, as the blood (oxyhaemoglobin) has not yet undergone metabolic transformation to a paramagnetic species (Fig. 2.26).

It is only in the acute period, after approximately 12 hours after the event responsible for the bleed, that the first of a series of haemoglobin breakdown products starts to form in amounts that will alter the MR signal. This new species, deoxyhaemoglobin, causes a shortening of T2 time, and, to a greater extent T2*, thus creating local inhomogeneities in the magnetic field generated by the MR unit. On the other hand, red blood cell lysis and the blockage of the respiratory chain in haemorrhages cause an increase in the quantity of free water and therefore an increase in T2 and proton density signal, with consequent balancing of the T2 shortening, effect and a possible concealment of the hypointensity linked to the presence of intracellular deoxyhaemoglobin. As the magnetic susceptibility effect and therefore T2* shortening is directly proportionate to the square of the intensity of the static magnetic field, by using high field MR appliances and sequences particularly sensitive to T2* (e.g., gradient echo sequences, echo-planar sampling techniques) it is possible to resolve the problem and achieve dominant T2 shortening effects on imaging (i.e., focal reduction of the MR signal within subacute haemorrhages).

Another limitation posed by MRI is the fact that it requires relatively longer examination times than does CT. Time is critical in the diagnostic management of critical cranial trauma patients. In addition, these patients frequently are unable to consciously cooperate for the long examination times inherent in MRI, thereby often resulting in motion artefacts. Recent progress in technology has largely made it possible to overcome such limits with the use of high field equipment having ultrafast acquisition sequences, that allows to obtain single slice images in less than one second (9, 20) (Fig. 2.27b).

However, it should be remembered that in acute head injury patients the fundamental question to be answered is whether emergency surgery is required. In almost all cases this question is answered by CT, which is efficient in depicting significant haematomas or fractures of surgical interest. MRI is doubtlessly more sensitive in identifying subtle haemor-

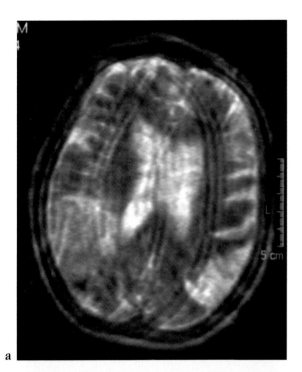

a

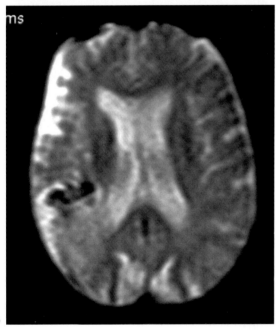

b

Fig. 2.27 - Multiple contusive and lacerative haemorrhagic cerebral foci in the acute phase. The T2-weighted sequence (**a**) shows multiple areas of signal hyperintensity within which haemorrhagic components cannot be distinguished. The long scan time often results in motion artefacts. The echo-planar sequence (**b**), which is more sensitive to T2*-weighted tissue, enables the identification of areas of hypointense signal caused by the presence of subacute haemorrhage (deoxyhaemoglobin). Motion artefacts can also be reduced by obtaining the acquisition in approximately 500 msec. [**a**) T2-weighted MRI; T2*-weighted MRI].

rhagic collections and small intraaxial lesions related to the traumatic incident, but such findings have no relevance with regard to emergency treatment (17, 23, 27). In any case, these minor imaging findings can be detected using MRI once the immediate life-threatening problems have been addressed and the patient has stabilized.

SEMEIOTICS

Primary intraaxial traumatic lesions

Contusions and *laceration-contusions* represent approximately 45% of all head injuries. They occur as a consequence of the impact of brain tissue against the inner table of the skull or dural insertion of the cranium. This trauma tends to cause related lesions in the poles of the frontal and temporal lobes and within the brainstem (22, 25). MRI is generally more sensitive in detecting these types of lesions than is CT due to the proximity of the traumatic alteration to the bony structures (i.e., CT beam hardening effects obscure this pathology) (15). A distinction must be made between simple non-haemorrhagic contusions and haemorrhagic or laceration-contusions.

Simple (non-haemorrhagic) contusions are areas of tissue characterized by the presence of oedema in the acute phase and by necrotic-encephalomalacic evolution in the chronic phase. MR is estimated to be up to 50% more sensitive than is CT in identifying simple contusions, which appear as hyperintense on T2-weighted sequences, typically affecting the surface layers of the cortical gyri. The sensitivity of MR is further increased by the use of FLAIR sequences; T1-weighted sequences by comparison are of little benefit in the acute phase in simple contusions (Fig. 2.28).

Laceration-contusions (haemorrhagic contusions) differ from simple contusions by the presence of a haemorrhagic zone within the contusion. In this type of lesion, CT can have greater specificity than MR, which is often not able to differentiate between haemorrhagic and non-haemorrhagic lesions (Figs. 2.26, 2.29, 2.30). As

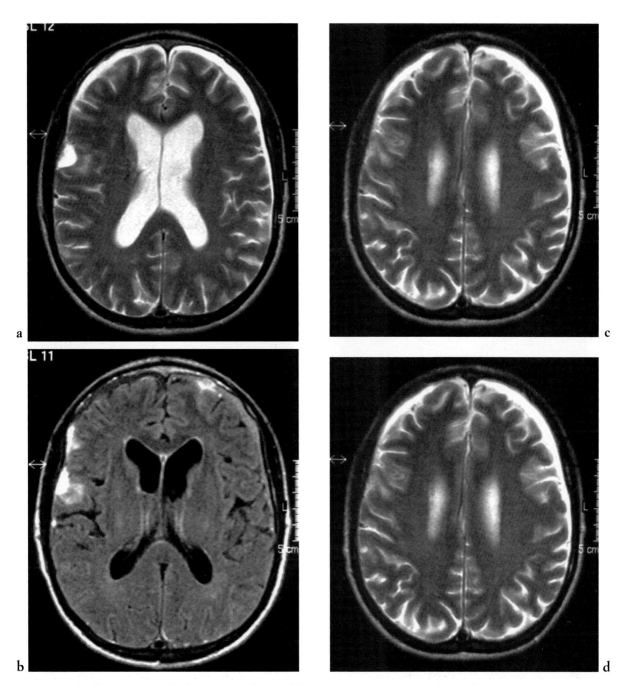

Fig. 2.28 - Cerebral contusions. T2 fast spin echo (FSE) and FLAIR sequences demonstrate that the latter prove more sensitive in identifying contusive foci, even of very small dimensions. The superior identification of the subdural haematoma with FLAIR sequences is also noted. [**a**), **c**), **d**) T2-weighted MRI; **b**) FLAIR MRI].

mentioned previously, the use of high field appliances with sequences sensitive to T2* increase MR's specificity, thereby enabling the identification of haemoglobin breakdown products within the haemorrhagic focus (Fig. 2.27).

Axonal injury is caused by axonal shear lesions that occur with linear or torsional inertial forces, which are common in instances of high speed trauma. They have preferential sites in specific areas of the brain that are particularly

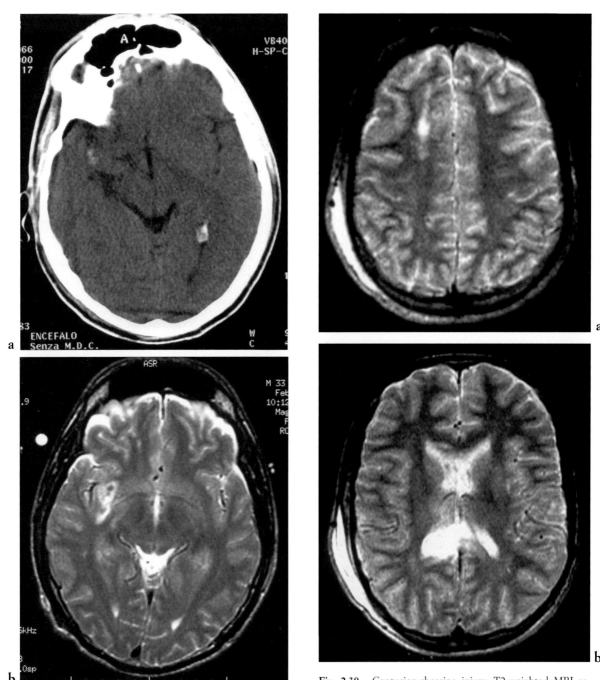

Fig. 2.29 - Hyperacute cerebral haemorrhage. CT and T2-weighted MRI images show that in the hyperacute phase only CT is capable of showing the haemorrhagic component of the right temporal-insular shear-contusive focus. [**a**) axial CT; **b**) axial T2-weighted MRI].

Fig. 2.30 - Contusion-shearing injury. T2-weighted MRI sequences highlight multiple grey-white matter junction axonal (**a**) callosal commissure lesions (**b**, **c**), lesions in the basal ganglia (**c**, **d**) and brainstem lesions (**e**). However CT alone is able to demonstrate the presence of any haemorrhagic component (**f**). [**a**)-**e**) axial T2-weighted MRI; **f**) axial CT].

sensitive to these kinds of force in trauma events, including: the white grey-white matter interface, the border between the superficial mantle and the deep grey matter structures (junctional lesions), the midline commissures (especially the corpus callosum: commissural

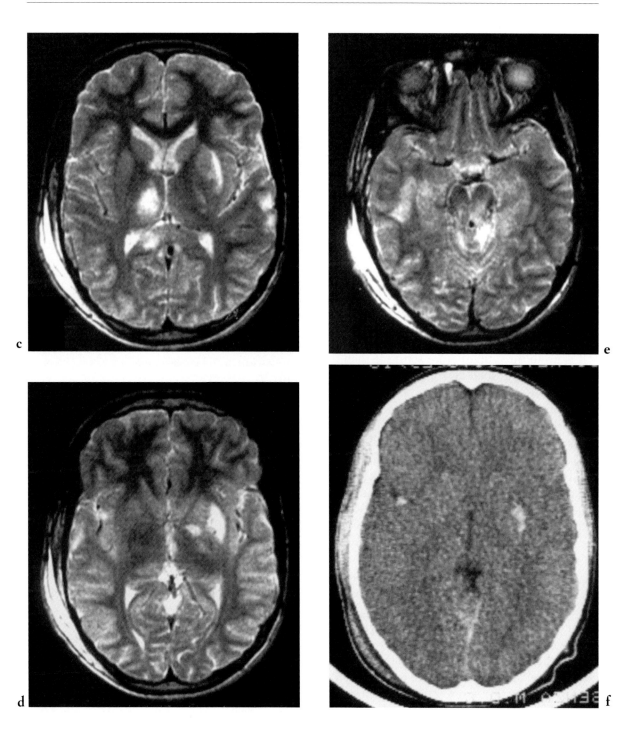

Fig. 2.30 (*cont.*).

lesions) and the brainstem (7, 13). These lesions are usually ovoid in shape with their longitudinal axis directed parallel to the direction of nerve fibre bundles, and having dimensions ranging from a few millimetres to 2 cm; these lesions are usually not haemorrhagic.

Junctional lesions are believed to be the most frequently observed type of traumatic cerebral injury and are usually located in the poles of the frontal and temporal lobes. Neuropathologically, the lesion is characterized by the transection of the nerve cell's axon, with subsequent Wallerian degeneration of the distal axon process and associated swelling of the nerve cell body. Junctional lesions only affect the grey-white matter interface in the basal ganglia in 4.5% of cases and usually have a focus in the thalamus; in these cases at least 50% of lesions are haemorrhagic, in part because of the rich vascularization of such tissue. The explanation for this preferential injury site lies in the difference between the relative kinetic energy of white matter versus grey matter, partly due to their different specific weights. Therefore, in the case of abrupt acceleration-deceleration, the two subcomponents come to a stop at different times, thus resulting in linear tears at their interface. MR is up to three times more sensitive than is CT in identifying such junctional lesions, typically demonstrating focal hyperintense areas on T2-weighted sequences having an ovoid shape and located at the border area between white and grey matter (Fig. 2.30). The sensitivity of MR can be further enhanced by the use of FLAIR sequences, which typically make it possible to visualize even the smallest lesions (Fig. 2.31). Once again, the use of high field magnets and T2*-dependent sequences makes it possible to detect haemorrhagic components when present (Fig. 2.32). However, it must be remembered that although the identification of this type of lesion is not important for reasons of emergency treatment, it can be a significant factor in later prognostic and legal analyses.

Commissural lesions affecting the axonal fibres of the corpus callosum typically occur in cases where the brain has been subjected to greater degrees of trauma, often of a torsional nature. This torsion injury results from differential forces applied to the corpus callosum when a different rotational kinetic energy obtains within one cerebral hemisphere as compared to the contralateral one during acceleration-deceleration trauma. The falx cerebri can act as a contributory factor in the traumatic effects, causing mechanical compression of the cingulate gyrus, by inducing vascular lesions via

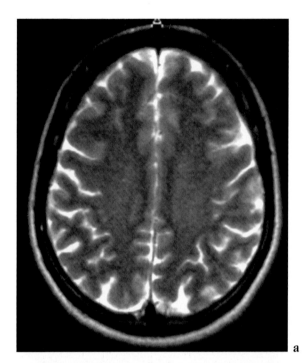

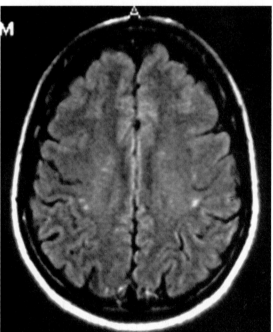

Fig. 2.31 - Shearing injury. The FLAIR MRI sequence (**b**) is more sensitive than the T2-weighted FSE sequence (**a**) in identifying even very small junction lesions (reprinted by M. Gallucci et al., 9)

trauma to the adjacent pericallosal artery or by direct contusion or even a slicing of the corpus callosum as it collides against the posterior ex-

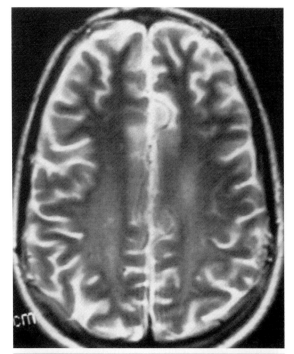

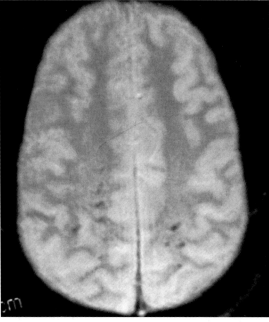

Fig. 2.32 - Haemorrhagic shearing injuries. Unlike FSE T2-weighted sequences, gradient recalled echo sequences which are more sensitive to T2* effects, are able to distinguish the presence of a haemorrhagic components within very small grey-white matter junction shearing injuries. [**a**) T2-weighted MRI; **b**) T2*-weighted MRI].

tent of the free edge of the callosum. The neuropathological picture is always that of a transection of the involved nerve fibres. The most common sites involved in this pathological process are the splenium and posterior body of the corpus callosum, in large part because of the proximity of these areas to the posterior free margin of the falx cerebri. The MR semeiotics are similar to those described for junctional lesions (Fig. 2.30).

Brainstem lesions constitute the clinically most serious form of axonal damage and can be divided into primarily non-haemorrhagic neuronal and primarily haemorrhagic microvascular lesions. Neuronal lesions, which are usually more severe from a clinical point of view, most frequently represent a transection of nerve fibres of the ascending sensory pathways, or more rarely, injuries of the fibres of the descending motor pathways. They are generally caused following torsion trauma due to the same mechanisms described for commissural lesions. These lesions tend to be round morphologically. The MR signal semeiology is typically identical to that seen in junctional lesions. These lesions are usually located in the dorsolateral portion of the pons and midbrain (Fig. 2.30). Primary haemorrhagic microvascular brainstem trauma, or Duret lesions, occur following the tearing of the perforating branches of the basilar artery or the proximal portion of the posterior cerebral artery. The most frequent location for this type of haemorrhagic lesion is the ventral midline portion of the brainstem. This type of lesion is often associated clinically with a "locked-in" syndrome. With regard to the MR signal characteristics, the same comments apply as those made above for haemorrhagic lesions.

The superior sensitivity of MR as compared to CT in the identification of brainstem lesions is further increased because of the obscuring effects of the beam hardening artefacts present on CT within the posterior fossa (Fig. 2.33).

Primary extraaxial traumatic lesions

Primary extraaxial traumatic lesions account for approximately 45% of all head injuries. Included in this category are subarachnoid haemorrhage, epi- and subdural haematomas, and subdural hygromas.

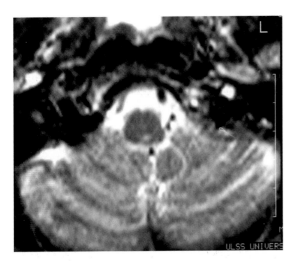

Fig. 2.33 - Shearing injury. Identified on this T2-weighted FSE sequence is a small posttraumatic lesion of the posterior medulla oblongata, following attempted suicide by hanging.

Subarachnoid haemorrhage consists of localized or diffuse haemorrhage within the subarachnoid space. These haemorrhages rarely occur as isolated lesions but instead are more frequently associated with extraaxial haematomas or cerebral laceration-contusions (3, 4, 28). A distinction can be made between primary and secondary subarachnoid haemorrhage. Primary subarachnoid haemorrhage results from the subarachnoid rupture of small pial-cortical surface vessels, from the tearing of bridging veins traversing the subarachnoid space or from the posttraumatic rupture of arteriovenous malformations or cerebral aneurysms. Secondary subarachnoid haemorrhage, on the other hand, is caused by the rupture of a subdural haematoma or a cerebral laceration-contusion into the subarachnoid space.

Routinely, CT is undoubtedly the examination of choice when subarachnoid haemorrhage is suspected. However, MR is more sensitive than CT in detecting the smaller subarachnoid bleeds, because it is able to identify the presence of small quantities of blood in the subarachnoid space if FLAIR sequences are used. In cases of massive primary subarachnoid haemorrhage, MR examinations performed in the acute phase combined with MR angiography (MRA) can potentially identify the AVM or aneurysm responsible for the bleed.

Subdural haematomas can be either primary, due to the rupture of superficial bridge veins or small, superficial cortical arteries, or secondary, when the presence of an intracerebral haematoma with a leptomeningeal margin results in a rupture of the blood into the subdural space (8). The rapid diagnosis of acute subdural haematomas in head injury patients is quite important, as surgical evacuation within the first 4 hours reduces the death rate in such patients by 30%. Yet again, when acute subdural haematoma is suspected, CT represents the technique of choice in head trauma patients. Subdural haematomas that are visualized on MRI but not seen on CT are usually small and of no surgical significance (Fig. 2.34). However, the discovery of small subdural haematomas can be important in distinguishing these lesions from other types of pathology, or alternatively in cases of legal or forensic interest, in which case MRI is the imaging technique of choice because of its higher relative sensitivity overall.

Acute subdural haematomas reveal characteristic MR signal, including isodensity on T1-weighted sequences and hyperintensity on PD and T2-weighted sequences indicating principally oxyhaemoglobin. The presence of clots within the subdural haematoma can be responsible for an inhomogeneity in the signal, these clots appearing hyperintense on T1 sequences and hypointense on T2-dependent sequences (i.e., the combined effects of clot consolidation and deoxyhaemoglobin).

Extradural or epidural haematomas are biconvex haemorrhagic collections with smooth, distinct margins, situated between the internal table of the skull and the dura mater. These haematomas are most commonly caused by the rupture of the middle meningeal artery or one of its branches, or less frequently, rupture of the posterior meningeal artery, one of the dural venous sinuses or the diploic vessels of the calvaria. Epidural haematomas are usually encountered at temporobasal or temporoparietal sites, and in most cases (85-90%) are associated with fractures of the adjacent skull. With re-

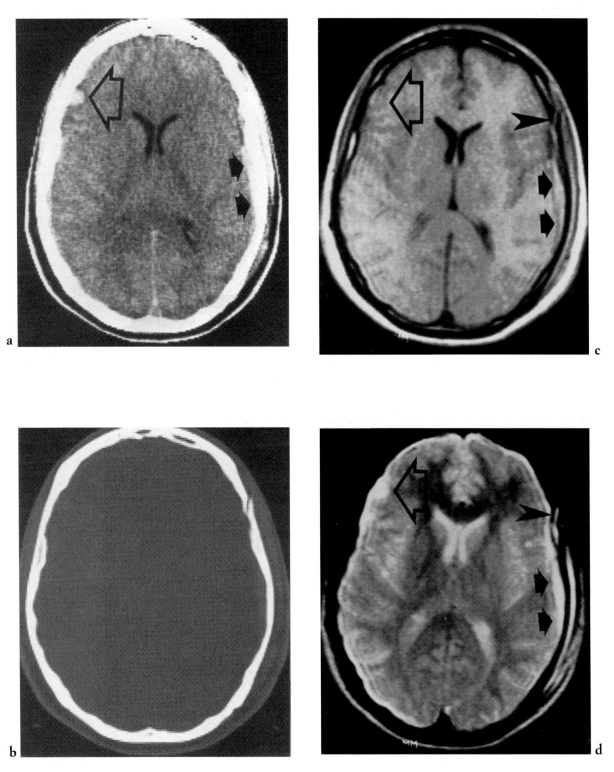

Fig. 2.34 - Haemorrhagic contusion, subdural haematoma and skull fracture. The CT examination (**a, b**) shows a haemorrhagic contusion associated with a small subdural haematoma (small solid arrows). The MRI conducted using T1- (**c**) and T2- (**d**) weighted sequences more clearly shows the thin subdural haematoma located adjacent to the overlying bone (small solid arrows). CT (**b**) allows more direct identification of small associated bony fractures, although fractures may also be visible on MRI (arrowheads). (reprinted from M. Gallucci, et al., 9) [see Fig. 2.36].

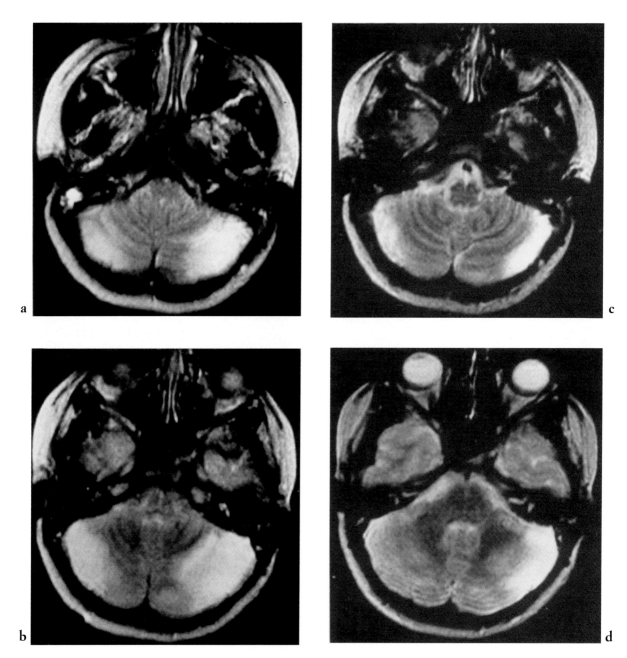

Fig. 2.35 - Left-sided cerebellar contusion. An MRI examination conducted in the hyperacute phase shows the presence of oedema in a left-sided cerebellar contusion (**a**, **b**). The MRI follow up conducted 15 days later documents the partial resolution of the oedema within the cerebellar contusion on the left. (**a**, **b**) (reprinted from M. Gallucci, et al., 9)

gard to the identification of extradural haematomas, the sensitivity MRI is similar to that of CT, but MRI is more accurate. This is principally due to the ability of obtaining multiplanar acquisitions on MRI that inherently have a greater probability of visualizing even small bleeds without artefact, and the difficulty encountered with CT in the detection of thin hyperdense collections of blood adjacent to bone (Fig. 2.29). However, CT does permit the simple identification of associated bone fractures when present. In any case, the thin ex-

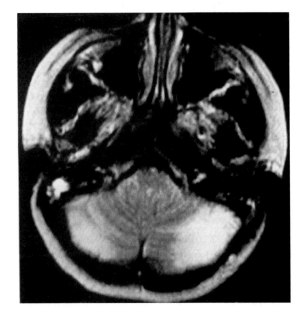

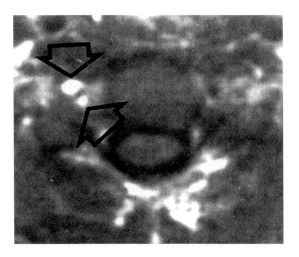

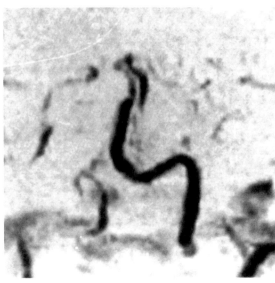

Fig. 2.36 - Posttraumatic right-sided cerebellar infarct. T2-weighted MRI shows the presence of a cerebellar infarct in the territory of the right posterior inferior artery. The frontal MRA examination reveals a thinned, string-like incomplete MRI flow signal within the right vertebral artery. A T1-weighted scan of the neck, carried out 4 days after the traumatic event, shows a dissection of the right vertebral artery with intramural hyperintensity (open arrows) due to the presence of methaemoglobin. (reprinted from M. Gallucci, et al., 9)

tradural collections that may be missed on CT but are visible on MRI do not require surgical intervention. Once again, legal and forensic interests may demand an MR examination in spite of these observations.

A tear of the leptomeninges and inner or meningeal layer of the cranial dural mater during head trauma can result in the passage of CSF into the subdural space. The resulting formation of a fluid collection, that is isointense with the fluid in all MR acquisitions, is known as a *subdural hygroma* (8). Subdural hygromas typically are not large and therefore produce little mass effect upon the underlying cerebral tissue, although exceptions are occasionally encountered.

Acute secondary traumatic lesions

These secondary complications arise at a fairly early stage in the evolution of head trauma, assume their own clinical importance and can eventually come to dominate the patient's clinical condition.

Cerebral swelling of a diffuse nature occurs in association with 10-20% of all severe head injuries, having a greater incidence in children. This type of brain swelling usually occurs in connection with a primary traumatic lesion of the cranium that in 85% of cases is a subdural haematoma. Diffuse cerebral swelling occurs as an isolated lesion in only 5% of cases of head trauma. It typically appears within 4-48 hours of the traumatic incident and represents an increase in cerebral volume in part due to diffuse vascular paralysis (i.e., loss of cerebrovascular self-regulation) with a consequential increase in

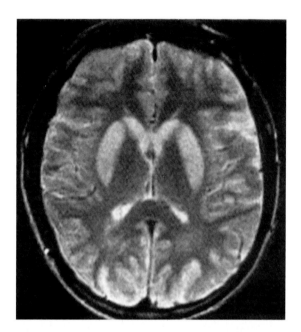

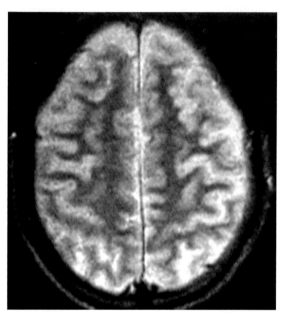

Fig. 2.37 (*cont. of 2.36*) - Basal ganglia cytotoxic oedema. T2-weighted MRI shows hyperintensity within the basal ganglia and cerebral cortex signal consistent with cytotoxic oedema in a case of brain death. (reprinted from M. Gallucci, et al., 9).

the cerebral blood pool. Cerebral swelling is therefore different from cellular or cytotoxic oedema (see below) of the cerebrum, which is caused by an increase in free water in the intracellular compartment, or vasogenic edema which is a result of leakage of fluid from the

vascular system into the extracellular compartment (21, 7, 27). The swelling can be monohemispheric or bihemispheric. Monohemispheric swelling tends to a more serious prognosis due to the greater incidence of internal cerebral herniation associated with this subtype. The overall mortality in cases of diffuse cerebral edema is approximately 50%. CT and MRI have similar sensitivity in diagnosing cerebral swelling. From a semeiological point of view, both techniques show a compression of the lateral ventricles and an effacement of the cerebral sulci over the cranial convexity. In the absence of complications or associated traumatic effects, no signal alteration on MRI can be identified in these cases on T2-weighted sequences.

Whether focal or diffuse, as it is linked to an increase in the amount of free water, cytotoxic and vasogenic *cerebral oedema* translates on MRI into a reduction of signal intensity on T1-weighted images and in an increase in signal intensity on PD- and T2-weighted sequences. The gradual resolution of the oedema in the days following the trauma can be well documented on MRI, with a parallel resolution of the T2-dependent hyperintensity of the oedematous brain tissue.

Vascular lesions. Trauma can cause the laceration, compression or dissection of the large vessels in the head and neck or of the intracranial vessels, and consequentially this can result in ischaemic or haemorrhagic lesions of the brain (9, 11, 13). The semeiotics of these secondary ischaemic traumatic lesions is no different than that described for primary ischaemic lesions. In such cases, MRI has an advantage over CT in that it is able to integrate into one basic examination the documentation of both the ischaemic lesion by means of MRI, as well as the responsible abnormality of the vascular system by means of MRA (Fig. 2.36).

Internal cerebral herniations typically occur in association with cases of posttraumatic haemorrhage in which the collections exert sufficient mass effect to result in the dramatic dislocation of brain tissue within the skull. Herniations are usually transfalcian, transtentorial, transphenoid or transalar in location, however, internal herniations can and do occur in the cerebellar tonsils and inferior vermis downwardly through the foramen magnum. The multiplanar capability of MRI and its more clear visualization of the posterior fossa structures routinely make it more informative than CT for the evaluation of this type of pathology.

Brain death. The literature contains some experiences with the MR angiography technique that demonstrate the absence of flow in the intracranial circle in the event of brain death (9, 21).

Our experience, associated with a review of the literature, identifies a number of imaging parameters seen in cases of *brain death* following cranial trauma. These findings include a loss of the gray-white matter distinction, low signal intensity within the cerebral cortex and basal ganglia related to brain oedema (Fig. 2.37), absence of vascular enhancement after IV contrast medium administration attributed to the absence of intracerebral flow, and an absence of MR flow signal in the main intracranial arterial structures (e.g., carotid siphons, middle cerebral arteries).

CONCLUSIONS

The observations in this chapter show that MRI is generally more sensitive than is CT in identifying the acute primary and secondary injuries associated with cranial trauma. However, this is counterbalanced by the intrinsic limits of the technique and the difficulties inherent in the clinical management of the patient with acute head trauma.

These limitations have recently been at least partially overcome by technological progress with regard to reduced MR scanning times and the better differentiation of haemorrhagic and non-haemorrhagic lesions on MRI in the acute phase of head trauma. This is in turn counterbalanced by the insurmountable incompatibility of many metallic life support appliances with the magnetic fields present in and near the MRI unit.

In summary, MRI is now more widely appropriately utilized in acute cases of cranial trauma than it was even a few years ago. Nevertheless, CT still remains the undisputed technique of choice for use in most acute phase trauma patients due to the relative rapidity with which it can be performed, the ready availability of the equipment required and its compatibility with the life support systems often required by trauma patients.

REFERENCES

1. Atlas SW, Mark AS, Grossman RI et al: Intracranial hemorrhage gradient-echo MR imaging at 1.5 T. Comparison with spin-echo imaging and clinical applications. Radiology 168:803-807, 1988.
2. Cirillo S, Simonetti L, Di Salle F et al: La RM in ematologia con particolare riguardo all'emorragia intracranica. In: Trattato delle malattie del sangue. Ed. P. Larizza pp. 563-568. Piccin, Padova, 1990.
3. Cirillo S, Simonetti L, Di Salle F et al: La RM nell'emorragia sub-aracnoidea: Parte 2, studio in vivo. Rivista di Neuroradiologia, 2:219-225, 1989.
4. Cirillo S, Simonetti L, Elefante R et al: La RM nell'emorragia sub-aracnoidea: Parte 1, studio in vitro. Rivista di Neuroradiologia, 2:211-217, 1989.
5. Elefante R, Cirillo S, Simonetti L et al: Confronto TC ed RM in patologia encefalica. In: La TC in Neuroradiologia, Microart's, Genova pp. 169-174, 1991.
6. Espagno J, Manelfe C, Bonsique JY et al: Interet et valeur prognostique de la TDM en traumatologie cranio-cerebrale. J Neuroradiol 7:121-32, 1980.
7. Espagno J, Tremoulet M, Espagno C: The prognosis of brainstem lesions in patients with recent head injuries. J Neurosurg Sci 20:33-50, 1976.
8. Fohlen ES, Grossman RI, Atlas SW et al: MR characteristics of subdural hematomas and hygromas at 1.5 T. Am J Neuroradiol 10:687-693, 1989.
9. Gallucci M, Bozzao A, Maurizi Enrici R: La Risonanza Magnetica nei traumi acuti. In: Pellicanò G, Bartolozzi A (eds): La TC nei traumi cranio-encefalici. Ed. del Centauro, Udine, pp. 129-153, 1996.
10. Gentry LR, Godersky JC, Thompson B et al: Prospective comparative study of intermediate-field MR and CT in the evaluation of closed head trauma. Am J Neuroradiol 9:91-100, 1985.
11. Gentry LR: Head trauma. In: Atlas S.W. Magnetic Resonance imaging fo the brain and spine. Lippincott Raven Press, Philadelphia 661-647, 1996.
12. Gentry LR: Imaging of closed head injury. Radiology 191:1-17, 1994.
13. Gentry LR, Godersky JC, Thompson B: MR imaging of head trauma: review of distribution and radiopathologic feature of traumatic lesions. Am J. Neuroradiol 9:101-110, 1985.
14. Gallucci M, Splendiani A, Bozzao A: Valutazione comparata RM-TC nel traumatizzato cranico. Eido Electa, 11-21, 1985.
15. Hesselink JR, Dowel CF, Healy ME et al: MR imaging of brain contusions: a comparative study with CT. Am J Neuroradiol 9:269-278, 1985.

16. Kelly AB, Zimmerman RD, Snow RB et al: Head trauma: comparison of MR and CT-experience in 100 patients. AJNR 9:269-78, 1988.

17. Lanksch W, Grumne T, Kazner E: Correlation between clinical symptoms and CT findings in closed head injuries. In: Frowein, Wilcke, Karini (eds): Advances in neurosurgery Vol 5: Head injuries. Springer-Verlag, Berlin, pp. 27-29, 1975.

18. Levin HS, Amparo E, Eisemberg HM et al: MR and CT in relation to the neurobehavioral sequelae of mild and moderate head injuries. J Neurosurg 6:706-713, 1987.

19. Ogawa T, Sekino H: Comparative study of MR and CT scan in cases of severe head injury. Acta Neurochir 55:8-10, 1992.

20. Orlandi B, Cardone G, Minio Paluello GB et al: Sequenze standard e sequenze veloci: bilancio di utilità su fantoccio ed in vivo. In: Neuroradiologia 1995, a cura di L. Bozzao. Ed del Centauro, Udine, 161-166, 1995.

21. Osborn AG: Diagnostic Neuroradiology. Mosby Year Book, St. Louis 1994. Cap. 8.

22. Passariello R: Elementi di tecnologia in radiologia e diagnostica per immagini. Cromac, Roma 1990.

23. Pierallini A, Pantano P, Zylberman R et al: Valutazione RM con sequenze FLAIR e FFE del carico lesionale in pazienti affetti da gravi traumi cranici chiusi. Rivista di Neuroradiologia 10:57-60, 1997.

24. Piovan E, Beltramello A, Alessandrini F et al: La Risonanza Magnetica nei traumi sub-acuti e cronici. In: Pellicanò G, Bartolozzi A (eds): La TC nei traumi cranio-encefalici. Ed. del Centauro, 153-171, Udine 1996.

25. Scotti G, Pieralli S, Righi C et al: Manuale di neuroradiologia diagnostica e terapeutica.

26. Sklar EM, Quencer RM: MR application in cerebral injury. RCNA 30(2):353-56, 1992.

27. Splendiani A, Gallucci M, Bozzao A et al: Ruolo della Risonanza Magnetica nello studio dei traumi cranici acuti e cronici: studio comparativo con tomografia computerizzata. In: Pardatscher K.: Neuroradiologia 1989. Ed. del Centauro, Udine 1989.

28. Yoon HC, Lufkin RS, Vinuela F et al: MR of acute subarachnoid hemorrhage. Am J Neuroradiol 9:404-5, 1988.

29. Zimmerman RA, Bilaniuk L, Gennarelli T et al: Cranial CT in the diagnosis and management of acute head trauma. Am J Radiol 131:27-34, 1975.

30. Zimmerman RD, Heier LA, Snow RB et al: Acute intracranial hemorrage. Intensity changes on sequential MR scans at 0.5 T. Am J Neuroradiol 9:47-57, 1985.

2.4

CT IN FACIAL TRAUMA

S. Perugini, S. Ghirlanda, A. Fresina, M.G. Bonetti, U. Salvolini

INTRODUCTION

Head injuries in the industrialized world constitute an important growing social and medical problem. On the basis of the clinical picture, these injuries are divided into major and minor. Unfortunately, the severe type accounts for a large part of all head injuries and most frequently affects the younger sector of the population, otherwise characterized by the highest life expectancy. The improvement of diagnostic techniques, especially Computed Tomography (CT), as well as neurosurgical techniques, have greatly reduced the death rate associated with this type of trauma, thus underlining the importance of early and accurate diagnosis in patient outcomes.

In emergencies involving facial trauma, many conventional radiological techniques have been replaced by spiral CT, which can be performed more rapidly, achieved with greater accuracy and with reduced patient discomfort, and accomplished at lower overall cost (8). The efficiency with which spiral CT examinations can be performed makes it possible to examine patients with serious facial injuries in accident and emergency wards. This is an important aspect in the instance of polytrauma patients, where several CT scans can be performed in succession within a very brief timeframe. The superior quality of spiral CT over alternative techniques is also due in part to the reduction in motion artefacts (including breathing artefacts), the use of safer intravascular contrast agents and the better quality of multiplanar reconstructions achieved from high resolution primary spiral image sets. Spiral CT is a reliable and rapid method of obtaining vital information and therefore improving treatment planning in seriously ill patients; this has resulted in a reduction in the utilization of traditional radiography in examining the head and neck in cases of trauma.

TECHNIQUES

For a diagnostic approach in acute and non-acute head trauma cases, it can be useful to divide patients into three groups based upon the severity of the clinical condition, each of which has a different diagnostic procedure associated with it: the patient in high grade coma with assisted breathing; the non-cooperative patient in low grade coma; and the awake and co-operative patient with or without focal neurological deficits.

1) *Patient in high grade coma with assisted breathing*

The patient must be laid supine on the imaging examination table, with the head in a position that keeps the cervical spine slightly hyperextended without forcing. When possible, the CT study should begin with a lateral scanogram (Fig. 2.38a) that includes both the facial structures as well as the cervical spine. The cervical spine is included because severe head injuries are often associated with traumatic lesions of the spine, an area that is difficult to evaluate clinically due to the presence of coma (Fig. 2.38b).

It has been proposed by some practitioners that several scanograms with different projections (anterior-posterior and right and left 45°obliques) be acquired in addition to the lateral in order to exclude the possibility of finding gross vertebral fracture-dislocations that may influence patient care (10). The wide-scale introduction of the spiral CT technique has encouraged this practice, where it has in part replaced conventional x-rays in screening investigations of head and neck trauma patients. It is important to emphasize that in some subjects with facial injuries, associated spinal trauma may be overlooked. A recent study conducted on 582 consecutive patients revealed 6 cases of cervical spine injury (approximately 1%), most of which were clinically unsuspected at the time of initial patient investigation (5).

In cases where the cervical spine is suspected of injury, systematic examination of the cervical spine can be undertaken with spiral CT at the same imaging session during which the facial structures are being analysed (1). In two published reports evaluating polytrauma involving the head and neck, 32 patients out of 88 (9) and 20 patients out of 58 (34%), respectively, were found to have traumatic cervical spine lesions.

Another reason why spiral CT is being increasingly used in facial injuries is because the multiplanar and 3D reconstructions made possible with this technique are very useful in studying the facial skeleton and skull (2-4). Spiral CT also makes it possible at the same time to demonstrate foreign bodies in more than one

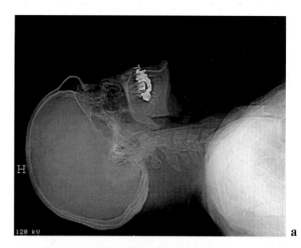

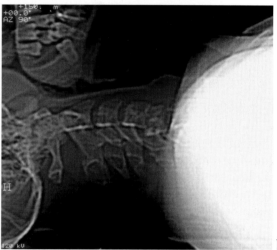

Fig. 2.38 - Cervical spine fracture. **a**) A scout view of the cervical spine. **b**) The CT scanogram identifies a C5 fracture.

plane using these multiplanar reconstructions (6). Finally, spiral CT is important because of its association with CT angiography.

These additional advantages offered by the spiral technique have reinforced CT's role in screening facial injuries, even in the era of MRI (7). This is especially true with regard to the high definition analysis of complex bony anatomy such as that found in the orbits. Spiral CT is also considered a suitable technique for the screening of facial injuries due to its relative low cost (11). As always, however, CT studies must not overshadow the importance of the physical examination, in order not to obtain results that could prove to be misleading (12).

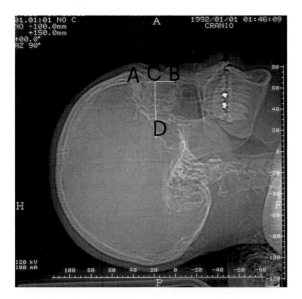

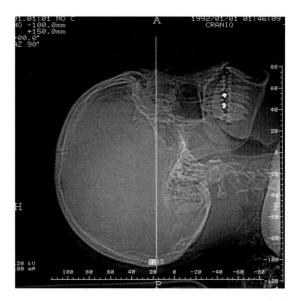

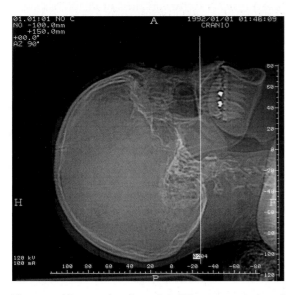

Fig. 2.39 - Neuro-ocular plane. **a**) A CT scanogram in lateral projection with indication of the neuro-ocular plane. A-B = line joining the orbital roof and floor. C-D = line joining the median point of A-B with the sphenoid jugum (neuro-ocular plane). **b**) The line that passes through the ocular lens, optic nerve, optic canal and occipital cortex in the neuro-ocular plane. **c**) Note that the neuro-ocular plane virtually coincides with that of the hard palate.

The preferable scan plane is the neuroocular plane (Fig. 2.39), which usually coincides with the plane of the hard palate or with the Frankfurt plane. This plane can almost always be determined from the lateral scanogram. It is preferable for the following reasons:

1. Simultaneous craniofacial imaging is possible: the facial skeleton, to include the orbits, can be scanned at the same time as the brain. As traumatic lesions of the face are frequently associated with concomitant injuries to the brain, this technique avoids having to delay a detailed study of the facial skeleton to the days subsequent to the initial patient imaging evaluation in the emergency room.

2. This plane allows for a more accurate examination of the frontobasal and cervicooccipital regions, frequent sites of associated traumatic lesions.

The scans can begin at the vertex of the cranium and proceed downwards toward the skull base, to include the cervical-occipital junction. Contiguous 10 mm-thick slices are utilized making it possible to identify the presence of intracranial lesions potentially requiring surgical intervention (e.g., extradural haematoma, subdural haematoma, hydrocephalus). The scan then proceeds with the study of the structures of the posterior cranial fossa and the orbitofacial area, using 5 mm-thick contiguous slices.

2) The non-cooperative patient in low grade coma

This is the most frequent clinical condition encountered in acute trauma patients. Because patients in low grade coma are not cooperative or are unable to cooperate, performing the

CT examination is a challenge and may require patient sedation or even general anaesthesia. It therefore follows that the clinical physician must determine whether performing the imaging examination is essential for management of the patient before proceeding. Patient condition permitting, a rapid CT examination should be conducted with contiguous 10 mm-thick scans, starting in the lowermost aspect of the posterior cranial fossa and using very short scan times. The images thus obtained, although not high resolution, do make it possible to exclude large intracranial space-occupying processes related to the trauma.

3) *The awake and cooperative patient with or without focal neurological deficits*

This clinical category tends to be seen in patients with minor head or facial injury and sequelae. Once again, the use of the neuroocular plane is preferable for the examination of the frontal and temporal lobes as well as for the study of the orbitofacial region. Slice thickness can vary from 2-10 mm: 10 mm for studying the supratentorial compartment of the cranium, 5 mm for the posterior fossa structures and 2 mm for the orbitofacial region.

The spiral CT technique recommended for the study of the facial skeleton is as follows: slice thickness: 3 mm; interval: 3 mm (pitch of 1); reconstruction slice thickness: 1.5 mm (alternatively for lower resolution reconstructions: 5 mm slice thickness); interval: 5 mm (pitch of 1); interval layer reconstruction: 2.5 mm.

In CT studies of the facial skeleton it is also possible to perform a more rapid study using low mA. This low technique yields good spatial information at the expense of densitometric data. However, the latter is typically of little practical importance in cases of facial injury.

The CT study of the facial skeleton must ideally include a direct coronal scan. This scan should be performed with caution due to the possibility of associated but unsuspected or undiagnosed injuries of the cervical spine. Especially in acute trauma patients, it is therefore better to use coronal reconstructions, reformed from the high resolution axial image

section set. The information thus obtained is less detailed than that obtained with direct coronal scans, but it is usually diagnostic in all but the most subtle cases of injury to the facial skeleton.

One must not underestimate the importance of a complete series of reconstructions in three dimensions, reformed from the high resolution axial image section set. While the diagnosis of specific trauma can be made from the axial sections, the reconstructions show the most severe fractures and dislocations of the face in multiple planes, thereby greatly assisting in surgical planning.

Of course, in awake and cooperative patients, the imaging investigations must be guided by clinical information. Any ocular or facial posttraumatic deformity, loss of vision, diplopia, ocular reflex disorder, and/or facial anaesthesia or hyperaesthesia merits an imaging study of the facial skeleton and cranium.

Most CT examinations are performed without the administration of intravascular contrast agents. Using contrast media only lengthens the time required to perform the examination, usually without adding any information in the trauma patient. Contrast is only administered in highly selected cases, for example: in the presence of considerable mass effect without the demonstration of a focal mass lesion; when extracerebral collections are suspected that are isodense to the cerebral parenchyma (e.g., subacute subdural haematoma); in cases of trauma complicated by a cerebral and or meningeal infectious process; or in instances of posttraumatic carotid-cavernous fistulae having a characteristic clinical picture.

Finally, it must be emphasized that the direct CT scans as well as the reconstructions should be filmed and examined utilizing both bony and soft tissue windows.

SEMEIOTICS

Traumatic craniofacial pathology can be divided into two separate but related groups: cranial injuries, and facial injuries. In clinical practice, the association between these two subtypes of head injury is quite frequent. Cranial trauma has been dealt with previously in a separate chapter.

FACIAL INJURIES

Fractures of the facial skeleton can involve the mandible or the maxilla. Fractures of the latter can be divided into isolated or complex subtypes. Isolated fractures involve one facial component only and are typically caused by low energy trauma, whereas complex fractures involve more than one component and are usually associated with high energy trauma.

1. Fractures of the mandible

Due to its anatomical position, the mandible is often the site of trauma caused by either direct or indirect forces. Mandibular trauma can either be isolated or associated with other head injuries. The most widely used of the many fracture classification systems makes a distinction between simple, compound, comminuted, complicated, ingrained, greenstick and pathological fractures.

By definition, simple fractures do not communicate with the external environment, unlike compound fractures, that have an external or open surface with the mouth and/or the skin. Comminuted fractures have more than one fracture line and consist of one or more bony fragments. A fracture is termed complicated when it affects nerves, vessels or the temporomandibular articulation. Ingrained fractures indicate that there is no dislocation of the various fracture fragments. Greenstick fractures are defined by a bony structure having a frank distracted fracture on one cortical surface, while the opposite side presents a bent but not fractured cortex; these fractures are most frequently encountered in children in the subcondylar region. Lastly, a fracture is classified as pathological when it occurs in an area that has been weakened by past abnormality (e.g., infectious, neoplastic), or when it occurs spontaneously or in the face of minor trauma.

Descriptions of mandibular fractures must always focus on the substructure of the mandible under discussion: the condyle (intra- or extracapsular, subcondylar); the choronoid process; the neck, the angle, or the body; the incisor (parasymphyseal); the symphysis; or the alveolar process. The direction of the fracture and any dislocation of fragments should also be recorded.

Traditional radiography (e.g., mandibular x-rays, pantomography, intraoral radiographs) is usually sufficient for diagnosing traumatic mandibular lesions. However, CT is suitable as a complementary imaging technique, especially in the study of the temporomandibular joint, as it provides good visualization of dislocations of the mandibular condyle and the condition of the masticatory muscles.

CT examinations are usually performed in the axial plane with thin slices, and supplemented with multiplanar reconstructions (e.g., coronal, sagittal, oblique and three-dimensional). Reconstructions are necessary for the diagnosis of fractures in the axial plane, such as those of the glenoid cavity. As noted in the foregoing sections, direct coronal scans should be avoided in acute trauma patients because of the frequent association of head and face injuries with instability of the atlanto-axial articulation or traumatic cervical spine lesions.

2. Simple fractures of the maxilla

The most frequently encountered simple fractures are those of the nasal bone, the orbito-malar-zygomatic complex and those of the bony orbit.

Fractures of the nasal bones

Nasal fractures are the most common of all facial fractures. Traditional radiography is sufficient for obtaining all the information necessary in these cases, although CT is also sensitive in the demonstration of nasal fractures, and can be useful if posttraumatic surgical reconstruction is being considered (Fig. 2.40).

Fractures of the zygomatic arch

Zygoma fractures are also frequently encountered, due to the prominent superficial position within the face and its relatively delicate constitution. The fractures of this region can be divided into isolated fractures of the zygomatic arch or so-called "tripod" fractures.

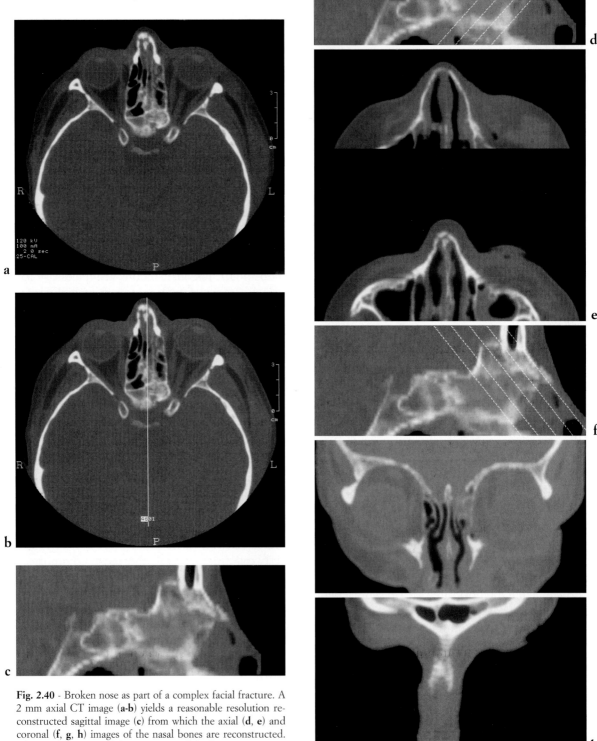

Fig. 2.40 - Broken nose as part of a complex facial fracture. A 2 mm axial CT image (**a-b**) yields a reasonable resolution reconstructed sagittal image (**c**) from which the axial (**d, e**) and coronal (**f, g, h**) images of the nasal bones are reconstructed. This results in optimal demonstration of the fractures.

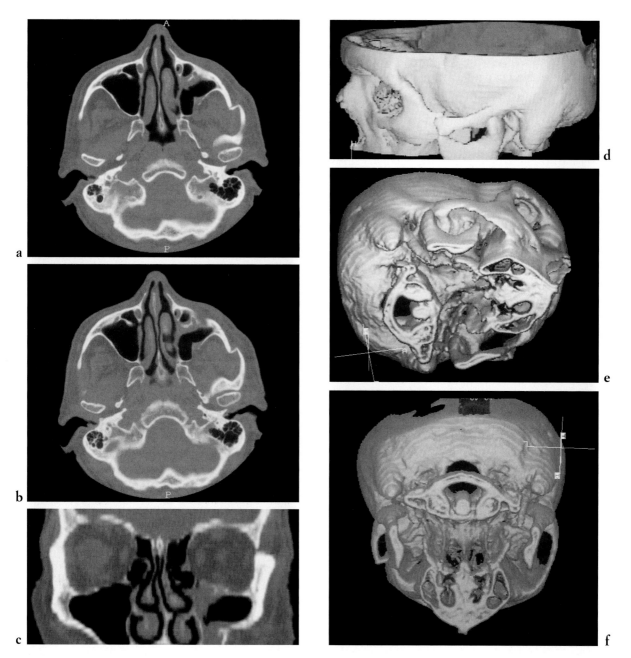

Fig. 2.41 - Tripod fracture of the left cheekbone, with medial and inferior displacement of the orbital-malar-zygomatic complex. Axial CT images (**a**, **b**), reconstructed coronal CT section (**c**) and three-dimensional reconstructions (**d**, **e**, **f**) show the mildly depressed, fractured zygomatic arch and lateral orbital-maxillary sinus walls.

Fractures of the zygomatic arch

The zygomatic arch is constituted by the zygomatic process of the temporal bone and the zygomatic process of the zygomatic (i.e., malar) bone. The traumatic involvement of this structure is well documented by both standard radiography as well as CT, which makes it possible to view the depression or dislocation of fracture fragments, the relationships of the arch to the deep structures (e.g., masticatory muscles and choronoid process) and to exclude the involvement of the nearby structures (e.g., the glenoid cavity of the temporal bone, orbit and maxillary sinus).

Tripod fractures

These are also termed malar fractures, fractures of the zygomatic-maxillary complex or fractures of the zygomatic complex and are characterized by the fracture and/or diastasis of the zygomatic-maxillary, zygomatic-frontal and zygomatic-temporal sutures or the underlying bony components. Therefore, these fractures affect the orbital structures and the maxillary sinus (Fig. 2.41a-c). This type of fracture can be composed or decomposed, with lateral, medial, posterior and/or inferior dislocation of the orbito-malar-zygomatic complex (i.e., depressed fracture).

CT performed in the axial plane must be supplemented with direct coronal acquisitions or reconstructions from a high resolution axial slice set in order to see the in-

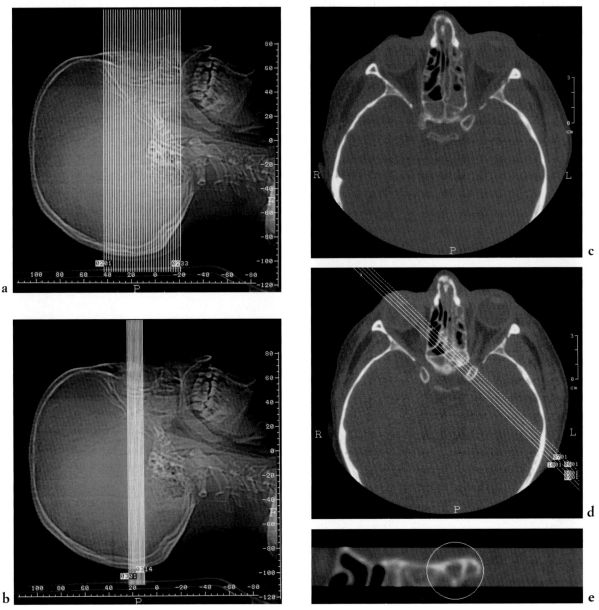

Fig. 2.42 - Orbital study technique. 2 mm (**a**) or 1mm-slices (**b**). The optic canal (**c**) may be documented well with high resolution oblique-coronal reconstructions (**d, e**).

volvement of the adjacent soft tissues (e.g., extraocular orbital muscles, structures within the pterygomaxillary fossa) and bony structures as well as to better define the dislocation of the orbito-malar-zygomatic complex in the three spatial planes (Fig. 2.41d-f). Among other clinical manifestations, the involvement of these nearby structures can cause: limitation of mandibular motility due to interference of the orbito-malar-zygomatic complex with the choronoid process; limitation of ocular motility; loss of vision with the optic nerve at the orbital apex.

Fractures of the bony orbit

Orbital trauma can cause: visual compromise due to involvement of the optic nerve; diplopia caused by lesions to the extraocular muscles or due to alterations of the oculomotor nerves; cosmetic alterations (e.g., exo- and enophthalmus). The mechanism of the orbital trauma includes: direct trauma; extension of a fracture of the adjacent connected bony structures; and "blow-out" fractures, which involve the thinner orbital wall structures, in particular the medial wall and floor.

Orbital fractures can involve a part or the entire rim of the bony orbit. CT is without doubt the single imaging examination that provides the largest amount of information on both the bony as well as the intra- and extraorbital soft tissue components of the orbit. A CT investigation angled to the neuroocular plane is preferred for studying the optic nerve and canal and is fundamental to imaging of the orbit as a whole. The CT slice thickness should be 2 mm, with 1 mm sections acquired at the level of the optic canal (Fig. 2.42); fast scanning times and low mA can be used to obtain good spatial definition.

The CT examination must be supplemented with direct or reconstructed coronal sec-

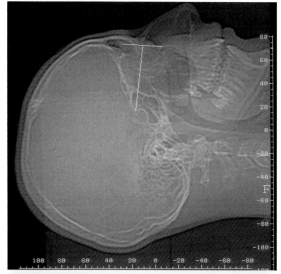

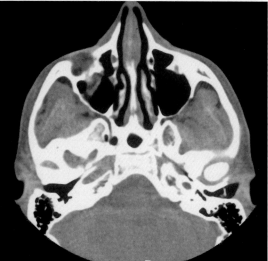

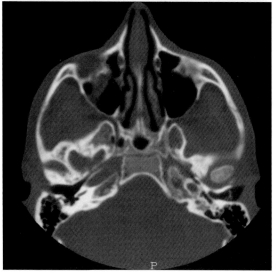

Fig. 2.43 - Orbital floor blow-out fractures. **a)** neuro-ocular plane of study; **b, c)** axial CT sections passing through the orbit show discontinuity of the right orbital floor and soft tissue within the roof of the right maxillary sinus.

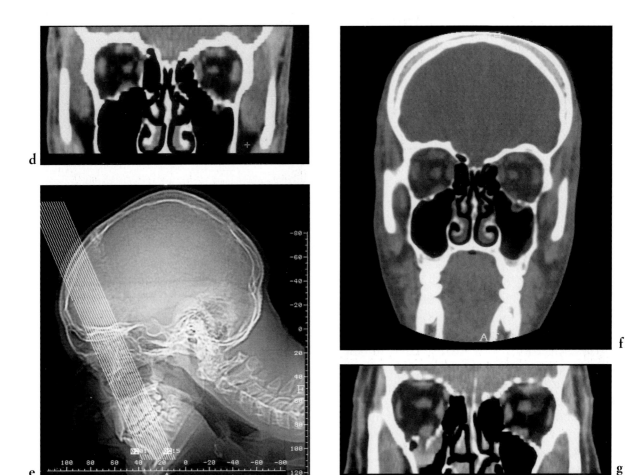

Fig. 2.43 (*cont.*) - **d**) A reconstructed coronal CT section shows the soft tissue within the roof of the maxillary sinus adjacent to the inferior rectus muscle. **e**), **f**) Direct coronal sections better show the orbital floor and the herniation of orbital material into the subjacent maxillary sinus. **g**) A second case showing a larger orbital floor fracture on the right side with depression of bone and soft tissue into the roof of the maxillary sinus.

tions in order to visualize the orbital floor and roof and to better document their relationship to the extraocular muscles (Fig. 2.43), and to exclude the entrapment of these muscles within a linear fracture (esp. orbital floor blow-out fractures). In this manner, diplopia when present can be clinically considered to be from other causes. CT also makes it possible to identify intraorbital or intraocular foreign bodies, orbital emphysema (Fig. 2.44) and intraorbital haematomas.

3. Complex fractures of the maxilla

This type of fracture can be divided into Le Fort fractures and nasal-ethmoid midface fractures.

Le Fort fractures

Horizontal complex facial fractures are classified according to Le Fort criteria, which are as follows:

a. Le Fort 1: involves the lower portion of the midline anteriorly and the posterior-lateral wall of the maxillary sinus(es), with extension into the distal part of the pterygoid processes.

b. Le Fort 2: involves the medial nasofrontal region, the maxillary sinuses (with the zygomatic bone spared), and the base of the pterygoid plates posteriorly.

c. Le Fort 3: involves the medial nasofrontal region and the orbito-malar-zygomatic complex laterally.

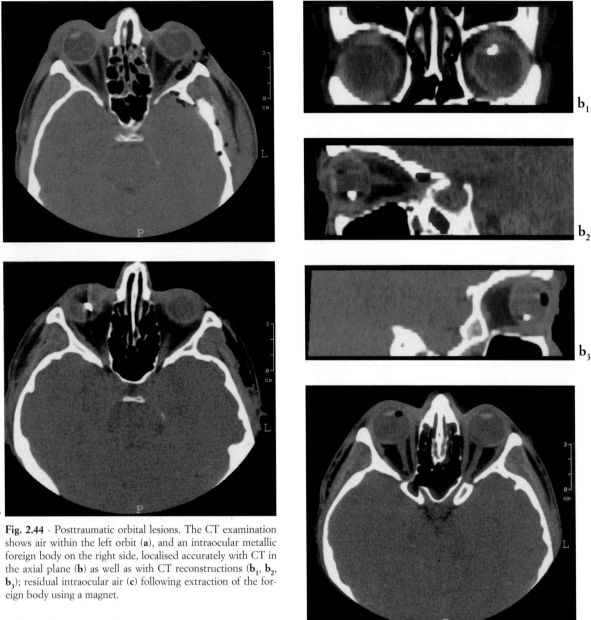

Fig. 2.44 - Posttraumatic orbital lesions. The CT examination shows air within the left orbit (**a**), and an intraocular metallic foreign body on the right side, localised accurately with CT in the axial plane (**b**) as well as with CT reconstructions (**b₁**, **b₂**, **b₃**); residual intraocular air (**c**) following extraction of the foreign body using a magnet.

In clinical practice, these fracture types tend to be more complicated, but they can always be traced back to one of these three categories. To make this more interesting, a Le Fort fracture of one type may involve one side of the face only, and be associated with a different type of Le Fort fracture on the opposite side.

Direct axial CT with multiplanar reconstructions without doubt offers an accurate spatial representation of bony fracture-dislocations while also analyzing involvement of the adjacent bony and soft tissue structures.

Nasal- ethmoid midface fractures

Vertical fractures of the face are usually complex, involving the facial midline structures from the nasal bone junction with the planum ethmoidale through to the hard palate. As described above, high resolution axial CT with multiplanar reconstructions makes it possible to clearly visualize such fractures as well as any related cerebral complications (Fig. 2.45).

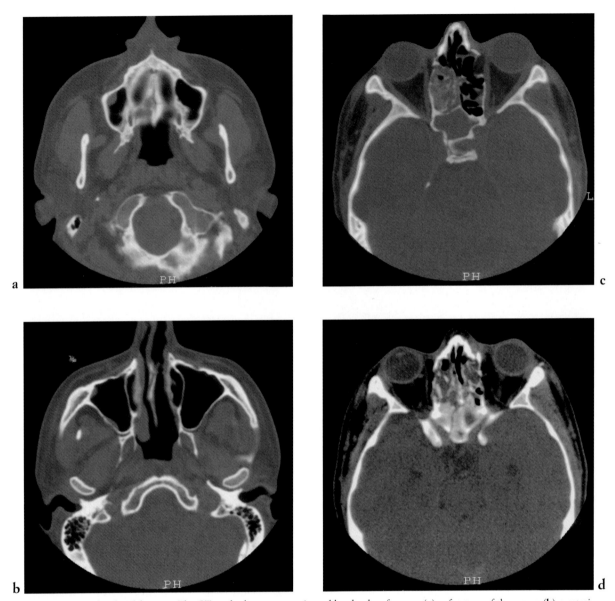

Fig. 2.45 - Complex facial fracture. The CT study shows a comminuted hard palate fracture (**a**), a fracture of the vomer (**b**), posterior extension of the fracture as far as the medial wall of the cavernous venous sinus on the right (**c**) and a right paramedian sagittal fracture of the ethmoid bone, extending into the optic canal (**d**).

REFERENCES

1. Beirne JC, Butler PE, Brady FA: Cervical spine injuries in patients with facial fractures: a 1-year prospective study. Int J Oral Maxillofa Surg, 24(1 Pt):26-29, 1995.
2. Buitrago-Tellez CH, Wachter R, Ferstl F et al: 3-D CT for the demonstration of findings in compound skull injuries. Rofo Fortschr Geb Rontgenstr Neuen Bildgeb Verfahr, 160(2):106-112, 1994.
3. Gentry LR, Manor WF, Turski PA et al: High-resolution CT analysis of facial struts in trauma: 2. Osseous and soft-tissue complications. AJR , 140(3):533-541, 1983.

4. Kassel EE, Noyek AM, Cooper PW: CT in facial trauma. J Otolaryngol, 12(1):2-15, 1983.
5. Kirshenbaum KJ, Nadimpalli SR, Fantus R et al: Unsuspected upper cervical spine fractures associated with significant head trauma: role of CT. J Emerg Med, 8(2):183-198, 1990.
6. Mauriello JA Jr, Lee HJ, Nguyen L: CT of soft tissue injury and orbital fractures. Radiol Clin North Am, 37(1):241-252, 1999.
7. Maya MM, Heier LA: Orbital CT. Current use in the MR era. Neuroimaging Clin N Am, 8(3):651-683, 1998.
8. Novelline RA, Rhea JT, Rao PM et al: Helical CT in emergency radiology. Radiology, 213(2):321-339, 1999.

9. Nunez DB Jr, Zuluaga A, Fuentes-Bernardo DA et al: Cervical spine trauma: how much more do we learn by routinely using helical CT? Radiographics, 16(6):1307-1318, 1996.

10. Perugini S, Bonetti MG, Ghirlanda S et al: Technical note: CT scout views of the cervical spine in severely head-injured patients. Skeletal Radiol, 25:247-249, 1996

11. Rhea JT, Rao PM, Novelline RA. Helical CT and three-dimensional CT of facial and orbital injury. Radiol Clin North Am, 37(3):489-513, 1999.

12. Thai KN, Hummel RP 3rd, Kitzmiller WJ et al: The role of computed tomographic scanning in the management of facial trauma. J Trauma, 43(2):214-217, 1997.

III

INTRACRANIAL HYPERTENSION

3.1

PATHOPHYSIOLOGY AND IMAGING

M.G. Bonetti, T. Scarabino, R. Rossi, A. Ceddia, U. Salvolini

INTRODUCTION

The skull and bony structures of the spine and cranium combined with the cerebral and spinal meninges form a relatively rigid construction of protection for the brain, cerebrospinal fluid (CSF) within the subarachnoid space and the craniospinal arteriovenous system. Alterations in the form of an increase in the volume of brain parenchyma, the CSF or the vascular components, or alterations of the bony compartment that contains them can give rise to a progressive increase in intracranial pressure.

The terms intracranial hypertension (ICH) and hydrocephalus do not define the same entity, but rather refer to a variation in the container-content relationship in the first case, and in the second case to an accumulation of CSF with a dilation of the cerebral ventricles; however, in the latter instance, there will also be some degree of necessarily associated ICH. ICH patients usually present the classic sign-symptom triad of headache, vomiting and papillary elevation (7, 9).

The headache has particular semeiologic characteristics, as it usually occurs upon awakening and has a frontal location. It is believed to be caused by the traction exerted on the meningeal neural structures both within the meninges as well as within the related vascular structures. Not only the parietal meningovascular structures are involved, but also innervated are the dura mater of the skull base, the walls of the dural venous sinuses and the bridging veins.

Vomiting is also manifested clinically in the morning, similarly upon awakening, and before the patient has eaten. It is not preceded by vegetative signs such as nausea or ptyalism (excessive flow of saliva) and is almost always associated with headache. The pathogenic mechanism responsible for the vomiting in cases of ICH is still unknown, however it has been observed that the headache subsides partially after the episode(s) of vomiting.

Bilateral ocular papillary elevation is caused by hypertension of the CSF pathways, accompanied by an increase in the CSF pulse pressure transmitted to the optic nerve head. This pulsatile pressure increase is directly broadcasted to the optic nerve trough of the optic subarachnoid space via the meningeal sheaths that coat the entire length of the optic nerve, thereby causing a progressive vascular compression-congestion of the optic nerve head and outward physical bulging of the optic papilla into the rear of the globe.

Minor signs and symptoms of ICH include:

1) Diplopia: Diplopia is caused by a paresis of the 4th cranial nerve as a consequence of the pressure increase, which injures the fragile abducens nerve;

2) Eyesight impairment: Protracted oedema, compression and expansion of the optic nerve head cause regressive phenomena entailing permanent damage and resultant atrophy, ultimately terminating in an impairment of eyesight. In extreme cases amaurosis occurs, a process that is almost always irreversible.

3) Endocrinological alterations: Chronic ICH is associated with a reduction in function of the hypophysis, with resultant alterations in hormone production (e.g., FSH, LH, TSH, ACTH, GH) and changes in the gland's response to physiological and pharmacological stimuli.

4) Disorder of recent memory: This nonspecific sign is almost always present in patients with long clinical histories of minor intracranial pressure elevations. The deficit would seem to affect the recall of recent events, rather than memory of chronological order or long-term memory.

There is a wide range of possible underlying pathological conditions responsible for the ICH, such as neoplastic, vascular, inflammatory, toxic, metabolic, traumatic or hormonal causes. This chapter deals with the physiopathology of intracranial hypertension, cerebral oedema, pseudotumor cerebri and hydrocephalus.

THE PATHOPHYSIOLOGY OF INTRACRANIAL HYPERTENSION

The intracranial space is divided by the tentorium cerebelli into the supratentorial and subtentorial compartments, which communicate with one another via the tentorial incisura. This intracranial space is completely occupied by solid or fluid components, including the brain, the subarachnoid space and cerebrospinal fluid, and the blood and attendant vascular walls; its content is considered uncompressible: variations in intracranial pressure are closely de-

pendent on and correlated with variations in these solid and fluid subcomponents.

Over a wide variety of pathological as well as normal physiological situations (normal health, changes of posture, some forms of illness, etc.) the quantity of blood present in the intracranial space does not undergo significant overall volume alterations. The blood exiting the cranium via the outgoing venous system guarantees sufficient space for the arterial blood that enters the skull with each systolic cycle, thus constituting a self-regulating mechanism of cerebral blood flow. This flow self-adjusts to intracranial pressure changes in order to guarantee steady blood flow to the brain.

Normal intracranial pressure

In order to clearly understand normal variations in intracranial pressure (ICP), a few simple models will be discussed as examples (10). Fig. 3.1a illustrates a patient in the lateral decubitus position, with a spinal tap needle within the lumbar subarachnoid space. The plane of the needle passes through the midsagittal plane of the spine and skull. In the case of the cranium being open to atmospheric pressure, the fluid pressure measured in the spine is equal to the distance between the middle sagittal plane and the uppermost lateral wall of the cranial meninges.

When the patient is in the vertical position (Fig. 3.1b) the hydrostatic column of CSF approximately equals the distance between the point in which the spinal tap is positioned and the top of the cranial meninges if it is open to the influence of atmospheric pressure. However, if the skull is excluded from the direct action of atmospheric pressure but instead is imagined to be completely closed, there is no change in pressure on the passage from the horizontal to the vertical position (Fig. 3.1c), because in this case the spinal portion of the system alone is subject to the action of atmospheric pressure.

Fig. 3.1d illustrates a normal person in a sitting position with the same lumbar subarachnoid needle in place. One can observe how the measurement of pressure reaches that expected of the cervico-thoracic junction level, thus showing to be lower than it would have been if the intracra-

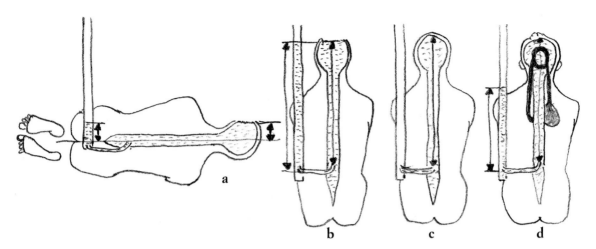

Fig. 3.1 - See text.

nial space had been open to the direct influence of atmospheric pressure, and greater than it would be were the system completely closed.

This series of experiments demonstrates that the intraarachnoid craniospinal system cannot be considered a completely closed system, as it is in contact with atmospheric pressure through the craniocerebral blood vessels. For the most part this pressure effect is transmitted through the veins that lead from the skull base or from the peridural venous plexus at the level of the foramen magnum.

When measuring CSF fluid pressure, the values recorded at lumbar level are greater than those obtained from the cervical area, which are, in turn, higher than those recorded directly at an intracranial level. In normal subjects, the balanced hydrostatic point is situated at the cervical-thoracic junction: it remains the same when measured in either the horizontal or vertical position. The zero pressure point is situated craniad to this in the cervical region of the spine. Normal intracranial pressure values fall between 9 and 13 mm Hg, and therefore values higher than 15 mm Hg are considered pathological.

The pressure-volume ratio

The various phenomena that occur in the volumetric alterations of the intracranial components are linked to physical laws expressed by the pressure-volume ratio (4).

Intracranial hypertension is the result of an increase in the total absolute intracranial volume of the contained soft tissue and fluid components. This volume increase may be caused by expansions in the volume of the cerebral parenchyma, circulating blood or CSF, either singularly or in combination. ICH does not appear immediately in response to a gradual, minor increase in volume of one of these constituents, as the other components of the system are able to compensate to a certain degree, thus maintaining the total volume at a constant level.

The Monro-Kellie doctrine establishes that because the volume within the skull is not able to increase, there is a fixed relationship between the various intracranial constituents. Therefore, if normal intracranial pressure is to be maintained, an increase in volume of one or more of these components or the development of a space-occupying lesion can only take place if there is a reduction in the volume occupied by the others.

As alterations in the volume of the intracranial nerve tissue can only be very slight, it follows that the larger compensatory alterations take place at the expense of the volume of the CSF and/or the circulating blood within the craniospinal system. It is estimated that the supratentorial structures can absorb approximately 50% of such volume alterations, the subtentorial structures 20% and the spinal compartment 30%. Any pathological process that alters the volume of these compartments reduces their total compensatory power.

Generally speaking, the CSF compartment in particular has a relatively high capacity for absorbing increases in intracranial pressure. However, this capacity is contingent on the condition that the pressure increase takes place gradually and slowly. In part this is due to the high resistance of the arachnoid villi to CSF filtration; when this CSF-venous drainage rate limit is reached, the intracranial pressure will rise. The system's fluid reabsorption capacity can at the most guarantee a CSF drainage rate of 1 ml/per minute. It therefore follows that an expansion, for example, of a subdural haematoma may not precipitate signs of intracranial hypertension if it forms sufficiently slowly.

The opposite is true for the vascular compartment, which has very little reserve space without circulatory insufficiency arising within the brain. However, what reserve there is adapts very rapidly, thanks to the direct connection of the cerebrovascular network with the systemic circulation.

Fluctuations in cerebral blood flow are governed by a number of factors such as carbon dioxide levels, adenosine, potassium, prostaglandins and anaesthetics. Numerous medicines, such as xantine, hypertonic saline solutions and hyperosmotic solutions can also increase cerebral blood flow. After a certain point is reached, an increase in cerebral blood flow causes an increase in intracranial pressure.

In healthy subjects, intracranial pressure appears to be controlled and maintained within a relatively narrow range from moment to moment by minor alterations of CSF volume. However, when intracranial hypertension is long-standing and considerable (e.g., cerebral oedema, intracranial space-occupying lesion, etc.), the resulting hypercapnia induced by these conditions causes an increase in intracranial pressure in part due to the reduced amount of fluid available for reabsorption.

To summarize, the abovementioned compensation mechanisms therefore have a varying role in intracranial pressure homeostasis. The intracranial volume occupied by pathological alterations can be obtained at the expense of the CSF volume, the amount of endovascular blood or, to a lesser extent, the brain's intracellular and interstitial water content. However, whereas prolonged mass effect upon the brain can produce a reduction in the amount of brain tissue water, variations in the parenchymal cellular tissue component are practically negligible. Moreover, although intraparenchymal blood volume can represent a small buffer reserve, realistically it is the intracranial CSF fluid content that is the most important buffer volume when intracranial alterations occur.

Intracranial pressure waves

Temporary intracranial pressure readings are not accurate in revealing the real characteristics of pressure waves. However, measurements recorded over a long period of time show a minor pulse-type pattern, due primarily to the effects of breathing and cardiac activity (5).

Three types of pressure wave alterations are described in patients with intracranial hypertension. The smallest waves, termed subtypes B and C, are accentuations of physiological phenomena: the C wave represents the breathing component, whereas the B wave is an expression of cardiac activity. The A wave, the only one of pathophysiological importance, can be divided into two forms:

1) rhythmic pressure fluctuations, with intervals of 15-30 minutes;

2) plateau waves, which last for longer periods of time.

The former have a frequency of 2-4 cycles per hour, they begin spontaneously from an average or moderately high pressure base and reach levels of 60-100 mm Hg, before returning to their baseline values. The latter often exceed a value of 100 mm Hg and represent, like rhythmic waves, a serious prognostic index of imminent serious cerebral consequences.

The relationship between intracranial pressure and CSF production

The CSF produced by the choroid plexuses is not a mere plasma filtrate, but rather an active fluid body tissue (e.g., certain electrolytes have higher concentrations than does the systemic blood) that functions in part via the action of carriers and pumps.

Increases in intracranial pressure cause a reduction in the cerebral perfusion pressure, which in turn results in a reduction of superfiltrate production by the choroid plexuses by hindering the activity of the active transport carriers and fluid pump. CSF production ceases at an intracranial pressure of 22-25 mm Hg.

The consequences of intracranial hypertension on cerebral circulation

Intracranial hypertension has a direct effect upon cerebral perfusion. An increase in intracranial pressure would cause a halt of the blood cerebral blood flow when arterial and intracranial pressure become equal, were it not for the intervention of two compensatory mechanisms: arteriolar-capillary vasodilatation and an increase in systemic arterial pressure.

The first of these mechanisms is a cerebrovascular self-regulation mechanism caused by a parietal vessel reflex that acts on the muscular fibres of the vessel wall, relaxing them when the pressure inside the vessels drops; a local increase in CO_2 and metabolic acids have a vasodilatory effect.

The increase in systemic pressure is a result of a bulbar (i.e., brainstem) reflex triggered by brainstem ischaemia and would only seem to come into play once the cerebrovascular self-regulation mechanisms have failed. The latter are efficient up to intracranial pressure values of 50-60 mm Hg, beyond which passive vasodilatation occurs. Increases in intracranial pressure then take place until complete circulatory arrest ultimately occurs.

Mechanical consequences of intracranial hypertension

By altering the mechanisms that keep intracranial pressure within normal limits, intracranial space-occupying lesions have an effect on cerebral perfusion but my also induce displacements of the cerebral tissues within the cranial cavity.

In childhood, intracranial hypertension takes longer to manifest itself than it does in adults because of the elasticity of the immature skull. The absence of cranial suture closure allows a degree of expansion of the bony structure of the calvaria of the skull when an increase in intracranial pressure occurs, whereas this adaptability no longer exists in adults having a rigid skull.

The matters discussed thus far may suggest that an increase in intracranial pressure is distributed uniformly inside the skull and is therefore borne equally by the various parts of the neuraxis. However, this is not true for two reasons: the majority of lesions causing intracranial hypertension are focal in nature, and, the cerebral parenchyma has mechanical properties that are similar to both those of elastic solids as well as those of viscous fluids.

The nervous tissue adjacent to a mass undergoes deformation, and the pressures are distributed in various ways: they are high in the vicinity of the lesion and gradually diminish with distance, thus creating pressure gradients under which the nervous tissue is displaced. These shifts of the nervous tissue, favoured by the oedema that reduces the viscosity of the parenchyma, may result in internal cerebral herniations. Neoplasia, abscesses, haematomas and other space-occupying lesions may cause these dislocations of the contents of the cranium.

When intracranial hypertension associated with mass formation occurs, initially the most important factor to recognize clinically is not the nature of the cause, but rather the presence or absence of internal cerebral herniation. The manner in which these shifts occur is more or less similar irrespective of their cause, although they vary with the site, size and rapidity with which the space-occupying lesion evolves.

In the initial stages, any expanding lesion exerts uniform pressure on the surrounding tissues. These forces are opposed by others, for example the cerebral tissue itself and the hydrodynamic resistance of the CSF-containing ventricles that oppose resistance to deformation from compressive forces. Another opposing force is the cerebral vascular system and the contained arterial pressure, as these arteries constitute a sort of skeleton for the surrounding cerebral tissue. In addition to the arteries, the veins, nerves and meninges also oppose this type of pressure.

It should also be remembered that the falx cerebri and the tentorium cerebelli divide the skull into three compartments and provide further opposition to the dislocating effects of mass lesions. This division of the intracranial space allows displacements of the brain parenchyma under the effect of space-occupying processes only in certain directions, including: within the same compartment, from one supratentorial compartment to another, beneath the falx cerebri, downward or upward through the tentorial hiatus, and from the posterior cranial fossa downward into the spinal canal through the foramen magnum.

In the presence of a space-occupying lesion, a sequence of compensation mechanisms can be described. Initially, the subarachnoid spaces adjacent to the lesion are compressed, with a flattening of the superficial gyri, distortion of the ventricular cavities and a deformation and dislocation of the nearby arteries and veins. This is followed by a second phase in which the volume of the brain tissue involved increases due to oedema, and the CSF spaces are no longer able to compensate for the primary and secondary mass effect. Any further compensation requires a shift of parenchymal tissue from one anatomical compartment to another, with the consequent development of internal cerebral herniation.

Subfalcian herniations are observed in association with dominant hemicranial lesions; the degree of brain dislocation beneath the falx varies according to the original site and size of the mass lesion. For example, masses that originate in the frontal regions are more frequently associated with this kind of herniation as the falx cerebri is less broad anteriorly and consequently the free space below is greater than that posteriorly, where the falx and the splenium of the corpus callosum are in closer proximity. This type of cerebral herniation involves the supracallosal and cingulate gyri, the corpus callosum, the anterior cerebral arteries and their branches, the frontal horns of the lateral ventricles and the midline cere-

bral veins. The third ventricle is also shifted across the midline.

Axial herniations take place through the tentorial hiatus in either an upward or downward direction. This type of internal herniation causes a distortion and compression of the brainstem. When downward and the mass effect is sufficiently large, the herniation may also affect the lower cerebellum, which can be displaced through the foramen magnum.

Temporal herniations involve the medial part of the temporal lobe and in particular the hippocampus and the uncus, which can herniate either unilaterally or bilaterally. This herniation stretches the oculomotor nerve, compresses the posterior cerebral artery and can impinge on the cerebral peduncle on one or both sides. These events are followed by secondary lesions including oedema and haemorrhage.

Temporal herniations therefore threaten functions regulated by the brainstem, including vigilance, muscle tone, voluntary motion and vegetative functions. A unilaterally expanding temporal mass lesion is less favourable than a bilateral one because it can cause temporal herniation at an earlier stage in the mass forming process.

Downward cerebellar herniations are observed as a complication of expanding processes in the posterior cranial fossa and may occur in two forms that are often associated. In the first type, the cerebellar tonsils are thrust towards the upper spinal canal through the foramen magnum. In the second type, the upper part of the cerebellar vermis (i.e., culmen) herniates upwards through the tentorial hiatus, thus pushing the lamina quadrigemina and the midbrain forwards. The resulting injury to the brainstem depends in part upon vascular compression and secondary ischaemia of the upper brainstem.

Finally, internal cerebral herniations can obstruct the subarachnoid cisterns, thus preventing the free circulation and proper drainage of CSF. Above the level of the herniation, intracranial pressure tends to increase, whereas below it it is normal or only slightly raised. These differentials in CSF pressure add to the vector of thrust and thus worsen the herniation.

This in part explains why in such cases a lumbar puncture can precipitate a worsening of the clinical status.

The relationship between intracranial pressure and cerebral function

Many patients with obstructive hydrocephalus or pseudotumor cerebri show modest signs of cortical compromise in the presence of high intracranial pressure, the degree of which depends in part upon whether or not the cerebrum in such patients was normal prior to the onset of the pathological event. The situation is somewhat different in patients with pre- or co-existent parenchymal lesions, such as neoplasia or contusions. In addition, an increase in ICP due to the volume of the mass, cerebral oedema and/or vasodilatation secondary to hypercapnia combine with local cerebral hypoperfusion, the function of the brain adjacent to the expanding lesion can be compromised with even relatively low elevations of ICP (e.g., 15-25 mm HG).

In summary, an increase in ICP causes malfunction of cerebral function through four related mechanisms: a generalized reduction of cerebral blood flow, a compression of the tissue surrounding the focal mass with local cerebral microcirculatory compromise, brainstem compression and an internal herniation of brain tissue.

PATHOPHYSIOLOGICAL CLASSIFICATION

The general causes of intracranial hypertension can be summarized as an increase in volume of one or more of the intracranial soft tissue components: the parenchyma, the CSF volume and the blood volume.

ICH Resulting From Cerebral Oedema

Cerebral oedema (13) is defined as an increase in the volume of the encephalon caused by an increase in its water content. This content may be focal or generalized. When widespread and severe it can be associated with neurological signs and may ultimately result in internal cerebral herniation. Cerebral oedema can be divided into a number of different types, including: vasogenic, ischaemic, cytotoxic and interstitial related to hydrocephalus. Cerebral oedema is usually accompanied by intracranial hypertension, but there are exceptions, especially when the degree is minor.

On CT scans cerebral oedema is characterized by an area of hypodensity as compared to the parenchyma. On MR oedema is hypointense on T1-weighted images, more intense than CSF and less than the parenchyma. On T2-weighted scans, the relative hyperintensity of oedema varies, and, depending on the protein content, it can appear more or less intense relative to CSF.

Vasogenic oedema

Vasogenic oedema is the most common form of cerebral oedema and is typically associated with neoplasia, abscesses, intraparenchymal haematomas and traumatic contusion. It is caused by an increase in the permeability of the blood-brain barrier and usually affects the white matter with a resulting increase in density/intensity between white and grey matter on medical imaging. These alterations are due to an increase in the volume of the extracellular fluid.

Vasogenic oedema is easily discernible in the white matter as it generally spares the grey matter and exerts mass effect on the ventricular structures (Fig. 3.2). After IV contrast medium administration, a curvilinear or gyral pattern of enhancement can often be observed also related to the increase in blood-brain permeability.

Ischaemic oedema

Ischaemic oedema is the result of a cerebrovascular accident. The pathological process involves both white and grey matter with a loss of differentiation on imaging between the two

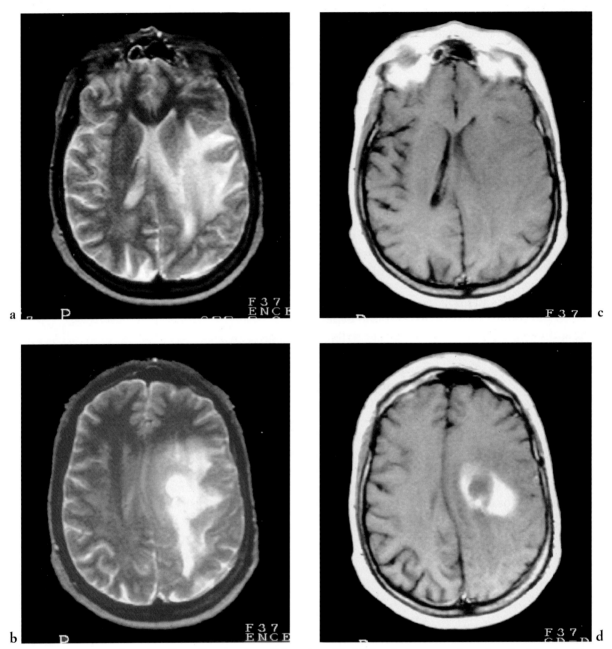

Fig. 3.2 - Vasogenic oedema caused by malignant cavitary glial neoplasm. The MRI study shows extensive oedema involving the white matter surrounding the neoplasm. Note the mass effect upon the lateral cerebral ventricles and the irregular mural contrast enhancement. [**a**), **b**) T2-weighted, **c**) unenhanced T1-weighted, **d**) and T1-weighted MRI following IV gadolinium (Gd) administration].

(Fig. 3.3). It causes the nerve cells to swell and an increase in the permeability of the blood-brain barrier. This type of oedema is both intra- and extracellular and consists of a plasma ultra-filtrate that includes proteins. On imaging these alterations demonstrate peripheral contrast enhancement and mass effect.

Cytotoxic oedema

Cytotoxic oedema is most frequently caused by an ischaemic-hypoxic insult such as preceding cardiopulmonary arrest. Less frequently it may be related to water intoxication, the decompensation syndrome in dialysis patients, di-

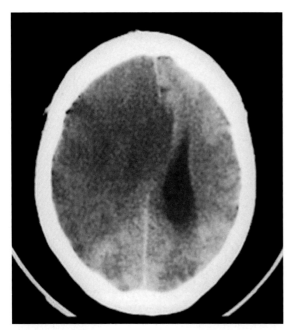

Fig. 3.3 - Hemispheric cerebral infarction. Unenhanced axial CT demonstrates a large hypodense area in the vascular distribution of the right anterior and middle cerebral arteries associated with mass effect.

abetic ketoacidosis, purulent meningitis, severe hypoglycaemia and methanol intoxication.

Brain swelling occurs within all cellular components of the cerebrum (e.g., neurons, glia, ependyma, endothelial cells), in both white and grey matter, with an increase in the total intracellular water content. Neuroradiologically, findings are most frequently observed in the cerebral and cerebellar cortex, the basal ganglia, the hippocampus and the vascular watersheds. The thalami and brainstem tend to be spared.

Mass effect when present results in ventricular compression and the effacement of the CSF spaces (e.g., sulci, basal cisterns). Due to reduced cerebral perfusion, there may be no enhancement after IV contrast medium administration.

Interstitial oedema related to hydrocephalus

This type of oedema is observed in obstructive hydrocephalus and is caused by the transependymal passage of fluid from the ventricles to the periventricular white matter, with consequent interstitial oedema. It is typically symmetric surrounding the anterolateral portion of the lateral ventricles (Fig. 3.4).

The grey matter is normal, and there is no abnormal enhancement after contrast medium administration. These periventricular alterations regress following proper ventricular shunting or spontaneous resolution of the hydrocephalus.

ICH RELATED TO ABNORMAL CSF PHYSIOLOGY

Pseudotumor cerebri

Pseudotumor cerebri is a condition (13) having an undefined pathogenesis that usually affects young, obese patients with or without hypercorticism and menstrual disorders. It is typically observed in females that are otherwise healthy. Electroencephalograms are normal, and the mental status is intact.

Signs and symptoms associated with pseudotumor cerebri include headache, nausea, vomiting and diplopia. Bilateral papilloedema is present, and visual loss is documented in one-third of cases, which becomes permanent in one of eight patients. The diagnosis is determined from lumbar punctures showing an increase in CSF pressure and from neuroradiological studies that exclude the presence of hydrocephalus, mass-forming processes and thrombosis of the dural venous sinuses.

In approximately 36% of cases, CT and MRI are negative; in the remainder, the following findings may be seen: a small ventricular system and a failure to visualize the basal cisterns; small ventricular system with normal visualization of the basal cisterns; empty sella turcica; and enlargement of the sheaths of the optic nerves. With normalization of fluid pressure, the ventricular and periencephalic fluid spaces return to normal.

HYDROCEPHALUS

CSF (3) is secreted by the choroid plexuses, especially those within the lateral cerebral ven-

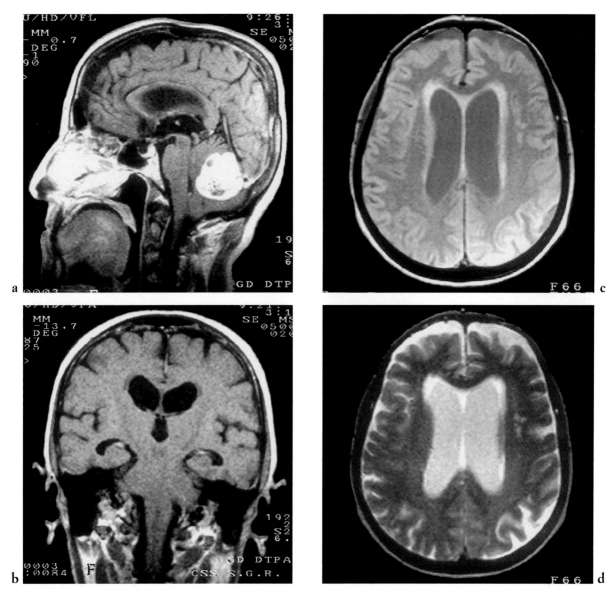

Fig. 3.4 - Neoplasm of the cerebellar vermis with obstructive hydrocephalus. The MRI examination shows a contrast enhancing mass (**a**) likely originating within the cerebellar vermis that compresses the 4th ventricle and has resulted in obstructive hydrocephalus (**b**). The T2-weighted images reveal transependymal extravasation of CSF into the periventricular white matter (**c, d**).

tricles. CSF is a clear, colourless fluid containing very few cells (approximately 2 per mm³) and little protein (normal range: 25-40 mg/100 ml). It has a different ionic composition as compared to plasma, as active secretion mechanisms such as carriers and pumps contribute to its production.

Interposed between the capillary blood of the choroid plexuses and the intraventricular CSF is a blood-fluid barrier, which is permeable to water, oxygen, carbon dioxide and to a lesser degree to electrolytes, but is imperme-

able to cellular and protein components of the blood. Certain drugs (e.g., acetazolamide, furosemide) and metabolic and respiratory alkalosis reduce CSF production.

Once produced, CSF passes from the lateral ventricles, through the foramina of Monro into the 3rd ventricle and from there through the aqueduct of Sylvius into the 4th ventricle. From the 4th ventricle, the CSF passes through the foramina of Luschka and Magendie, to reach the subarachnoid spaces of the skull base.

Thereafter the CSF passes into the anterior pericerebellar cisterns and surrounds the brainstem. CSF therefore generally follows two pathways, one medial and one lateral.

Along the medial pathway, it reaches the prepontine, interpenducular, suprasellar, chiasmatic and terminal laminar cisterns, until arriving at the subfrontal regions. Then it reaches the superior sagittal sinus, through the interhemispheric spaces. Simultaneously, it flows upward through the pericerebellar, lamina quadrigemina and pericallosal cisterns until reaching the region surrounding the superior sagittal sinus. Along the lateral pathway, the fluid passes from the interpeduncular, prepontine, ambient and suprasellar cisterns into the Sylvian fissures, and from there through the subarachnoid spaces over the cranial convexity.

In these locations over the cranial convexity are the arachnoid villi of the Pacchionian granulations, which are essential for the proper reabsorption of CSF into the venous blood of the dural venous sinuses. This absorption partly depends upon the hydrostatic pressure gradient between the CSF and blood of the dural sinuses. When this gradient is sufficient, the microtubules of the granulations remain open and permit the passage of CSF towards the bloodstream. If, however, the difference in pressure is very high, the tubules close, thus preventing the reabsorption of fluid.

In addition to this reabsorption mechanism, limited absorption apparently takes place along the perineural sheaths of the cranial and spinal nerves, through the surfaces of the neuraxis bordering upon the subarachnoid space and through the ventricular ependyma.

The total volume of CSF within the subarachnoid spaces in normal adults is approximately 120-160 ml, and 30-40 ml is present within the cerebral ventricles. The intraventricular CSF pressure is 712 cm of water, and the lumbar pressure is 8-18 cm of water.

Hydrocephalus: diagnostic morphological aspects

The term hydrocephalus is used to describe any condition in which an abnormal increase in the volume of CSF occurs within the cranium. There are four possible types (1, 8, 11).

In *obstructive* hydrocephalus, there is a blockage to the passage of CSF through the ventricular cavities and outlets, with a dilation of the ventricular spaces proximal to the obstruction. Frequent causes are neoplastic and nonneoplastic mass-forming lesions; another relatively common aetiology is fibrotic adhesions secondary to inflammatory and haemorrhagic processes. The CSF obstruction may occur at the level of the foramina of Monro (e.g., neoplasia, inflammatory processes), the 3rd ventricle (usually neoplasia), the cerebral aqueduct of Sylvius (e.g., congenital atresia, inflammatory stenoses), posthaemorrhagic adhesions, or in the 4th ventricle (e.g., neoplasia, craniocervical malformation, infection or subarachnoid haemorrhage).

From an imaging point of view, obstructive hydrocephalus is characterized by a symmetric dilation of the ventricular system proximal to the point of obstruction. Characteristic is the rounded appearance of the dilation of the frontal horns, with a reduction of the angle between the medial walls of the frontal horns themselves (<100 degrees). If involved in the process, the 3rd and 4th ventricle are also dilated. The basal subarachnoid cisterns are either normal or mildly encroached upon, as are the superficial cerebral sulci, which are either absent or smaller than usual.

Unilateral obstruction of one of the foramina of Monro causes the distension of one lateral ventricle only. Such obstructions may be intermittent if the obstructive process is valvular, with clinical manifestations of headache, nausea and vomiting. Characteristically, these episodes resolve rapidly when and if CSF drainage is restored. On the other hand, if both foramina of Monro are involved, the obstructive hydrocephalus is limited to the lateral ventricles.

An obstruction of the aqueduct of Sylvius causes supratentorial triventricular dilation (i.e., the 3rd ventricle and lateral ventricles). Aqueductal stenosis is a frequent cause of hydrocephalus in infancy and the early stages of childhood. As at this age the cranial sutures are not yet fused, macrocrania develops. If, however, hydrocephalus develops in late childhood after closure of the sutures, the enlargement of the skull is absent or at most modest. In adults the aqueduct is more frequently compressed by a tumour (e.g., periaqueductal astrocytoma) (Fig. 3.5).

If the 4th ventricle or its outlets are obstructed, all the other parts of the ventricular system are distended. Obstruction of the foramen of Magendie can be caused by a developmental

malformation (e.g., Arnold-Chiari malformation [Fig. 3.6], platybasia and basilar invagination, atlantooccipital fusion, etc.) or alternatively a peri- or intraventricular tumour. The foramina of the 4th ventricle can also become nonpatent due to a granulomatous ependymitis, caused for example, by the tubercle bacillus. An *entrapped* 4th ventricle refers to a simultaneous obstruction of the aqueduct of Sylvius and the foramina of Luschka and Magendie, with a consequent distension of its cavity (Fig. 3.7).

In decompensated obstructive hydrocephalus, the transependymal passage of fluid is more evident in the anterior-lateral portion of the frontal horns, and on CT has a reduction in periventricular density with regular margins (or an increase of signal on T2-weighted MR images, Fig. 3.4).

In *communicating hydrocephalus* there is a lack of fluid reabsorption due to the thrombosis of the venous sinuses, malfunction of the arachnoid granulations or poor circulation within intracranial subarachnoid spaces due to meningitis, meningeal carcinomatosis or following a subarachnoid haemorrhage. Blood, pus, meningeal metastases or adhesions may mechanically obstruct the fluid circulation path-

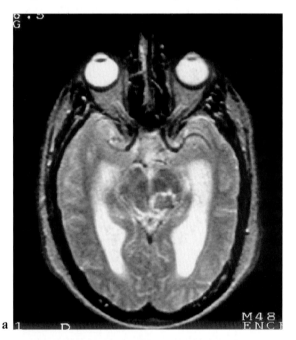

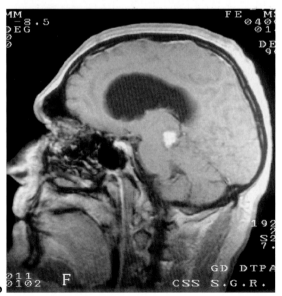

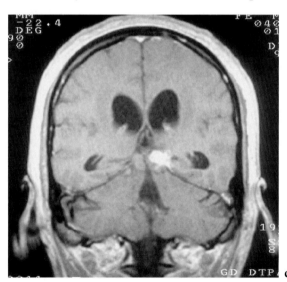

Fig. 3.5 - Mesencephalic tuberculoma with obstructive hydrocephalus. The MRI shows a contrast enhancing mass lesion of the posterolateral midbrain resulting in stenosis of the aqueduct of Sylvius and obstructive hydrocephalus. [**a**) axial T2-weighted and **b**) sagittal T2-weighted MRI; **c**) coronal T1-weighted MRI following IV Gd].

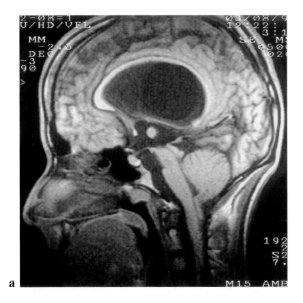

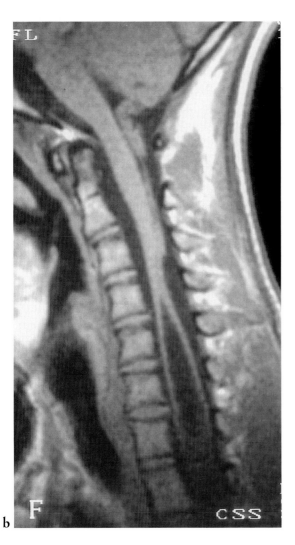

ways in the basal subarachnoid cisterns and/or involve the arachnoid granulations. The connection of the cranial subarachnoid space to the spinal subarachnoid space may remain patent.

After a certain time, chronic inadequate fluid reabsorption can produce an enlargement of the ventricles without an attendant increase in fluid pressure (normotensive hydrocephalus). In acute hydrocephalus, the CSF is reabsorbed vicariously by the minor resorption systems, firstly by the transependymal pathway, with the appearance of typical findings of hypodensity on CT and hyperintensity on T2-weighted MRI in the periventricular white matter (Fig. 3.8). This absorption pathway is more permeable than the normal one and permits the passage through the periventricular white matter of even large protein molecules.

In communicating hydrocephalus, the dilation starts from the anterior and temporal horns, followed by the occipital horns and the 3rd ventricle. The 4th ventricle is not necessarily dilated. Occasionally, dilated sulci can also be observed in hydrocephalus associated with a block of the subarachnoid spaces over the cranial convexity.

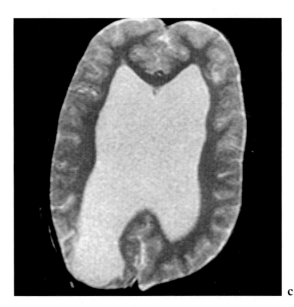

Fig. 3.6 - Type II Arnold Chiari malformation with obstructive hydrocephalus The MRI examination demonstrates cerebellar tonsillar ectopia, fourth ventricular outlet obstruction and hydrocephalus. In addition, there is right occipital encephalomalacic porencephalic cyst and cervicothoracic syringohydromyelia. [**a**) sagittal T1- weighted cranial MRI; **b**) sagittal T1-weighted cervical MRI; **c**) axial T2-weighted cranial MRI].

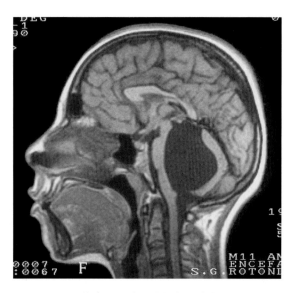

Fig. 3.7 - Trapped 4th ventricle with hydrocephalus. T1-weighted MRI showing a trapped 4th ventricle associated with obstructive hydrocephalus in a patient with tuberculous meningitis.

In *hypersecretory hydrocephalus,* there is an increase in the production of CSF (beyond the normal 0.3-0.4 ml/minute) in the choroid plexuses due to infection or the presence of a choroid plexus papilloma.

Lastly, in *ex-vacuo ventricular enlargement* there is a passive increase in the ventricular and extraventricular CSF spaces without an increase in the intraventricular fluid pressure. This type of ventricular enlargement is due to a generalized atrophy of the brain parenchyma (Fig. 3.9). Generalized atrophy results in a symmetric dilatation of the ventricular system, which may principally involve the lateral ventricles although the 3rd ventricle may also be affected. If there is atrophy of the structures of the posterior fossa, the 4th ventricle will also be passively enlarged. The angle between the frontal horns is always greater than 110 degrees. The basal subarachnoid cisterns and the superficial cerebral sulci can be normal, however they more frequently are widened in synchrony with the overall atrophy.

Functional diagnosis

CT and MRI are excellent techniques for illustrating the morphological characteristics of hydrocephalus as well as the presence of the underlying pathology when this pathological change is a mass. However, both techniques have limitations in their ability to directly demonstrate the obstructing element to CSF circulation resulting from adhesions of inflammatory or haemorrhagic origin.

Radionuclide myelocisternography (12) or myelocisternal-CT with water-soluble contrast medium can be used to study CSF circulation, subject to the intrathecal spinal introduction of the tracer or contrast agent (e.g., 111-In DTPA and Iopamiro 300, respectively) and subsequent serial imaging in order to follow the progress of the agent through the subarachnoid spaces of the cranium.

In normal subjects, the basal subarachnoid cisterns show presence of the tracer or contrast by the first to third hour, and the Sylvian fissures at the fourth to sixth hour. The subarachnoid spaces over the cranial convexity are normally opacified by the 12th hour, and more completely at the 24th hour. In normal subjects, the cerebral ventricles are never opacified. The imaging appearance of the cerebral ventricles in normal subjects depends in part upon the age of the patient. CSF opacification is more rapid in children, typically disappearing by the 24th hour, than in the elderly, in whom opacification over the convexity can persist beyond the 48th hour.

The radioisotopic technique can also be used to study CSF/plasma clearance of the tracer by means of a series of blood samples. In normal subjects, this will give the following haematological activity values as a percentage of the dose injected: 2nd hour: 1.6%; 6th hour: 10%; 24th hour: 33%; 48th hour: 41%.

The study of cerebrospinal fluid circulation and CSF/plasma clearance in normotensive hydrocephalus enables some prognostic indication for the efficacy of the treatment with surgically placed shunts. This shunt operation proves to be effective in clinical practice in patients with normotensive hydrocephalus, in whom myelocisternal scintigraphy shows a constant, early and persistent opacification of the cerebral ventricles after the 48th hour.

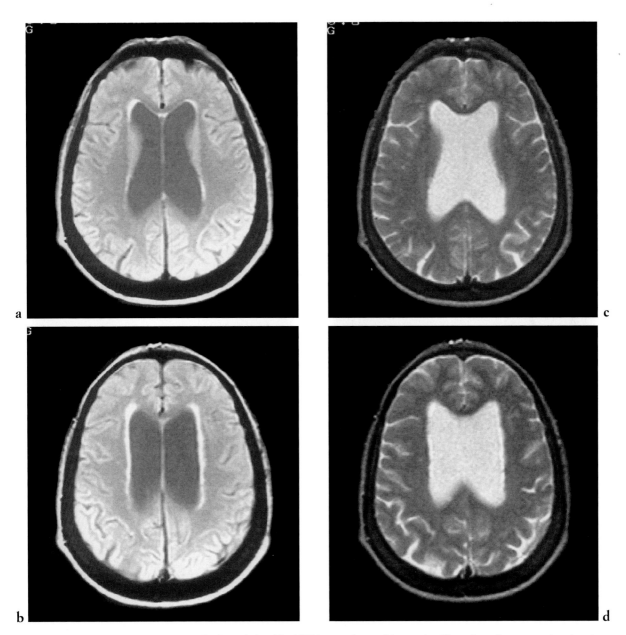

Fig. 3.8 - Normotensive communicating hydrocephalus. The MRI images show a thin margin of hyperintensity representing chronic gliosis surrounding the lateral ventricles in a patient with clinically diagnosed chronic normotensive communicating hydrocephalus, not transependymal extravasation of CSF. [**a**, **b**) proton density-weighted MRI; **c**, **d**) T2-weighted MRI].

Potentially important diagnostic information can also be supplied by prolonged and continuous pressure monitoring of ventricular fluid using a catheter or by Katzman's lumbar infusion test. The latter technique involves the continuous infusion of the lumbar subarachnoid space with a physiological solution at a speed of 0.8 ml/minute; in normal subjects there is an increase in fluid pressure up to a plateau of approximately 20 mm Hg after about 30 minutes. In CSF reabsorption disorders such as hydrocephalus there will be a marked and early increase in CSF pressure values.

If the subarachnoid spaces, typically at a spinal level, are isolated from one another due to a blockage of CSF circulation at some point, the CSF below the blockage will undergo an

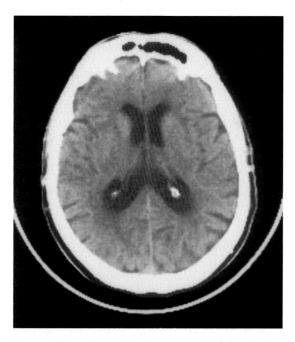

Fig. 3.9 - Ventriculomegaly with passive cerebral atrophy. Axial CT shows passive cerebral atrophy associated with ventriculomegaly.

abnormal increase in cells (i.e., Froin's syndrome), while that above the obstruction will have a normal cell and protein content.

Clinically, the Queckenstedt test (i.e., jugular compression test) (2) is usually sufficient to establish whether there is a partial or total CSF obstruction. With the patient in a lateral decubitus position, a lumbar puncture is performed and fluid pressure is measured. In normal conditions this pressure alters in synchrony with pulse and breathing. In normal subjects CSF pressure alters in a very marked and rapidly reversible manner with abdominal compression. The mechanism for this is via an increase in intraabdominal pressure originating from a temporary blockage of the spinal veins, in turn resulting in an increase in intraspinal fluid pressure; this demonstrates that there is no obstruction in the subarachnoid space at the spinal level.

If this abdominal compression test confirms that the subarachnoid space is not obstructed, and in the absence of intracranial hypertension and an intracranial mass, one can perform the Queckenstedt manoeuvre by compressing both internal jugular veins simultaneously. This will

cause an increase in intracranial venous pressure with a resulting increase in intracranial fluid pressure, which in normal conditions will be transmitted along the spinal subarachnoid spaces to the lumbar level of CSF pressure measurement. However, if there is a blockage in the spinal canal or at the cranio-cervical junction, the expected pressure increase will not reach the pressure gauge. If the increase in CSF pressure at the level of the pressure gauge is slow and incomplete in returning to normal once the pressure on the jugular veins has been removed, an incomplete blockage can be assumed.

MRI is also capable of supplying important information on spinal and intracranial fluid spaces and its circulation. In sectors of the subarachnoid space with high pulsatile CSF speeds, the MR signal normally disappears due to the flow void phenomenon. This can typically be observed in the aqueduct of Sylvius, the foramina of Monro, the 3rd ventricle and in the region of the foramen of Magendie.

A circulation blockage with CSF stasis will bring about a disappearance of this phenomenon. Using gradient-echo sequences combined with ECG gating, these phenomena can also be studied dynamically with CSF flow measurements (6).

ICH RELATED TO VASCULAR CAUSES

A third cause of ICH is a relative increase in the amount of blood contained in the cranial cavity. This form of ICH may involve the venous or the arterial system. ICH may have a venous cause when the circulation of the returning blood is obstructed, which can occur in cases of venous thrombosis associated with thrombophlebitis of the dural venous sinuses, or in instances of mediastinal compressive pathology. In this type of ICH, the venous congestion results in a partial inhibition of normal CSF drainage.

Increases in intracranial blood volume may also affect the arterial capillary sector of cerebral circulation. In active vasodilatation, the effect is usually due a local increase in CO_2, which, irrespective of its origin ultimately results in a vicious circle arising once intracranial hypertension has begun. In passive vasodilatation there is a loss of cerebrovascular autoregulation as a consequence of a systemic acidosis. In this situation, the vessels become passively distended by the systemic blood pressure.

AETIOLOGICAL CAUSES OF INTRACRANIAL HYPERTENSION

Intracerebral tumours represent the most frequent cause of intracranial hypertension. Beyond the size of the mass itself, the principal pathophysiological mechanism involved in ICH production in many neoplasms is oedema. However, not all tumours are equally productive of oedema, the most oedema-inducing being glioblastomas and neoplastic metastases. Low degree gliomas by comparison cause little or no oedema, and when present it remains localized to the immediate area around the lesion. Extracerebral tumours such as meningiomas, on the other hand, may become quite large before causing ICH.

Expanding lesions localized to the subtentorial compartment can lead to intracranial hypertension in part by CSF obstruction. This tends to occur earlier in intraventricular tumours and those of the midline (e.g., medulloblastomas and ependymomas) than in laterally positioned tumours (e.g., neoplasia of the cerebellar hemispheres and the cerebellopontine angle), which typically cause a delayed increase in intracranial pressure.

Intracranial hypertension of a vascular cause is observed in a number of conditions. For example, in arterial hypertension, oedema can also occur as a result of paroxysmal hypertension. Subarachnoid haemorrhages are always accompanied by an initial episode of intracranial hypertension due to a blockage of the CSF reabsorption pathways by the haemorrhage. The subarachnoid blood usually reabsorbs without sequelae; however, if the haemorrhage has been widespread or is a rebleed, subarachnoid adhesions can form with the possible development of a secondary form of hydrocephalus. Intraparenchymal haematomas with perilesional oedema behave as a mass formation and can occasionally result in the onset of ICH. Intracranial pressure usually spontaneously returns to normal with resolution of the haematoma.

Among the types of intracranial hypertension of infectious origin, acute meningitis is typically associated with ICH. Pyogenic cerebral infections are almost always oedema-inducing, and ICH is rarely absent in the acute phase. Viral encephalitis can also be accompanied by considerable cerebral oedema and resultant ICH.

Serious cranial trauma is often associated with varying degrees of ICH, due both to the presence of an intraparenchymal haematoma in parenchymal contusion foci, as well as to related oedema and haemodynamic alterations. In fact, in the initial phase that follows trauma, an increase in cerebral blood volume plays an important role in the pathological increase in intracranial pressure.

ICH can also be observed in cases of intoxication from carbon dioxide, lead, arsenic or following allergic reactions.

In summary, while there are many potential causes of ICH, the majority are due to disorders of fluid dynamics that can be primarily attributed to mass-forming processes as well as to obstructions to CSF circulation due to haemorrhagic, infectious or neoplastic involvement.

REFERENCES

1. Butler AB, McLone DG: Hydrocephalus. In Grossmann, Hamilton eds.: Principles of Neurosurgery, pp. 165-177. Raven Press, New York, 1991.
2. De Myer W: Tecnica dell'esame neurologico, pp. 415-429. Piccin ed., Padova, 1980.
3. Duus P: Diagnosi di sede in Neurologia. Casa ed. Ambrosiana, pp. 337-353, Milano, 1988.
4. Langfitt TW, Weinstein JD, Kassel NF et al: Trasmission of increased intracranial pressure. I. Within craniospinal axis. J Neurosurg. 21:989-997, 1964.
5. Lundberg N: Continuous recording and control of ventricular fluid pressure in neurosurgical practice. Acta Psychiat. Scand. 36 (S 149):1-193, 1960.
6. Mascalchi M, Ciraolo L, Tanfani G et al.: Cardiac-gated phase MR imaging of aqueductal CSF flow. J. C.A.T. 12:923-926, 1988.

7. Pagni CA: Lezioni di neurochirurgia. Cap. 13: Fisiopatologia e clinica della sindrome di ipertensione endocranica nei tumori cerebrali, pp. 203-214. Ed. Libreria Cortina, Torino, 1978.

8. Pagni CA: Lezioni di neurochirurgia. Cap. 11: L'idrocefalo, pp. 161-196. Ed. Libreria Cortina, Torino, 1978.

9. Papo I: Ruolo dell'ipertensione endocranica nella patogenesi del coma cerebrale traumatico. In Papo, Cohadon, Massarotti eds: Le coma traumatique, pp. 111-127. Liviana ed., Padova, 1986.

10. Pollock LJ, Boshes B: Cerebrospinal fluid pressure. Arch. Neurol. Psychiatry 36:931-974, 1936.

11. Rao KCVG: The CSF spaces (Hydrocephalus and Atrophy). In Lee, Rao, Zimmermann eds.: Cranial MRI and CT. 3rd ed., pp. 227-294, McGraw-Hill, Inc. New York, 1992.

12. Staab EV: Radionuclide cisternography. In Freeman, Johnson eds.: Clinical radionuclide imaging, pp. 679-703. Grune and Stratton, New York, 1986.

13. Weisberg L, Nice C: Cerebral computed tomography. A text atlas. Cap. 13: Increased intracranial pressure, pp. 241-253. 3rd ed. W.B. Saunders Co., Philadelphia, 1989.

3.2

NEOPLASTIC CRANIOCEREBRAL EMERGENCIES

T. Tartaglione, C. Settecasi, G.M. Di Lella , C. Colosimo

INTRODUCTION

The clinical onset of intracranial neoplasia is typically subacute and progressive, or characterized by episodes of epilepsy; however, it is not infrequent for a tumour to present with an acute clinical syndrome, requiring emergency diagnostic imaging. This need arises in cases associated with an abrupt onset of intracranial hypertension, seizure or focal neurological deficit. This acute onset can be caused by alterations that result in a progressive mass effect of the neoplasia upon the adjacent nervous tissue and subarachnoid spaces, including the changes of perilesional oedema, haemorrhage and hydrocephalus.

The volume of the tumour can vary suddenly in response to involutional intrinsic tumoral phenomena such as necrosis or haemorrhage. These effects usually take place secondary to the inadequacy of the neoplastic vascular architecture, but can also be a result of the effects of radio- or chemotherapy. In addition, in certain tumours such as astrocytomas, primitive neuroectodermal tumours (PNET) and craniopharyngiomas, the formation and/or distension of an internal cyst may take place very quickly.

Perilesional vasogenic oedema, a result of the primitive nature of the neovasculature of the tumour, the intratumoral degenerative effects described above and the effects of these phenomena upon the surrounding neural tissue, increases the overall volume of the area involved and therefore causes an increase in the so-called tumoral mass effect. The most severe consequence of neoplastic mass effect is internal cerebral herniation. Perilesional vasogenic oedema is variably proportionate to the size of the tumour, its speed of growth, its internal constitution including its vascular supply, and the effects of the lesion upon the surrounding tissue. Therefore, small intraparenchymal metastatic lesions are typically accompanied by substantial vasogenic oedema, whereas benign tumours such as meningiomas, which are slow-growing and extraaxial, often have no perilesional oedema unless they have grown through the overlying pia mater of the underlying brain or have internal complication (e.g., intrinsic necrosis).

Hydrocephalus, which can also be limited to one or more ventricular cavities (i.e., caused by entrapment), is usually a result of the mass effect of the neoplasm; a typical example is monoventricular hydrocephalus secondary to the distortional parenchymal effect that causes effacement and ultimate obstruction of the foramen of Monro. Certain intraventricular tumours, or those adjacent to critical points of CSF outflow (aqueduct of Sylvius), can be the direct cause of subarachnoid space obstruction. However, in such cases the hydrocephalic condition usually sets in slowly and symptoms have a subacute although progressive pattern.

In this summarized introduction dedicated to neoplastic emergencies, we will briefly consider examination technique, the key points of imaging findings and certain particular posttraumatic clinical and diagnostic situations.

IMAGING EXAMINATION TECHNIQUE

True radiological emergencies are usually imaged first using CT due to the considerable speed with which examinations of uncooperative patients with serious conditions must be carried out. In addition, when the ictal symptomatology points to a haemorrhage, CT is the imaging technique having the greatest sensitivity.

However, in the case of cooperative patients, and where available, MRI using fast sequences could become the technique of choice in neurological emergencies. Wide user agreement attributes clear superiority to MRI over CT in recognising the lesion site, probable type, relationship to the adjacent structures and therefore the true extent of the pathological process, in part due to its multiplanar nature and greater definition of contrast resolution. When useful, MRA sequences, with or without paramagnetic contrast media, make it possible to obtain a general vascular map of the area non-invasively, which is helpful for differential diagnostic purposes as well as for surgical planning (2, 13, 16). Nevertheless, MRA today is scarcely sensitive to neoplastic vasculature. Finally, the use of functional MR sequences may be beneficial in some patients preoperatively, especially when the lesion is near neurologically sensitive areas such as the motor areas of the cerebrum (2).

SEMEIOTICS

a) *Recognition of the neoplastic nature and definition of the site/origin of the lesion*

The radiologist must be able to recognize the neoplastic nature of the lesion and to define its site with accuracy. In particular, the intra- or extraaxial site of the tumour and the relationship of the lesion with the surrounding subarachnoid spaces, the nervous and the vascular structures must be discerned. Neoplastic lesions are defined by the density/signal alterations as compared to the surrounding neural tissue, the degree and pattern of enhancement after IV contrast administration and its marginal characteristics. The further definition of the supra- or subtentorial position of the lesion guides the differential diagnosis and treatment planning (5, 13, 16).

b) *Characterization of the pathological tissue*

The majority of neoplastic lesions are characterized by an increase in free water and therefore a relative hypointensity on T1-weighted MRI, hyperintensity in PD- and T2-dependent sequences and a relative hypodensity on CT. Exceptions to these rules are those tumours with a high cellular and a high nucleus/cytoplasm ratio (e.g., PNET, germinoma, lymphoma) that present signal degeneration in T2-dependent images and a relative hyperdensity in CT (Fig. 3.10). IV contrast medium administration is almost always used in the examination of cerebral tumours and is only of somewhat limited value in generally haemorrhagic lesions (2, 13, 16).

c) *Detection of "acute" intraneoplastic alterations*

Cystic and necrotic areas are often present within tumours, and it can sometimes be impossible to distinguish between the two subtypes. The cyst CT density and MR signal characteristics depend on their content and can vary greatly, although they are typically characterized by marked hypodensity on CT and generally iso- hypointensity as compared to CSF on MR sequences; the signal and density generally increase with a rise in protein content. As noted above, the dis-

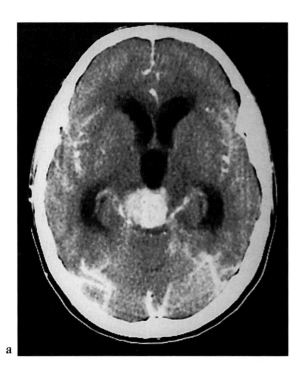

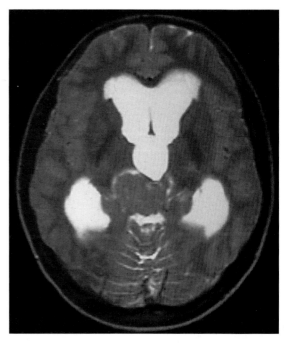

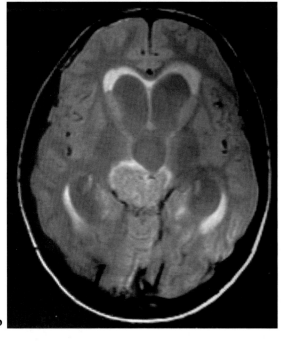

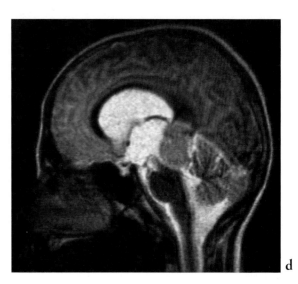

Fig. 3.10 - Pineal region germinoma with obstructive hydrocephalus. A solid mass is seen in the pineal region characterised by marked, homogeneous contrast enhancement. There is compressive obstruction the aqueduct of Sylvius resulting in obstructive hydrocephalus. Also identified are associated signs of CSF hypertension revealed as transependymal extravasation of the CSF signalled by the broad margin of hyperintensity within the periventricular white matter on T2-weighted sequences. [**a**) axial CT following IV contrast; **b**, **c**) axial proton density-, T2-weighted MRI; **d**) sagittal T2-weighted MRI].

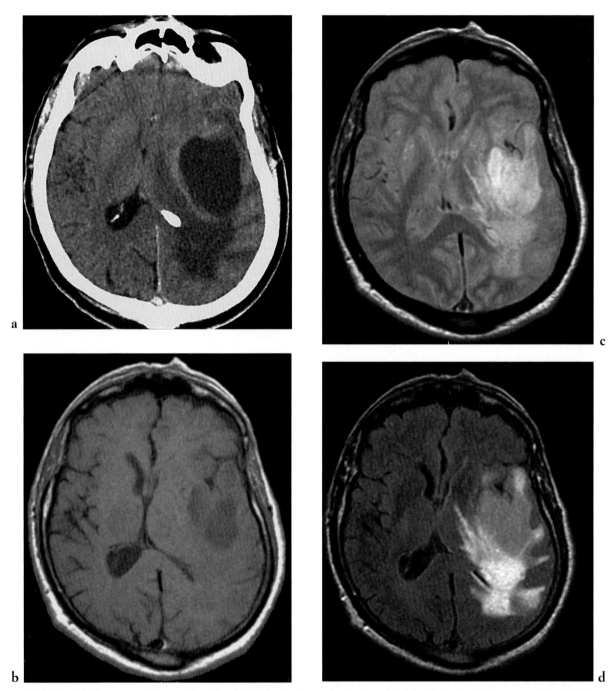

Fig. 3.11 - Glioblastoma multiforme. The CT and MRI studies show a large, necrotic left hemispheric glioblastoma associated with extensive perilesional vasogenic oedema resulting mass effect and lateral subfalcian herniation. [**a, b**) unenhanced axial CT; **c, d, b**) PD-, FLAIR, T2-weighted MRI; **f, g**) T1-weighted axial and coronal MRI following IV Gd].

tinction between tumour cysts and necrosis is not often possible and is not always useful. That being said, necrosis is generally characterized by a heterogeneous content with irregular, nodular walls and markedly inhomogeneous contrast enhancement (Fig. 3.11) (2, 13, 16). Intraneoplastic haemorrhages include both microhaemorrhages and

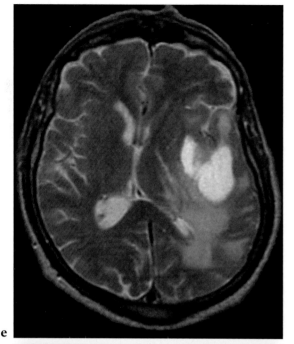

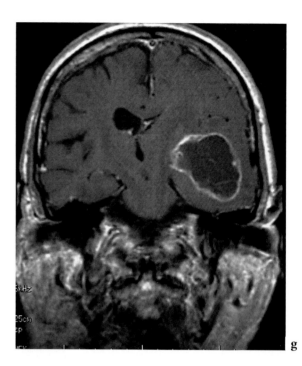

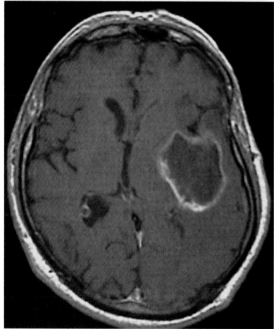

Fig. 3.11 (cont.).

macroscopic haemorrhages; these larger haemorrhages occur in approximately 1-15% of all neoplasias (2, 16, 20). This haemorrhagic frequency tends to increase within the subgroup of malignant tumours and especially in cases of metastases and malignant gliomas (2, 10, 12, 19, 23). There are a number of possible intraneoplastic causes of haemorrhage; among these are: primitive tumoral neovascularization with a disorderly endothelial proliferation and formation of arteriovenous shunts, rapid tumour growth with subsequent ischaemic necrosis, release of plasminogens and vascular infiltration by the tumour (2, 6, 11, 23, 24). The metabolism within haemorrhagic neoplasia is variable, but is generally lower than that observed in "benign" haemorrhages (1, 2).

Deoxyhaemoglobin, which is usually only found in the acute phase of haematomas between 7-72 hours from onset, can persist for weeks in intratumoral haemorrhages. Methaemoglobin, which forms in the subacute phase (i.e., 4-30 days), remains along the peripheral rims of haematomas for months in neoplastic haemorrhages. Haemosiderin, observed in the final stage of haemorrhage evolution, is typically absent. It is theorized that this altered evolution of the haemoglobin derives from the low oxygen tension obtaining in tumours on which the persistence of methaemoglobin depends (1, 7, 8, 14, 15, 21). Therefore, the density character-

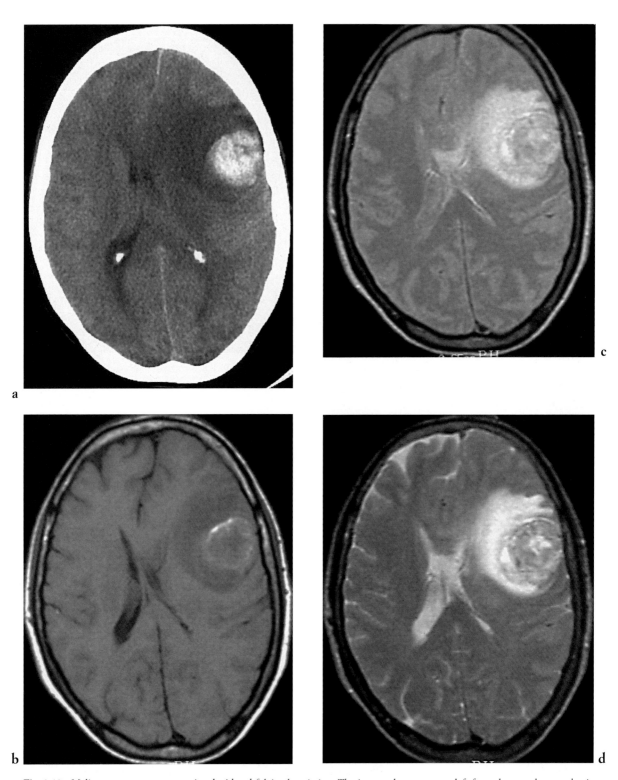

Fig. 3.12 - Malignant astrocytoma associated with subfalcian herniation. The images demonstrate a left frontal cortex haemorrhagic lesion with marked perilesional vasogenic oedema that compresses the ipsilateral ventricle and results in subfalcian herniation of the contralateral midline structures. There are cystic, necrotic components with various haemoglobin species in different stages of breakdown. After IV contrast medium administration irregular enhancement of the margins of the lesion is observed. [a] unenhanced axial CT; b, c, d) axial T1-, PD-, T2-weighted MRI.

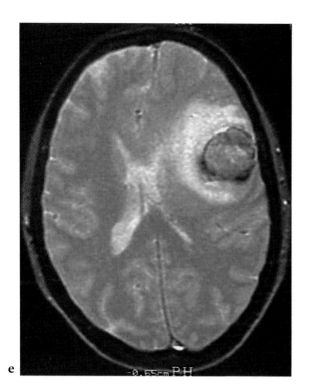

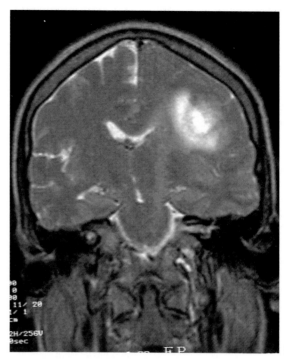

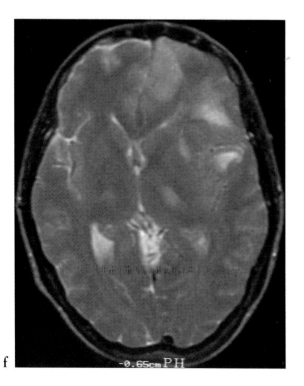

Fig. 3.12 (*cont.*) - **e**) Axial T2*-weighted, **f**) axial T2-weighted and **g**) coronal T2-weighted MRI.

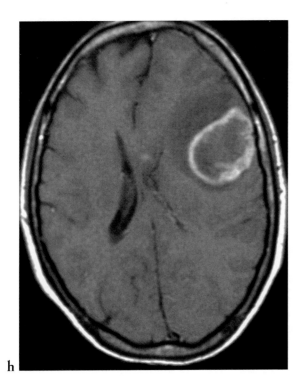

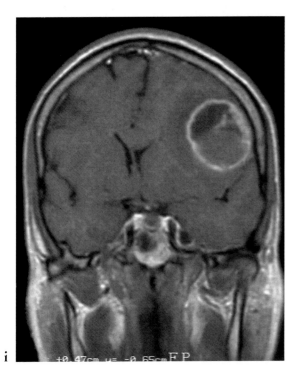

Fig. 3.12 (*cont.*) - **h**, **i**) axial and coronal T1-weighted MRI following IV Gd].

istics on CT and signal intensity on MRI of intratumoral haemorrhages differ somewhat from those of benign haemorrhages. In addition, neoplastic haemorrhages tend to appear more heterogeneous and complex (Fig. 3.12). Non-haemorrhagic areas of solid tumour and cystic-necrotic components with blood-fluid levels may also coexist with tumour enhancement after IV contrast medium administration. Finally, one last fundamental characteristic of many tumours is the persistence on imaging in the chronic phase of a marked hyperintense band of signal intensity surrounding the haemorrhage on long TR images due to vasogenic oedema (1, 2, 16, 18).

d) *Vasogenic oedema*

The most frequent observation within the cerebral nervous tissue surrounding a neoplasia is vasogenic oedema. Vasogenic oedema causes an increase in intracranial volume as well as that of the affected neural tissue. This oedema is hypodense on CT, hypointense in T1-weighted sequences and hyperintense on PD- and T2-weighted images. As mentioned previously, the origin of the oedema does not depend so much on the size of the neoplastic lesion as it does upon the speed with which the tumour grows, the fundamental nature of the intrinsic angiogenesis and the integrity of the blood-brain barrier (2, 5, 13, 16) (Fig. 3.12).

e) *Internal cerebral herniation*

The localized increase in cerebral volume caused by the neoplasia itself, as well as by associated haemorrhages, cysts, intratumoral necrosis and/or vasogenic oedema can determine the displacement of adjacent structures (cerebral, ventricular, subarachnoid spaces). The skull is divided by two large relatively rigid meningeal structures, the falx cerebri and the tentorium cerebelli, into three subcompartments. Depending upon the focus of the mass effect in relation to the tentorium, a distinction is made between supra- and subtentorial space; the falx represents an incomplete separation between the cerebral hemispheres in the midline. The cerebral struc-

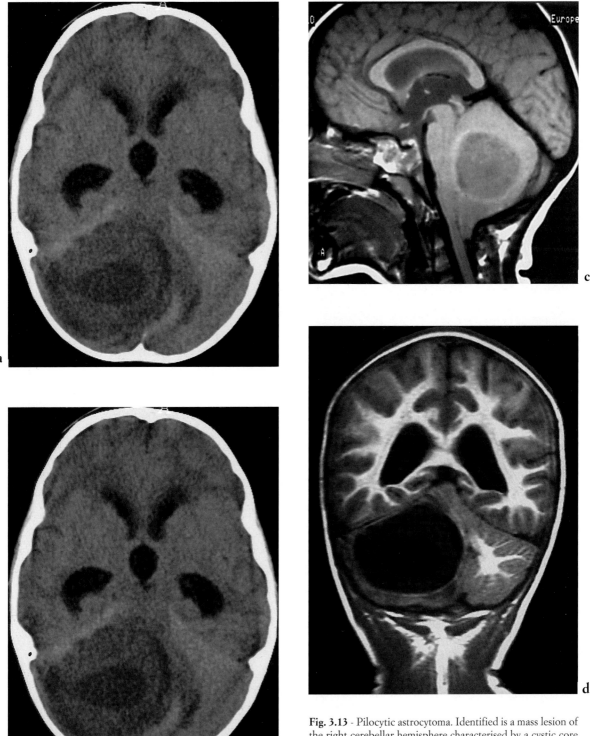

Fig. 3.13 - Pilocytic astrocytoma. Identified is a mass lesion of the right cerebellar hemisphere characterised by a cystic core and thick rim of solid tissue. The neoplasm compresses the 4th ventricle and brainstem resulting in obstruction of the aqueduct of Sylvius aqueduct and obstructive hydrocephalus. This in turn results in herniation of the midline inferior cerebellar structures caudally into the foramen magnum and cranially through the tentorial hiatus. [**a, b**) unenhanced axial CT; **c**) sagittal T1-weighted spin echo MRI; **d**) coronal inversion recovery T1-weighted MRI].

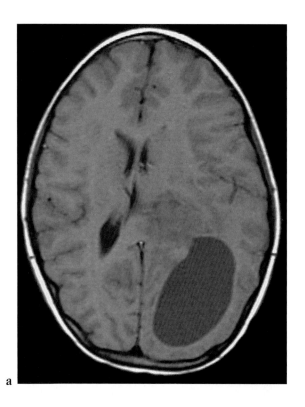

a

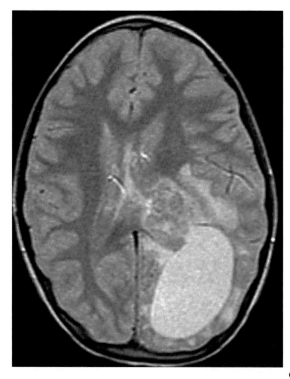

c

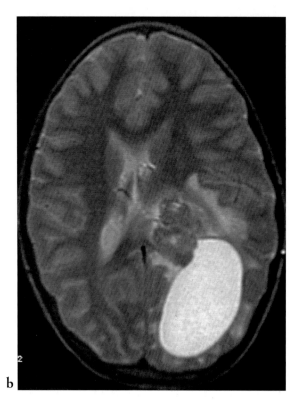

b

Fig. 3.14 - Anaplastic choroid plexus papilloma. The imaging studies show an inhomogeneous mass lesion whose epicentre is located within the left lateral ventricular trigone, characterised by an enhancing solid nodule and a cystic component with thin mural contrast enhancement. There is some associated perilesional vasogenic oedema. The sum mass effect results in minor lateral herniation of the midline supratentorial structures beneath the falx cerebri. [**a, b, c**) axial T1-, T2-, PD-weighted MRI].

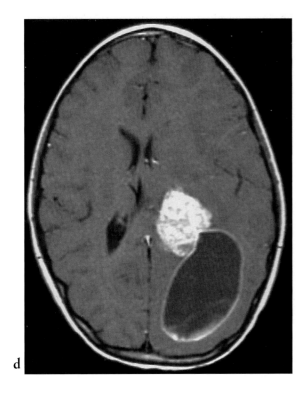

d

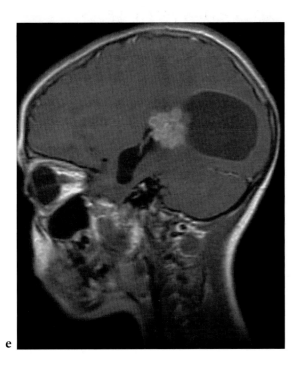

e

tures adjacent to a mass are pushed towards regions of lesser resistance and tend to move towards the pathways of communication between the various endocranial subcompartments, resulting in so-called internal cerebral herniations. The compressive effect of an expanding hemispheric lesion can cause herniation of the paramedian cerebral structures, the lateral ventricles, the 3rd ventricle and the anterior cerebral artery and its immediate branches below the falx cerebri towards the contralateral hemicranium causing a subfalcian herniation (Fig. 3.11, 3.12). A subfalcian herniation can in turn become complicated by an infarction of the territory of the anterior cerebral artery branches involved. In addition, uni- or biventricular hydrocephalus may ensue due to the obstruction of the foramina of Monro as a result of parenchymal distortion phenomena.

An expanding process situated in one cerebral hemicranium, especially if positioned in the middle cranial fossa, may push the uncus of the temporal lobe medially and downward between the free edge of the tentorium cerebelli and the ipsilateral cerebral peduncle into the perimesencephalic cistern; in the most severe cases, the brainstem, ipsilateral posterior cerebral and anterior choroid arteries and basal vein(s) of Rosenthal are compressed. This type of internal cerebral dislocation is termed descending transtentorial herniation.

An expanding cerebellar hemispheric lesion can compress the upper midline and paramedian structures of the posterior fossa, pushing them upward towards the tentorial incisura, ascending transtentorial herniation, and simultaneously may dislocate the cerebellar tonsils and lower vermis downward through the foramen magnum, descending foramen magnum herniation (Fig. 3.13).

Transtentorial herniations, be they descending or ascending, may cause the infarction of tissue in the distribution of the posterior cere-

Fig. 3.14 (*cont.*) - **d, e**) Axial and sagittal T1-weighted MRI following Gd].

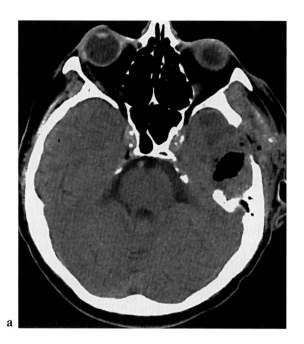

a

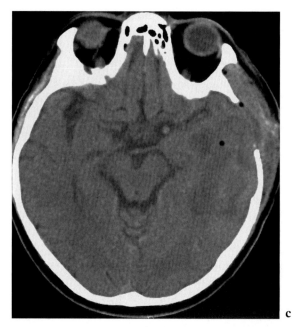

c

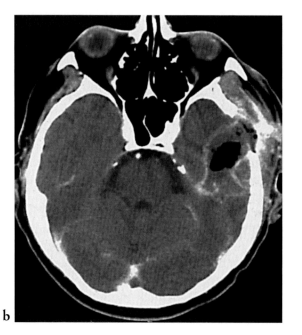

b

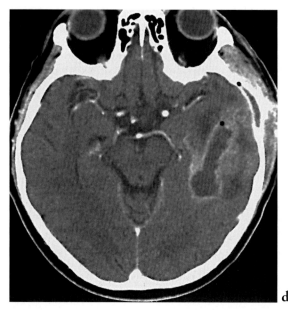

d

Fig. 3.15 - Postsurgical infection of surgical site. The surgical cavity demonstrates air with irregular contrast enhancement along the resection margins; hypodensity persists in the adjacent white matter due to persistent vasogenic oedema. The CT findings described are of uncertain significance, as they are still compatible with expected postsurgical alterations, however the associated clinical findings (headache and high fever) suggest a probable infection of the surgical site. [**a**, **b**) unenhanced axial CT; **c**, **d**) axial CT following IV contrast].

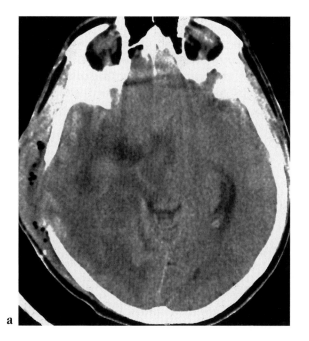

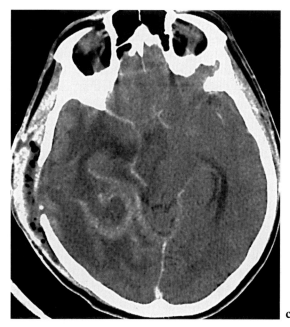

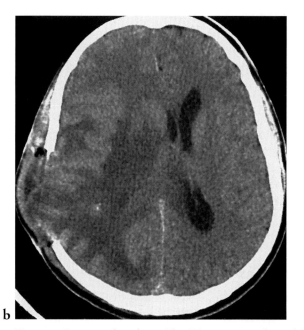

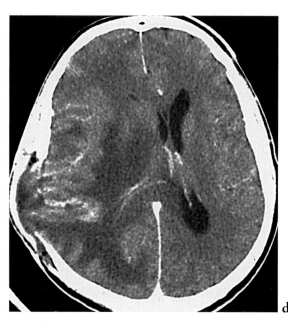

Fig. 3.16 - Postsurgical cerebritis. The CT examination shows diffuse hypodensity of the subcortical and deep white matter of the right cerebral hemisphere consistent with oedema, with inhomogeneous contrast enhancement and marked mass effect. The mass results in compression of the ipsilateral ventricle, subfalcian herniation of the midline supratentorial structures and early dilation of the contralateral ventricle caused by obstruction at the level of the foramen of Monro on the left side. The ipsilateral perimesencephalic cistern is obliterated due to downward internal herniation of the uncus of the temporal lobe. [**a, b**) unenhanced axial CT; **c, d**) axial CT after IV contrast].

bral arteries, the perforating arteries of the midbrain and the upper cerebellar arteries. In addition, obstructive triventricular hydrocephalus may occur as a result of the parenchymal compression/distortion of the aqueduct of Sylvius by the herniative process.

Internal cerebral herniation is a serious complication that may bring about a rapid escalation of clinical signs and symptoms, and therefore its neuroradiological recognition can profitably alter the therapeutic approach. It must be underlined that the clinical expression of severity of the herniation is in part directly proportional to the rapidity with which it forms; in the presence of a herniation into the foramen magnum or a descending transtentorial herniation, lumbar punctures are to be considered absolutely contraindicated in that they can result in a fatal compression of the brainstem (4, 5, 17).

f) Hydrocephalus

The effect of a tumour on CSF dynamics must be evaluated and, in particular, hydrocephalus must be recognized. The site of the obstruction must be established. The portion of the ventricular system situated proximal to the obstruction undergoes distension which can be acute. The level of the obstruction is usually the foramina or pathways of communication between the ventricles (e.g., foramina of Monro, aqueduct of Sylvius), which are compressed by the parenchymal distortion (Figs. 3.10, 3.13). In certain cases, neoplasia can cause an entrapment of a small section of the ventricular section; one typical example is a neoplasm located within or near the ventricular trigone (Fig. 3.10), which causes entrapment of the temporal horn of the lateral ventricle (5, 13).

POSTTHERAPEUTIC NEOPLASTIC EMERGENCIES

a) Postsurgical complications

In the postsurgical period, including after stereotaxic biopsy, neuroradiological evaluation is often required to exclude early complications that may occur, including haemorrhage (9), postsurgical oedema, acute hydrocephalus and infection. In such cases the diagnosis is often problematic because of the difficulties in distinguishing between neoplastic residue, aseptic postsurgical reactive phenomena, and frank infection with cerebritis (Figs. 3.15, 3.16), which may evolve into an abscess (3, 9).

b) Postventricular shunting complications

The complications of hydrocephalus shunts include:

1) Recurrence of hydrocephalus: A failure of the shunt may be secondary to an obstruction of the shunt catheter, for example due to a blood clot, or to an interruption to the shunt system's continuity due to a disconnection of a coupling or a fracture of the line.

2) CSF sequestration with a failure of drainage: Sequestration may occur in cases in which the tumour excludes part of the ventricular system on the proximal end, or when a loculation of the drainage fluid occurs on the distal end (i.e., the peritoneal cavity).

3) Hyperfunction of the shunt: This condition precipitates an "overshunting" syndrome; this is associated with a considerable reduction in the dimensions of the ventricles, which are sometimes nearly completely collapsed (i.e., "slit ventricle" syndrome). This situation can further be complicated by the formation of hygromas, and, in the most severe cases, subdural haematomas that are often bilateral.

4) Infection: Infection may consist of simple ependymitis with periventricular enhancement after IV contrast medium administration or of meningitis with generalized enhancement of the cranial leptomeninges.

REFERENCES

1. Atlas SW, Grossman RI, Gomori JM: Hemorragic intracranial malignant neoplasms: spin-echo MR imaging. Radiol 164:71, 1987.
2. Atlas SW: MRI of the brain and spine. Spell Checking, Thesaurus and Dictionaries, 1994.
3. Bayston R: Hydrocephalus shunt infection. Chapman and Hall Medical, London, 1989.
4. Blinkov SM, Smirnov NA: Brain displacements and deformations. Plenum Press, New York-London, 1971.

5. Cittadini G: Manuale di Radiologia clinica, 2nd. ECIG, Genova, 1983.

6. Davis JM, Zimmerman RA, Bilaniuk LT: Metastases to the central nervous system. Radiol Clin North Am 20:417, 1982.

7. Destian S, Sze G, Krol G et al: MR imaging of hemorragic intracranial neoplasms. AJNR 9:1115, 1988.

8. Gatenby RA, Coia LR, Richter MP: Oxygen tension in human tumors: in vivo mapping using CT-guided probes. Radiology 156:211, 1985.

9. Horwit NH, Rizzoli HV: Postoperative complications in intracranial neurological surgery. Williams and Wilkins, Baltimore-London, 1982.

10. Leeds NE, Elkin CM, Zimmerman RD: Gliomas of the brain. Semin Roentgenol 19:27, 1984.

11. Little JR, Dial B, Belanger G, et al: Brain hemorrhage from intracranial tumor. Stroke 10:283, 1979.

12. Mandybur TI: Intracranial hemorrhage caused by metastatic tumors. Neurology 27:650, 1977.

13. Marano P: Diagnostica per immagini, II vol. Casa Editrice Ambrosiana, Milano, 1994.

14. Neill JM: Studies on the oxidation-reduction of hemoglobin and methemoglobin. III. The formation of methemoglobin during the oxidation of autooxidizable substances. J Exper Med 41:551, 1925.

15. Neill JM: Studies on the oxidation-reduction of hemoglobin and methemoglobin. IV. The inhibition of spontaneous methemoglobin. J Exper Med 41:561, 1925.

16. Osborne AG: Diagnostic Neuroradiology. Mosby Year Book, Inc, 1994.

17. Pagni CA: Lezioni di neurochirurgia. Edizioni Libreria Cortina, Torino, 1984.

18. Potts DG, Abbott OF, von Sneidern JV: National Cancer Institute Study: evaluation of computed tomography in the diagnosis of intracranial neoplasms. III. Metastatic tumors. Radiol 136:657, 1980.

19. Russel DS, Rubinstein LJ: Pathology of tumors of the nervous system, 5th ed. Williams and Wilkins, Baltimore-London, 1989.

20. Scott M: Spontaneous intracerebral hematoma caused by cerebral neoplasm: report of eight verified cases. J Neurosurg 42:338, 1975.

21. Sze G, Krol G, Olson WL et al: Hemorragic neoplasms: MRI mimics of occult vascular malformations. Am J Radiol 149:1223, 1987.

22. Zimmerman H: The pathology of primary brain tumors. Semin Roentgenol 19:129, 1984.

23. Zimmerman RA, Bilaniuk LT: Computed tomography of acute intratumoral hemorrhage. Radiol 135:355, 1980.

24. Zulch KJ: Brain Tumors. Their Biology and Pathology, 3rd ed. Springer-Verlag, Berlin, 1986.

3.3

ANGIOGRAPHY IN BRAIN TUMOURS

C. Piana, U. Pasquini

INTRODUCTION

Cerebral angiography in the evaluation of cranioencephalic tumours has a role that is determined to a great extent by CT and MRI as it is no longer required to diagnose the existence of a lesion (7). However, selective cerebral angiography is still utilized in cases where the neurosurgeon is considering emergency surgery or another aggressive form of treatment.

Modern angiography is very different from the past, as the evolution in cauterization materials and angiographic equipment have brought about vast improvements in the quality of the images obtained while drastically reducing patient risk. The innovations in equipment have witnessed the introduction of digital acquisition, storage and image display, thereby making the resulting examination yet more practical to perform and review (1-4, 6, 8).

The evolution of the imaging instrumentation has coincided with the enormous technical progress made in angiographic materials, such as increasingly small catheters with ever greater torsion control and thin walls with extremely high mechanical resistance. It therefore follows that what was once considered a procedure associated with some degree of risk has now become quite safe, benefiting from the use of new contrast media, appliances and instruments.

Neovascular architecture is characterized by certain semeiological signs deriving from traditional angiography, including: alteration of the calibre, morphology and course of the vessels; presence of haemodynamic alterations; the presence of arteriovenous microshunts; and presence of a characteristic arteriolar-capillary parenchymal blush. There are three possible subtypes of angioarchitectural alteration in neoplasia: typical pathological vascularization (e.g., meningiomas, gliomas); atypical pathological vascularisation and avascular lesions (5).

Pathological vascularization can originate from the intraaxial vasculature (e.g., internal carotid and vertebrobasilar artery branches) or the meningeal vessels (e.g., branches of the external carotid artery). The type of vascularization depends on tumour type, however it should be stressed that angiography, like all other imaging techniques, is not able to provide a precise tissue diagnosis.

The table below shows a general classification of brain tumours as published by the WHO:

– *Neuroectodermal tumours* (gliomas, medulloblastomas, ependymomas, papillomas, neurinomas)

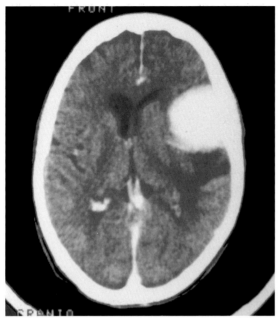

a

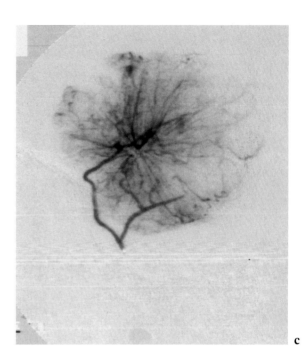

c

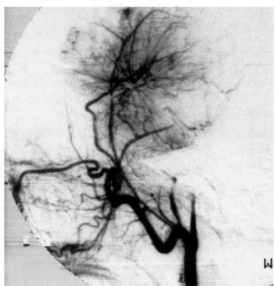

b Fig. 3.17 - Meningioma of the left pterion. The imaging studies reveal a left frontoparietal homogenously enhancing, broad dural based mass with perilesional oedema and neovascularity originating from the left middle meningeal artery. [a) unenhanced CT; b, c) left external carotid, left middle meningeal arteriogram].

- *Ectodermal tumours* (craniopharyngiomas, hypophyseal adenomas)
- *Embryogenic tumours* (epidermoids, dermoids, teratomas)
- *Mesodermal tumours* (meningiomas, angiomas, fibromas, chordomas, lipomas, osteomas, sarcomas).

This angiographic discussion of brain tumours cannot exhaustively deal with all the various types that can occur and will only detail the most frequently encountered.

MENINGIOMAS

Semeiotics

Statistically, meningiomas are most frequent in females, with a ratio of 3:1 as compared to males. With regard to other intracranial neoplasias, they are the most common type with an overall relative incidence that varies between 20-25%.

The angiographic characteristics of meningiomas vary with the histological type and specific degree of vascularization. Minor distinctions are made between skull base meningiomas and those of the convexity. Meningiomas have preferential sites with frontal, pterional and parietal locations being the most common, and they can be multiple.

During their development meningiomas deform and compress the overlying neural and vascular tissues, some of which, such as the internal carotid artery and cranial nerves within the cavernous sinuses, become enveloped within the confines of the tumour. They are supplied by arterial branches that are usually hypertrophic. These tumors demonstrate a pathological circulation fed principally from meningeal vessels that are usually quite regular with a diffuse and homogeneous tumour blush in the later phases of the serial angiographic study (Figs 3.17, 3.18). The neovascular tumour circulation can also be supplied from the pial arteries (i.e., internal carotid or vertebrobasilar arteries).

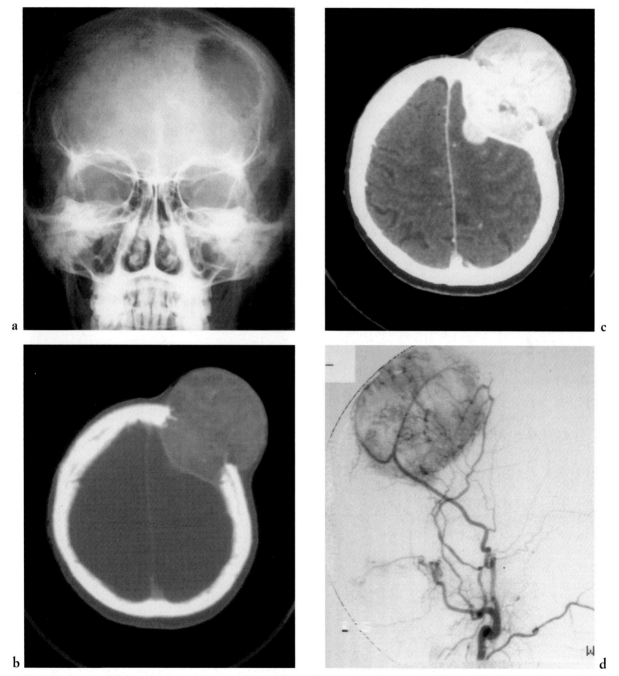

Fig. 3.18 - Invasive left frontal region meningioma. The skull x-ray demonstrates a large osteolytic lesion of the left frontal region. The CT shows a hyperdense lesion invading the overlying skull and extracranial soft tissues. The angiogram of the left external carotid artery reveals prominent neovascularity originating from branches of the left superficial temporal and middle meningeal arteries. [a) frontal radiograph; b), c) axial CT imaged with bone and soft tissue windows; d) left external carotid arteriogram].

In order to obtain a precise and complete documentation of the vascular contributions to the meningioma, it is mandatory to perform an angiographic examination that also includes all the meningeal arteries that might potentially contribute to this supply. Angiographic examinations must also include a thorough search for venous alterations (e.g., compressions and dural venous sinus invasion with stenosis or complete occlusion).

The circulation of meningeal sarcomas is quite different than that of benign meningiomas and is characterized by reduced circulation times, in part due to the presence of arteriovenous fistulae. Given their site of origin in the meninges, these tumours are also supplied by intra- and extracranial meningeal branches.

Olfactory groove (Fig. 3.19) and cavernous venous sinus meningiomas are less frequent and have typical appearances on CT and MRI. In the case of olfactory groove meningiomas, angiographic examinations rarely contribute additional information. However, in the case of cavernous venous sinus meningiomas, angiography can show an encasement and resulting stenosis of the carotid siphon and a neovascularization with parenchymal blush originating directly from branches of the carotid siphon itself. This observation points out the potential danger of surgical intervention and in some cases may suggest alternative treatment (radiotherapy).

One last characteristic location that bears discussion is the meningioma of the tentorium cerebelli. In such cases the angiographic picture is typical as it shows one or more hypertrophic tentorial meningeal arteries originating from the supraclinoid segment of the internal carotid that flow toward the central core of the tumour, where the characteristic hypervascularization is noted.

Discussion

From these brief considerations it would appear evident that the angiographic examination of a meningeal lesion must be performed not so much for diagnostic purposes, but rather to ob-

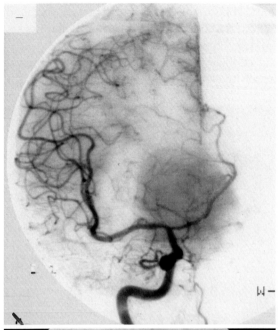

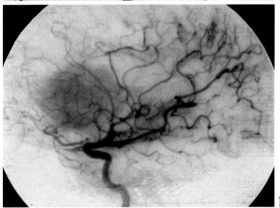

Fig. 3.19 - Olfactory groove meningioma. The right internal carotid arteriogram demonstrates neovascularity associated with a persistent parenchymal blush within a lesion in the anterior aspect of the skull base on the right side originating principally from ethmoid arterial branches. In addition, the right ophthalmic artery in hypertrophied as a result of the increased flow in transit to the neoplasm. [**a**) frontal projection right internal carotid arteriogram; **b**) lateral projection right internal carotid arteriogram].

tain an accurate angiographic map of the lesion and surrounding tissues. There are two fundamental reasons to accurately define this map: to demonstrate the type and degree of vascularization and to show the neurosurgeon the vessels that are to be isolated and coagulated.

Technological progress in recent years has brought about a new approach to the treatment of meningiomas: embolization. This technique typically precedes surgery, as it results in a devascularization of the tumour permitting a considerable reduction in the surgical time period, a reduction in intraoperative bleeding and therefore an overall reduction in surgical risk and complications. However, the embolic procedure must be performed by an expert team trained specifically in interventional radiology.

GLIOMAS

Semeiotics

CT and MRI have altered the indications for cerebral angiography somewhat by permitting a precise determination of the location of the lesion as well as a clear depiction of its various components and gross internal structure. However, visualization of the pathological neocirculation of the tumor still remains the province of conventional angiography.

On angiographic examinations gliomas have direct and indirect signs: direct signs are the actual vasculature of the neoplasm and the indirect signs are shifts of the vascular structures surrounding the tumour induced by its growth. This distinction between direct and indirect signs derives from conventional angiographic semeiology.

These direct angiographic signs are characterized by the specific afferent and efferent vessels, the appearance of the tumour vessels and the circulation time of the tumour. The evaluation of the efferent vessels is also quite important in the diagnostic angiographic analysis of brain tumours; for example, the detection of medullary veins and deep venous drainage virtually excludes the possibility of an extraaxial lesion.

The regularity of tumour neovessels can be an element in favour of the relative benignancy of a lesion. Conversely, the irregularity of the vessels is usually associated with malignancy, and the presence of arteriovenous shunts almost always indicates a malignant lesion.

Another distinctive characteristic of brain tumours is the tumour circulation time: in a number of lesions this circulation time is re-

duced due to the presence of arteriovenous shunts with early venous drainage. In other lesions the tumour circulation time appears increased and the tumour blush persists within the lesion. Tumour circulation times are also influenced by the presence of associated perilesional oedema, the presence or absence of vascular spasm and the degree of resistance of the draining veins (e.g., compression or complete obstruction of the draining venous structures).

Glioblastomas (Figs. 3.20, 3.21) are the subtype of glioma that has the most varied angiographic findings. In part due to their high biological activity, theses tumours typically reveal angiographic characteristics that define a malignant pathological circulation: a reduction in

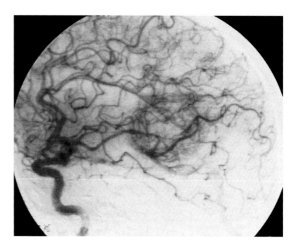

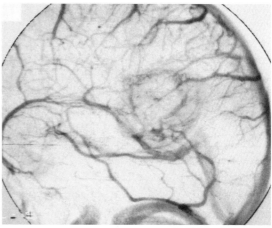

Fig. 3.20 - Left temporoparietal glioblastoma multiforme. Angiogram of the left internal carotid artery reveals a prominent parenchymal blush and arteriovenous shunting typical of malignant cerebral neoplasms.

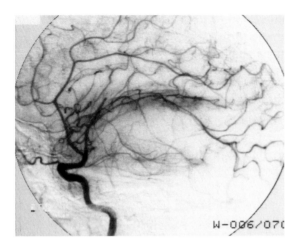

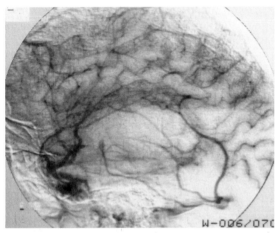

Fig. 3.21 - Left temporal lobe cystic glioblastoma. Angiogram of the left internal carotid artery shows mass effect in the elevation of the Sylvian vessels associated with a peripheral parenchymal blush.

OTHER CEREBRAL NEOPLASMS

Ependymomas and *medulloblastomas* can demonstrate a minor neovascularization; however, these are not characteristic elements that define these lesions. In *choroid plexus papillomas* (Fig. 3.23), the angiographic findings show a neocirculation composed of small vessels that give rise to a dense tumour blush. In these lesions one observes hypertrophy of the choroidal arteries from which the tumour vessels originate.

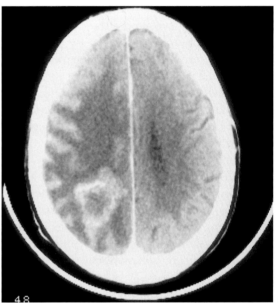

a

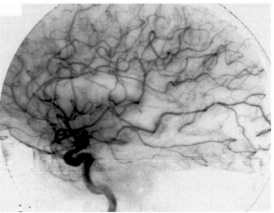

b

Fig. 3.22 - Right parietal lobe astrocytoma. Contrast enhanced CT shows mural enhancement within a right parietal lobe subcortical mass lesion surrounded by much perilesional oedema. The angiogram of the right internal carotid artery demonstrates no hypervascularity. [a) axial CT following IV contrast; b) lateral projection right internal carotid arteriogram]

circulation time, irregularity in the calibre of vessels with very disorderly patterns, arteriovenous fistulae and early venous drainage.

Other gliomas have different angiographic findings, some presenting with a picture that is more or less avascular. Even some quite hypervascular gliomas have areas that are avascular indicating necrosis or the presence of cysts or haemorrhage within the tumour.

Benign *astrocytomas* (Fig. 3.22) and *oligodendrogliomas* only rarely have significant macroscopic pathological neocirculation. However, in certain cases some intrinsic vascular elements can be detected. When present, such findings can be interpreted as a greater or lesser degree of lesion malignancy.

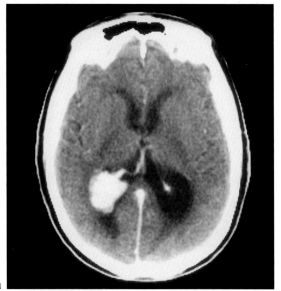

a

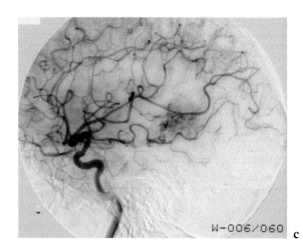

c

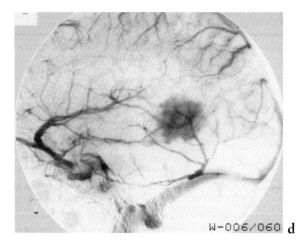

d

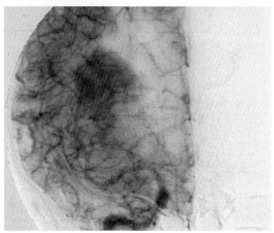

b

Fig. 3.23 - Papilloma of the right choroid plexus. The contrast enhanced CT shows a homogeneously enhancing intraventricular mass. The right internal carotid arteriogram reveals a mass lesion having neovascularity, associated with a tumor blush and arteriovenous shunting. [**a**) axial CT following IV contrast; **b**, **e**) frontal projection right internal carotid arteriogram; **c**, **d**) lateral projection right internal carotid artery arteriogram].

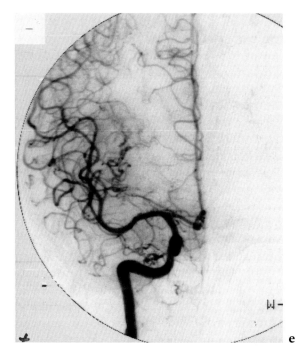

e

Discussion

The angiographic analysis of cranial neoplasia is important from the view point of the potential neurosurgical therapeutic implications. Emergency angiographic examinations implicate the intention to perform interventional procedures in order to reduce the vascularity of the lesion and are dictated by the patient's clinical situation.

The exact representation of the tumour vascularity permits a proper and careful approach to stereotaxic biopsy, as it shows the course of the vessels to be avoided and tumour vessels. These observations potentially reduce the risks of a possible intratumoral haemorrhage.

Complete angiographic examinations facilitate surgical intervention. However, in cases in which the lesion cannot be operated on, angiography may suggest alternative therapies such as radiotherapy and intraarterial chemotherapy. This latter technique is proving efficacious in the treatment of particularly hypervascular lesions; in such cases, the angiographic picture can be correlated with considerable biological activity, and therefore with greater pharmacological sensitivity.

Lastly, in cases where the neurosurgeon does not intend to intervene, angiographic evaluations are of little or no value as the combination of CT and MRI provide more than satisfactory information concerning the type and location of the lesion.

METASTASES

Given precise clinical and historical medical data, this type of lesion is usually not difficult to interpret using CT and MRI. From a statistical point of view, autopsy findings reveal brain metastases in 24% of patients suffering from tumours. The tumours that most frequently spread to the CNS include melanomas, lung carcinoma, breast carcinoma, thyroid tumours and leukaemia/lymphoma.

Although there is usually no diagnostic dilemma in diagnosing cerebral metastases on CT and MRI in the presence of multiple lesions, this changes in the case of isolated lesions that are often cortical-subcortical in location and may infiltrate the overlying meninges. In such cases, it may be necessary to perform an angiography in order to resolve differential diagnostic problems between metastasis and meningioma.

The angiographic picture of metastases (Fig. 3.24) is somewhat typical with the depiction of rather homogeneous neovascularity, which is most frequently supplied by a single arterial branch. This neovascular circulation

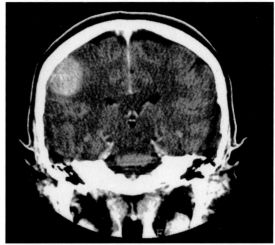

a

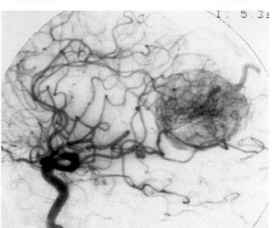

b

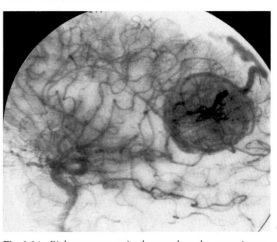

c

Fig. 3.24 - Right temporoparietal parenchymal metastatic neoplastic disease. Contrast enhanced coronal CT demonstrates an enhancing mass lesion adjacent to the skull on the right side. The right internal carotid arteriogram in the lateral projection reveals an intensely hypervascular cortical lesion associated with a tumor blush and arteriovenous shunting. [**a**] coronal CT following IV contrast; **b**, **c**] lateral projection right internal carotid arteriogram].

has well-defined margins and persists in time into the venous angiographic phase. Typically a single draining cortical vein is visible.

The lesion usually has a cortical or subcortical location. In cases where the lesion infiltrates the overlying meninges and bone of the skull, an examination of the meningeal branches is essential as the absence of supply of the tumour from these vessels permits differentiation from meningioma.

Discussion

This brief analysis highlights the fact that multiple metastases do not necessarily require an angiographic evaluation, as CT and MRI are sufficient for diagnosis. The principal exception is that of isolated cortical lesions that infiltrate the overlying meninges and skull. As noted above, angiography can provide valuable information in such cases in terms of differentiating a metastasis from a meningioma.

CONCLUSIONS

Cerebral angiography has precise indications in the light of new diagnostic and therapeutic considerations; presurgical angiographic investigations are always required in order to facilitate the surgical approach to the lesion by demonstrating the afferent and efferent vascular branches to the lesion. Angiographic studies may prove useful in subsequent intraarterial embolization or chemotherapy in conjunction with surgery or once it has been established that surgery is not possible.

Cerebral angiography is considered superfluous in the more benign or lower grade tumour types, in tumours of the posterior cranial fossa and in tumour follow-up; in most of these cases, CT and MRI are usually sufficient for diagnosis and treatment planning.

MRA has a complementary diagnostic role regarding information on hypervascular intracranial lesions. In particular, the recently developed techniques involving the injection of a contrast medium bolus in order to better identify the arterial vascularization may prove useful in the future. This makes it possible to visualize some degree of the pathological neovascularization present in many malignant tumours. However, bolus contrast enhanced MRA does not yet possess the sufficient definition to distinguish with certainty the smaller arteries; in addition, by its nature it lacks the ability to selectively differentiate the various vascular territories.

REFERENCES

1. Brant-Zawadki M, Gould R et al: Lane B.: Digital subtraction cerebral angiography by intrarterial injection: comparison with conventional angiography. AJR 140, 347-353, 1983.
2. Chilcote WA, Modic MT, Pavlicek WA et al.: Digital subtraction angiography of the carotid arteries: a comparative study in 100 patients. Radiology 130, 287-295, 1981.
3. Davis PC, Hoffman JC: Intraarterial digital subtraction angiography: evaluation in 150 patients. Radiology 148, 9-15, 1983.
4. Kelly W, Brant-Zawadzki M, Pitts LH: Arterial injection-digital subtraction angiography. J. Neurosurg. 58, 851-856, 1983.
5. Leeds NE, Rosenblatt R: Arterial wall irregularities in intracranial neoplams: the shaggy vessel brought into focus. Radiology 103, 121-124, 1972.
6. Modic MT, Weinstein MA, Chilcote WA et al.: Digital subtraction angiography of the intracranial vascular system: comparative study in 55 patients. AJR 138, 299-306, 1982.
7. Newton TH, Potts DG: Radiology of the skull and brain: angiography. Volume two/book 4. The CV Mosby Company Saint Louis 1974.
8. Weinstein MA, Pavlicek WA, Modic MT et al: Intra-arterial digital subtraction angiography of the head and neck. Radiology 147, 717-724, 1983.

IV

EMERGENCY NEURORESUSCITATION

4.1

TOXIC ENCEPHALOPATHY

M. Gallucci, M. Caulo, G. Cerone, A. Splendiani, R. De Amicis, C. Masciocchi

INTRODUCTION

Toxic encephalopathy arises following the interaction between a chemical compound and the Central Nervous System (CNS) (9). A wide range of chemical substances can be neurotoxic, having mechanisms that affect the CNS either directly or indirectly by means of alterations to cerebral or systemic homeostasis induced by the substance in question. The main causes of brain damage include: oxidative energy depletion, deficit of the substrate for cerebral activity, alterations in cell membrane integrity, enzyme deficit, alterations to the electrolytic equilibrium, and neurotransmission damage.

Toxic substances can be either *endogenous* or *exogenous*. Endogenous agents typically result from congenital cerebral errors in metabolism; exogenous substances are classified as *external* (i.e., when they are introduced into the organism from outside) and *internal* (when they are produced by systemic metabolism errors and come into contact with the CNS via the blood-brain barrier).

Neuroradiological emergencies are most frequently linked to external exogenous toxins. Intoxication requires immediate diagnosis and swift treatment in order to prevent brain damage becoming irreversible or fatal. Once the risk of death has been overcome, the contribu-

tion of diagnostic imaging and of MRI in particular consists in the possibility of monitoring treatment and the evolution of the neuroradiological picture over time.

In general, brain damage caused by toxins involves both hemispheres, as there is no side preference. It is still unclear why some CNS structures are affected to a greater extent than others, however it is probable that differences in vulnerability and/or tissue affinity to the toxic substance are implicated.

It should be underlined that the clinical and neuroradiological findings do not always match, and even in cases of neuropathologically proven brain damage diagnostic imaging techniques may provide falsely negative results.

ALCOHOLIC ENCEPHALOPATHY

Due to its low cost and ready availability, alcohol is by far the most widespread drug in the western world. Given its marked neurotoxic capacity, alcohol is probably the most commonly encountered CNS toxin. The neurological pathology seen in alcoholics can only partly be attributed to the direct toxic effect of alcohol and its metabolites, and some of the aetiological explanations are still unknown. The factors that are presumed to explain brain

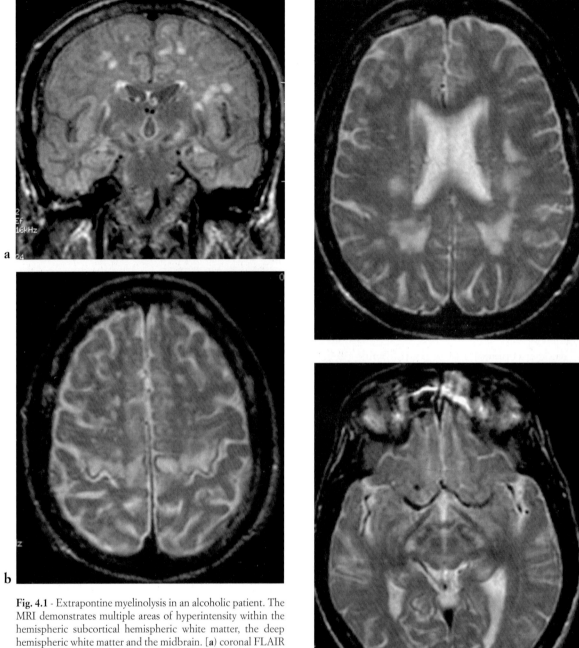

Fig. 4.1 - Extrapontine myelinolysis in an alcoholic patient. The MRI demonstrates multiple areas of hyperintensity within the hemispheric subcortical hemispheric white matter, the deep hemispheric white matter and the midbrain. [**a**) coronal FLAIR MRI; **b, c, d**) axial T2-weighted MRI].

damage include vitamin deficiency, hypoglycaemia, associated repeated cranial trauma, chronic liver failure and the presence of non-alcohol toxic substances that are present in alcoholic beverages. In chronic alcoholics, arterial hypertension, subarachnoid haemorrhage and strokes are also more common than in average age-matched controls. Although not all alcohol-related neurological pathology requires management in emergency conditions, some do require immediate diagnosis and treatment.

Osmotic myelinolysis

Osmotic myelinolysis is a demyelinating process that arises from a too rapid correction of an existing state of hyponatraemia, which, in the case of alcoholics, is induced by the impairment of ADH secretion caused by alcohol. On MRI, these lesions appear as areas containing "excess water" that result in high signal intensity areas in T2-weighted sequences and low intensity areas in T1-weighted sequences. These pure demyelinating forms do not manifest evidence of inflammation or blood-brain barrier damage. For this reason, MRI shows no enhancement following IV contrast medium administration.

A distinction is made between pontine and extrapontine myelinolysis. In the latter, the most frequent sites of demyelination are the putamen, caudate nucleus, thalamus and subcortical white matter. Less frequently, the mamillary body, the tegmen of the midbrain and the white matter of the cerebellum may also be involved (Fig. 4.1). Central pontine myelinolysis appears on MRI as a single symmetric lesion that spreads to the pontine raphe and involves the transverse pontocerebellar fibres and the long descending corticobulbar tracts (Fig. 4.2). The clinical aspect of this type of lesion is characterized by a flaccid quadraparesis that may regress or alternatively evolve into a subsequent spastic form with pseudo-bulbar paralysis. Osmotic myelinolysis is not always an alcohol-related pathology and may be caused by or connected to many conditions in which there is a too rapid correction of a water and electrolyte imbalance. For example, this may also occur in dialysis patients (3, 18, 19, 29).

Wernicke encephalopathy

Wernicke encephalopathy is the consequence of a thiamine deficiency resulting either from reduced intake or from intestinal malabsorption. This type of abnormal metabolism typically occurs in subjects with congenital transketolase activity deficits. Thiamine deficits

cause a reduced use of glucose in the brain. This condition has an acute onset characterized by ophthalmoplegia, ataxia and mental confusion. In the chronic phase patients may demonstrate a reduction in olfactory discrimination secondary to midbrain lesions, whereas memory disorders are related to injury to the mamillary bodies and the dorsomedial nuclei of the thalamus. Following thiamine therapy, the clinical situation may either improve or evolve into Korsakoff's syndrome. Korsakoff's syndrome is characterized clinically by the impairment of chronological fixation memory, learning ability and the appearance of confabulatory attacks (i.e., amnesia with the appearance of false recollections).

MR examinations using T2-dependent sequences show abnormal high intensity areas in the involved white and grey matter with a characteristic topographic distribution. The affected areas include those surrounding the 3rd ventricle: the massa intermedia, the floor of the 3rd ventricle, the mamillary bodies, the reticular formation and the periaqueductal region (Figs. 4.3, 4.4). In chronic forms one also observes a passive dilation of the third ventricle and atrophy of the mamillary bodies.

The involvement of the mamillary bodies has been demonstrated in 98% of autopsies performed on Wernicke sufferers. Using MRI it is possible to demonstrate the involvement of the mamillary bodies primarily in acute cases in which contrast enhancement of the mamillary bodies is observed. However, this finding is not constant and is probably only present in cases in which there is endothelial necrosis with atten-

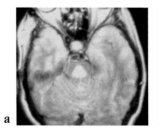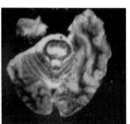

a   b

Fig. 4.2 - Two cases of pontine myelinolysis in alcoholic patients. T2-weighted MRI shows a single hyperintense lesion of the pons in each case. [**a**, **b**) axial T2-weighted MRI].

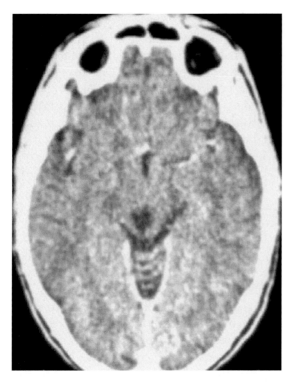

Fig. 4.3 - Wernicke's encephalopathy in alcoholic patient. CT only rarely shows an area of hypodensity in the midbrain in cases of Wernicke's encephalopathy, as in this case.

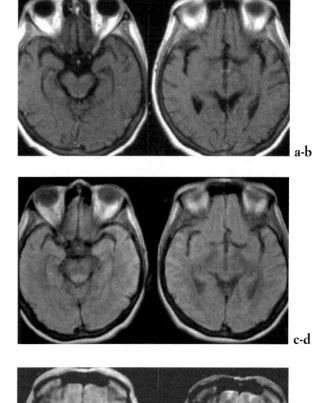

Fig. 4.4 - Wernicke's encephalopathy in an alcoholic patient. Enhanced MRI shows contrast enhancement within the mamillary bodies bilaterally. More craniad T2-weighted scans shows abnormal hyperintensity within the posteromedial aspect of the thalami bilaterally and the hypothalamus. [**a**), **b**) T1-weighted MRI following IV Gd; **c-e**) PD- and T2-weighted MRI].

dant blood-brain barrier disruption. Nevertheless, in such cases the finding of mamillary body enhancement can dispel diagnostic doubts (Fig. 4.4). Certain authors have also documented high signal intensity areas in the cortex of the central and precentral gyri.

In Korsakoff's syndrome the neuropathological and neuroradiological alterations are focused on the dorsomedial nuclei of the thalamus and the hippocampal formations. Injury to these structures is associated with amnesic symptomatology that defines the symptoms of Wernicke-Korsakoff syndrome (Fig. 4.5). Recent studies using PET and perfusion MR in the thalamic and temporal regions of patients with Korsakoff's syndrome have shown both reduced blood flow and metabolic activity in these areas. In a similar manner to osmotic myelinolysis, Wernicke's syndrome is not necessarily alcohol-related and can be encountered in other diet-related, deficiency-related or malabsorption pathology (Fig. 4.6) (1, 8, 10, 11, 25, 29).

Marchiafava-Bignami disease

This rare disorder was initially described in middle-aged and elderly drinkers of red wine having a high tannin content. For this reason for many years it was believed that the specific cause of the disease was Chianti wine, a theory that has now been rejected. The most probable

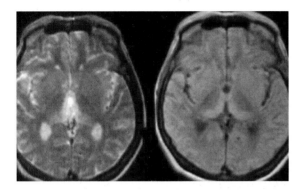

Fig. 4.5 - Wernicke-Korsakoff syndrome in alcoholic patient. T2-dependent SE **a**) and PD-dependent sequences **b**). Widespread signal alteration in the dorsal-medial region of the thalamus bilaterally and in the hypothalamus.

cause of the illness is an as yet unspecified nutritional deficiency. Clinical symptoms vary from convulsions to hallucinations and delirium, and in the terminal stages stupor and coma may be seen. The clinical diagnosis is problematic given the heterogeneity and non-specific

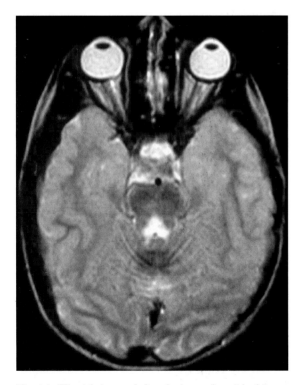

Fig. 4.6 - Wernicke's encephalopathy in a malnourished 8-year old child. T2-weighted MRI shows hyperintense periaqueductal MRI signal alteration.

nature of the symptoms, and for this reason the use of diagnostic imaging techniques is essential. Marchifava-Bignami disease is characterized by the necrosis and demyelination of the midline lamina of the corpus callosum and the injury of other commissural fibres and the hemispheric white matter. MRI performed in the sagittal plane in the chronic phase shows atrophy of the corpus callosum and the presence of multifocal necrotic areas characterized by low signal intensity in T1-weighted sequences and high signal intensity in T2- and PD-weighted sequences (Fig. 4.7) (2, 4, 22, 29).

Acquired hepatocellular degeneration (AHCD)

Acquired hepatocellular degeneration syndrome is a complex illness characterized by changes in consciousness, behaviour and personality often associated with acute or chronic kidney disease or liver cirrhosis. It would appear to be linked to alterations in the metabolism of nitrogenated substances and alterations of the glutamate-glutamine ratio, with an increase in the synthesis of aromatic amino acids and false neurotransmitters. The alterations visible on MRI are closely correlated with plasma ammonia levels, but do not seem to be linked to the degree of neuropsychiatric

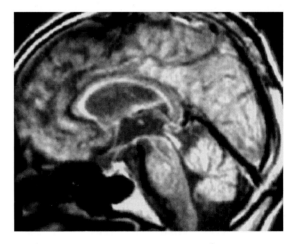

Fig.4.7 - Marchiafava-Bignami disease in alcoholic patient. Sagittal T2 weighted MRI shows marked thinning of the corpus callosum associated with abnormal signal hyperintensity along its entire course.

dysfunction or to electroencephalographic alterations. In most cases, there is a widespread shortening of the T1-dependent signal including hyperintensity of the basal ganglia; prominent involvement of the globus pallidus is typical (Fig. 4.8). The caudate nucleus, pineal gland, subthalamic region and the midbrain around the red nuclei may also be similarly involved. The reason for this signal alteration is not yet clear, but it is thought to be connected to a hyperplasia of the Alzheimer type II astrocytes in association with neuronal necrosis and the subsequent deposition of paramagnetic substances such as magnesium (10, 12, 23, 29).

METHANOL INTOXICATION

There are a number of sources of methanol, which can be present in solvents, industrial liquids, perfumes and counterfeit spirits, thus making methanol intoxication relatively common amongst alcoholics. It manifests clinically as general malaise and headache and may progress to stupor and coma. Necrotic areas are visible in the putamen as hypodense on CT scans and as high signal intensity on T2-dependent sequences in MR studies (Fig. 4.9). The appearance of these areas can also be affected by the presence of haemorrhagic infarction. Other related necrotic areas can be identified in the subcortical white matter and in the frontal cortex (12, 28, 29).

ETHYLENE-GLYCOL INTOXICATION

Ethylene-glycol is typically present in paints and glues but can also be encountered in food preservatives and as an alcohol substitute. Ingestion occurs accidentally or, more rarely, voluntarily in the case of alcoholics. Neurological clinical symptomatology sets in after approximately 12 hours of ingestion and is characterized by a sense of inebriation and convulsions progressing to coma.

As with methanol intoxication, the toxic effects are manifested as areas of necrosis that principally affect the frontal cortex, the thalami and the basal ganglia (Fig. 4.10) (28, 29).

INTOXICATION FROM NARCOTIC INHALATION

Toluene and methyl-ethylketone are lipophilic solvents that are used in the chemical industry and that may be accidentally inhaled during processing. These substances are capable of causing a similar neurological, neuropathological and neuroradiological picture to those caused by other voluntarily inhaled substances such as heroin and, more rarely, cocaine (in such cases the toxic effect may be related to the substances with which the drugs are diluted). In cocaine and

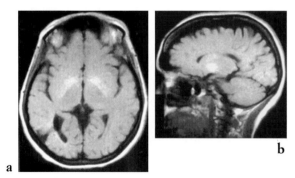

Fig. 4.8 - Hepatocerebral degeneration in patient with cirrhosis. The MRI demonstrates an abnormal area of high MRI signal intensity in the globus pallidus bilaterally. [a) axial, b) sagittal T1-weighted MRI].

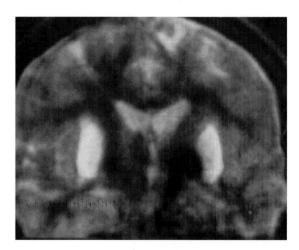

Fig. 4.9 - Alcoholic patient following consumption of a large quantity of methanol. Coronal T2-weighted MRI reveals high signal intensity within the putamena and in the frontal subcortical white matter bilaterally.

may also be possible to observe hypertensive encephalopathy (from cocaine) and hypotensive encephalopathy (from heroin) (Fig. 4.11), or rarer forms of vacuolating encephalopathy with foci of demyelination in the supra- and subtentorial white matter. Although in these cases the toxic agent has yet to be identified, it is theorized that a lipophilic substance present in the drug is responsible (7, 15, 21, 27-29).

INTOXICATION FROM MEDICINES

Many of the medicines currently available have neurotoxic characteristics, including chemotherapy drugs, which give can give rise to the most severe conditions.

Intoxication from Methotrexate

Methotrexate is usually administered intravenously or via subarachnoid catheter, the latter principally in the case of lymphoproliferative disorders of the CNS. Although its neurotoxicity has been proved, the pathophysiology

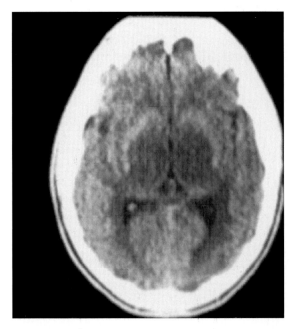

Fig. 4.10 - Glycol-ethylene intoxication. Axial CT shows marked hypodensity of the thalami bilaterally.

heroin sniffers, in an acute stage the neuropathological and neuroradiological manifestations include microinfarcts caused by toxic vasculitis. It

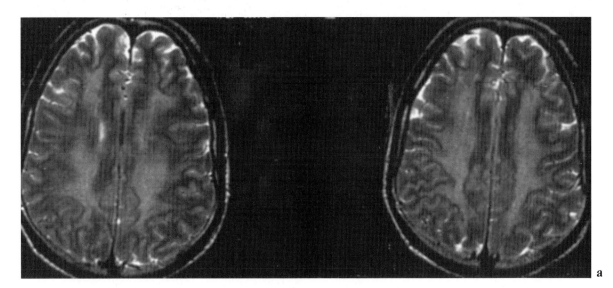

Fig. 4.11 - Delayed post-hypoxic leukoencephalopathy,. MRI examination performed approximately three hours following admission shows widespread MRI signal hyperintensity of the white matter of the centrum semiovale. Follow up MRI approximately 1 month later shows necrosis within the abnormal hemispheric white matter foci identified on earlier scans. This evolution is consistent with delayed post-hypoxic leukoencephalopathy. As in this case, this phenomenon has been described in heroine addicts following experiencing acute cardiorespiratory depression. [**a**), **b**) axial T-2 weighted MRI on admission; **b**) axial T1-weighted MRI on admission; **c**), one month follow up axial T2-weighted MRI; **d**) one month follow up T1-weighted MRI].

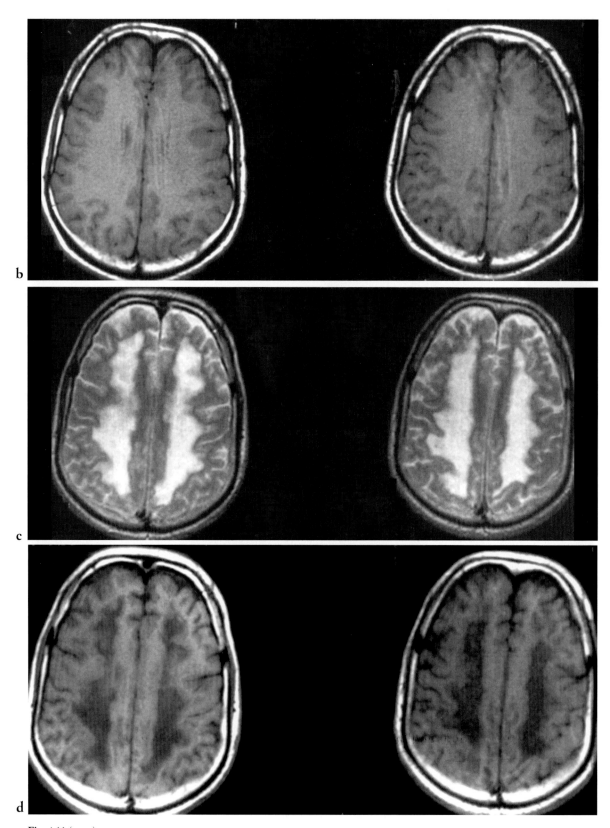

Fig. 4.11 (*cont.*).

of the neurological damage caused by this drug is still controversial. The most commonly accepted theory is that it causes a thickening of the endothelial walls of the cerebral vasculature, with consequent occlusion, ischaemia and necrosis of the served neural tissue. During chemotherapy, this condition is believed to be favoured by concomitant radiation therapy. The MRI semeiotics vary from focal lesions to diffuse alterations of the white matter signal, mainly the deeper areas of the brain, having high signal intensity on long TR sequences (Fig. 4.12). On CT, the lesions appear hypodense with the presence of hyperdense foci (i.e., calcified deposits) in the subcortical regions. The MR appearance of the lesions that are hyperdense on CT scans were evaluated using FLASH MRI sequences and were found to have low signal intensity. CT and MR findings therefore show a picture of leukoencephalopathy with calcified deposits that are typical of the disease (13, 17, 20, 23, 29).

Intoxication from Cyclosporin A (CsA)

Cyclosporin A is an immunosuppressive medicine used in the prevention of so-called graft vs. host disease. Although the neurotoxic effects of this drug have been determined, the pathophysiological mechanism is yet to be specified. One theories of the most widely accepted theories is that CsA causes arterial hypertension (90% of all patients treated), with consequent similar neuropathological and neuroradiological conditions to those of hypertensive encephalopathy; another, more recent theory states that CsA may cause damage to the capillary endothelium with consequent vasogenic oedema. This second theory would justify the reversibility of the clinical and neuroradiological situation in CsA intoxication.

Clinically CsA intoxication is manifested as headache, epilepsy, cortical blindness, visual hallucinations, trembling and cerebellar ataxia. MR examinations show areas of high signal intensity on T2-dependent and FLAIR sequences, most frequently observed in the subcortical white matter of the occipital lobes of the posterior por-

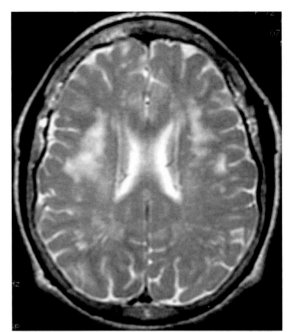

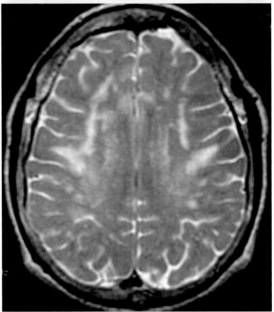

Fig. 4.12 - Methotrexate neurotoxicity. T2-weighted MRI, in a patient with disseminated cancer under treatment with methotrexate, shows widespread hyperintense MRI signal alterations within the hemispheric deep and subcortical white matter consistent with chronic treatment related neurotoxicity. [**a, b**) axial T2-weighted MRI].

tions of the temporal and parietal lobes (16). The lesions are frequently symmetrical, and they only rarely show enhancement following IV contrast agent administration. Recent observations performed using diffusion MR in cases of CsA

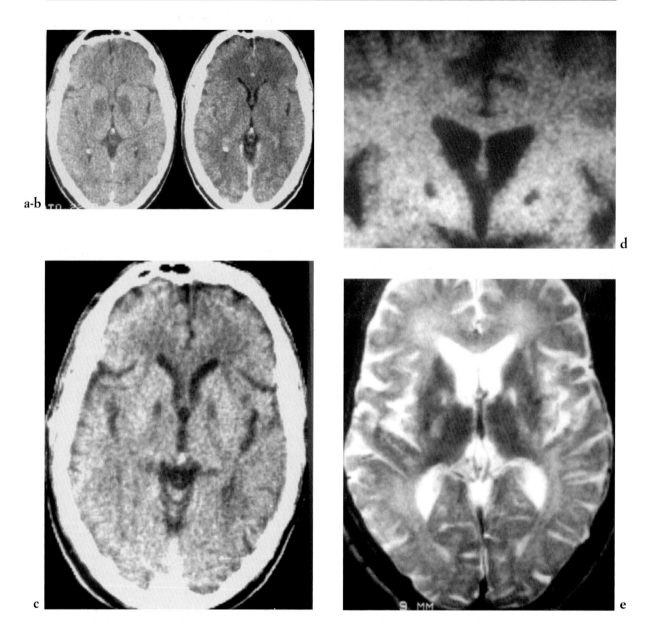

Fig. 4.13 - Acute carbon monoxide intoxication with cerebral necrosis. CT undertaken in the acute phase documents bilateral globus pallidus hypodensity and within the anterior frontal white matter on both sides. CT follow up approximately three weeks later reveals bilateral globus pallidus necrosis; MRI performed the same day as confirms globus pallidus necrosis and the frontal subcortical degenerative alteration. [**a**, **b**) acute phase axial CT; **c**) three week follow up CT; **d**) three week follow up T2-weighted MRI].

intoxication have shown that the altered signal areas are due to vasogenic rather than to intracellular oedema, thus supporting the direct endothelial damage theory. In 4 out of 14 cases of CsA intoxication, Schwartz, et al (24) observed the presence of cerebral haemorrhage, and in one case small focal areas of intraparenchymal haemorrhage in the occipital lobes. The grey matter is also rarely involved (5, 23, 24).

CARBON MONOXIDE (CO) INTOXICATION

CO intoxication causes ischaemia-based brain damage in preferential positions that have been known for some time. CO's affinity to haemoglobin is 250 times greater than that of the oxygen with which it competes, thus reducing haemoglobin's capacity to capture, trans-

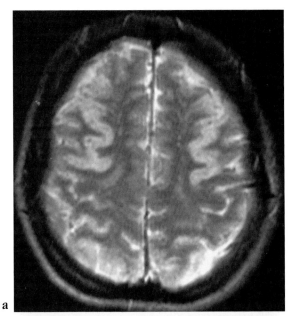

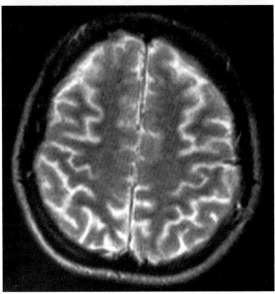

Fig. 4.14 - Acute carbon monoxide intoxication with clinicoradiologic resolution. T2-weighted MRI on patient admission shows swelling of the frontal lobe cortex, more prominent on the right side, resulting from cytotoxic oedema. Follow up MRI performed after clinical resolution reveals regression of the frontal swelling. [**a**, admission T2-weighted MRI; **b**) follow up T2-weighted MRI].

port and release oxygen. The presence of carboxyhaemoglobin shifts the haemoglobin's dissociation curve to the left, and CO hampers cellular respiration as it bonds with cytochrome oxydase and generates hypertension due to the myocardial dysfunction caused by the presence of carboxyhaemoglobin in the heart tissue.

In the brain, it is typically responsible for bilateral necrosis of the globus pallidus (Fig. 4.13) and the hippocampal structures, and for either diffuse or focal involvement of the white matter. The involvement of the white matter can be combined with that of the grey matter in the more distal vascular territories where capillary proliferation (Fig. 4.14) can be observed pathologically. CO intoxication may also have a specific direct toxic effect upon the globus pallidus, which would justify such selective involvement. This observation derives from the fact that in cases of non-CO-induced hypoxia, different structures such as the putamen, the caudate nucleus and the cerebral grey matter are typically involved. The interruption or delay in the transport of non-haematogenous iron through axonal structures damaged by the ischaemic insult is probably responsible for the low signal density detected in the basal ganglia on T2-dependent sequences (6, 14, 25, 26, 28, 29).

REFERENCES

1. Antunez E, Estruch R, Cardenal C: Usefulness of CT and MR imaging in the diagnosis of acute Wernicke's encephalopathy. AJR 171:1131-37; 1998.
2. Bracard S, Claude D et al: Computerized tomography and MRI in Marchiafava-Bignami disease. J Neuroradiol 13:87-94; 1986.
3. Brunner JE, Redmond JM et al: Central pontine myelinolysis and pontine lesions after rapid correction of hyponatremia: a prospective MRI study. Ann Neurol 27:61-7; 1990.
4. Chang KH, Cha SH et al: Marchiafava Bignami disease: serial changes in corpus callossum on MRI. Neuroradiology 34:480-2; 1992.
5. Debaere C, Stadnik T, De Maeseneer M: Diffusion-weighted MRI in cyclosporin A neurotoxicity for the classification of cerebral edema. Eur Radiol 9(9):1916-8; 1999.
6. Dietrich RB, Bradley WG: Iron accumulation in the basal ganglia following severe ischemic-anossic insult in children. Radiology 168:203-6; 1988.
7. Diez-Tejedor E, Frank A, Gutierrez M et al: Encephalopathy and biopsy-proven cerebrovascular inflammatory changes in a cocaine abuser. Eur J Neurol 5(1):103-7; 1998.
8. Donnal JF, Heinz ER, Burger PC: MR of reversible thalamic lesions in Wernicke syndrome. AJNR 11:893-5; 1990
9. Fazio C, Loeb C: Neurologia, Società Editrice Universo, Roma, 1994.
10. Gallucci M, Amicarelli I, Rossi A et al: MR imaging of white matter lesions in uncomplicated chronic alcoholism, J Comp Asst Tomogr 13:395-398, 1989.

11. Gallucci M, Bozzao A, Splendiani A et al: Wernicke encephalopathy: MR findings in five patients, AJNR 11:887-892, 1990.

12. Gallucci M, Caulo M et al: L'encefalopatia alcolica. Atti Meeting Scienze Neurologiche. Selva di Val Gardena, 1999.

13. Genevresse I, Dietzman A et al: Subacute encephalopathy after combination chemotherapy including moderate-dose methotrexate in a patient with gastric cancer. Anticancer Drug 10(3):293-4; 1999.

14. Horowitz AL, Kaplan R: Carbon monoxide toxicity: MR imaging in the brain. Radiology 162:787-8; 1987.

15. Ikeda M, Tsukagoshi H: Encephalopathy due to toluene sniffing. Report of a case with Magnetic Resonance Imaging. Eur Neurol 30(6):347-9; 1990.

16. Jansen O, Krieger D et al: Cortical hyperintesity on proton density-weighted images: an MR sign of cyclosporine-related encephalopathy. AJNR 17(2):337-44; 1996.

17. Kubo M, Azuma E, Arai S et al: Transient encephalopathy following a single exposure of high-dose methotrexate in a child with acute lymphoblastic leukemia. Pediatr Hematol Oncol 9(2):157-65; 1992.

18. Laubenberger J, Schneider B, Ansorge O et al: Central pontine myelinolysis: clinical presentation and radiologic findings. Eur. Radiol. 6:177-83; 1996.

19. Lohr JW: Osmotic demyelination syndrome following correction of hyponatremia: association with hypokalemia. Am J Med 96:408-12; 1994.

20. Lovblad K, Kelkar P et al: Pure methotrexate encephalopathy presenting with seizures: CT and MRI features. Pediatr Radiol 28(2):86-91; 1998.

21. Maschke M, Fehlings T, Kastrup O et al: Toxic leukoencephalopathy after intravenous consumption of heroine and cocaine with unexpected clinical recovery. J Neurol 246(9):850-1; 1999.

22. Mayer JW, De Liége P, Netter JM: Computerized tomography and nuclear magnetic resonance in Marchiafava-Bignami disease. J Neuroradiol 14:152-8; 1987.

23. Osborne AG: Diagnostic Neuroradiology. Mosby ed. St. Louis, Missouri, 1992.

24. Schwartz BR, Bravo MS, Klufas RA et al: Cyclosporine neurotoxicity and its relationship to hipertensive encephalopathy: CT and MR findings in 16 cases. AJR 165:627-31; 1995.

25. Shogry MEC, Curnes JT: Mamillary body enhancement on MR as the only sign of acute Wernicke encephalopathy. AJNR 15:172-4; 1994.

26. Silverman CS, Brenner J et al: Hemorragic necrosis and vascular injury in carbon monoxide poisoning: MR demonstration. AJNR 14:168-70; 1993.

27. Thuomas KA, Moller C, Odkvist LM et al: MR imaging in solvent-induced chronic toxic encephalopathy. Acta Radiol 37(2):177-9; 1996.

28. Valk J, van der Knaap: Toxic encephalopathy. AJNR 13 (2):747-60; 1992.

29. Valk J, van der Knaap MS: Magnetic resonance of myelin, myelination and myelin disorders. Springer edition 1995.

4.2

THE NEURORADIOLOGICAL APPROACH
TO PATIENTS IN COMA

G.M. Di Lella, M. Rollo, T. Tartaglione, C. Colosimo

INTRODUCTION

Coma is rightly considered to be the one of the most commonly occurring neurological emergency conditions. Coma can be the consequence of an entire spectrum of pathological conditions and thus requires equally varied but quite specific treatment (8, 15, 16). Neuroradiological studies are often the only real practical option for initial diagnostic patient investigation, as the clinician may have access to little or no information when the patient is admitted.

In such situations, it is almost always Computed Tomography (CT) that assumes the leading role in the initial diagnostic, prognostic and therapeutic approach. The fundamental question is whether or not there are documentable intracranial neuroanatomical alterations, which, if present, can be subsequently monitored after the patient is admitted to the intensive care suite.

We will not deal in detail here with the entire spectrum of the intracranial pathology responsible for causing coma, as they are dealt with separately in the various chapters of this volume; instead, we will briefly outline the optimal neuroradiological approach to be utilized in patients in coma including: a) the modes of investigation; b) the related technical variables; c) conditions causing acute focal lesions (9), and d) conditions causing diffuse brain impairment.

MODES OF INTRACRANIAL ANALYSIS

The neuroradiological evaluation can be divided into two clinical phases: the initial evaluation and the re-evaluation of the patient over time. The aim of the initial evaluation is to detect or exclude focal alterations and to define the overall status of the tissues within the intracranial compartment. As an example, the revelation of demonstrable focal cerebral lesions eliminates clinical suspicion of a metabolic or toxic cause of coma, while the opposite can prompt and direct swift specific medical or surgical treatment. A typical example of this is the demonstration of an extracerebral haematoma that requires immediate surgical evacuation.

We will ultimately go on to describe the elementary cerebral alterations implied in coma. However, first we intend to underline the importance of an overall evaluation of the in-

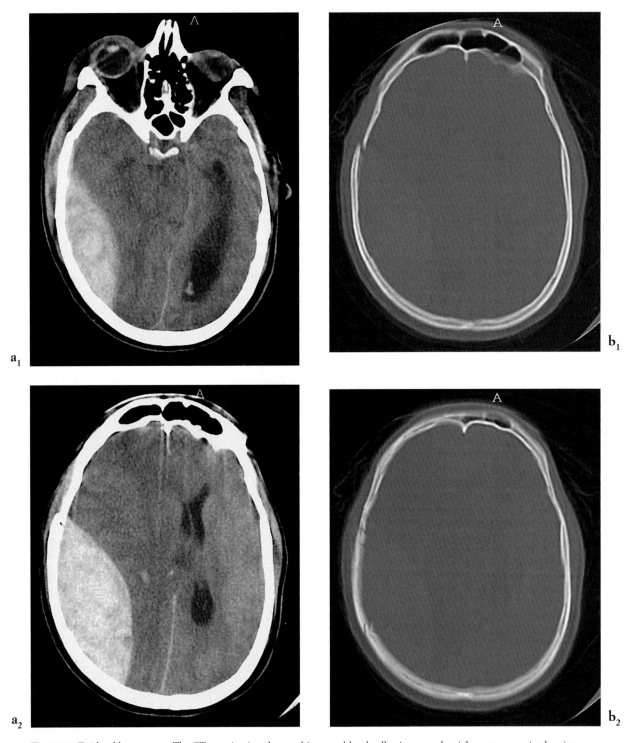

Fig. 4.15 - Epidural haematoma. The CT examination shows a biconvex blood collection over the right temporoparietal region associated with marked mass effect. Note the displacement of the surrounding parenchymal structures associated with leftward midline subfalcian herniation and compression of the right lateral ventricle. In the more caudal scan, ipsilateral downward herniation of the uncus is also clearly visible. In addition, there is a fracture in the right temporal bone, with minor fragment displacement. CT follow up three months later documents encephalomalacia of the posterior temporal lobe, perhaps as a result of infarction secondary compression-occlusion of the posterior cerebral artery caused by the uncal herniation. [a_{1-2}) initial axial unenhanced CT with brain windows; b_{1-2}) initial axial CT with bone windows; **c**) three month follow up axial CT].

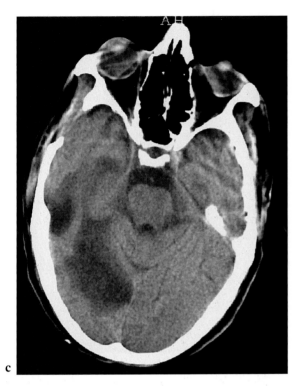

c

Fig. 4.15 (*cont.*).

tracranial compartment, which is subject to particular pressure balances, the alteration of which is often closely related to the patient's clinical evolution and prognosis.

The importance of the effects of relatively sudden changes upon the contents of the intracranial compartment hinges upon its being a "closed system" with a fixed volume. This compartment has a strict relationship between its rigid container (the skull) and its contents (cerebral parenchyma, CSF and blood). Any condition that creates a change in intracranial pressure (ICP) will have a direct effect on what is visualized on CT and/or MR studies. An increase in ICP can alter cerebral blood flow (CBF) and even completely obstruct it when cerebral perfusion pressure (PP) is exceeded. Any alteration that causes an increase in intracranial contents shows signs of mass effect on either CT or MRI. Mass lesions above all are defined by the effacement and displacement of the intracranial fluid-filled spaces. The mass effect

and their corresponding CT/MR findings are initially observed locally and subsequently in a more widespread manner. As cerebral swelling increases, the structures contained in the expanding intracranial compartment are displaced beyond the boundaries of that compartment. Ultimately this may result in internal cerebral herniation. In the case of monohemispheric swelling, this herniation may occur below or beyond the falx cerebri (i.e., subfalcian herniation) or downward through the tentorial incisura with dislocation of the uncus of the temporal lobe (i.e., descending uncal herniation). In the case of infratentorial compartment swelling, portions of the cerebellum and brainstem are pushed upward through the tentorial hiatus (i.e., ascending transtentorial herniation) or downward through the foramen magnum into the proximal cervical spinal canal (i.e., descending tonsillar herniation). This internal cerebral herniation represents the displacement, distortion and compression of the involved neural parenchyma and attendant vascular structures.

The most severe and sometimes fatal effect of these internal cerebral herniations is dysfunction of the brainstem, which can be impaired in any of the descending uncal, ascending transtentorial and descending forms of tonsillar herniation. The complete effacement of the cisternal spaces surrounding the brainstem, the distortion/dislocation of the brainstem and the direct demonstration of uncal herniation (Fig. 4.15) (i.e., medial and downward displacement of the uncus or unci) are quite common findings in patients in coma induced by acute, rapidly forming mass lesions, whatever the underlying cause. On axial CT, the signs of uncal herniation are typically easily recognized, whereas herniations caused by expanding subtentorial lesions may be less apparent; in this latter case the dislocation occurs in an upward caudocranial direction which has far less obvious findings on axial CT images (Fig. 4.16). In the case of ascending transtentorial herniations, one must search for the disappearance of the superior cerebellar cisternal spaces and for the inversion, distor-

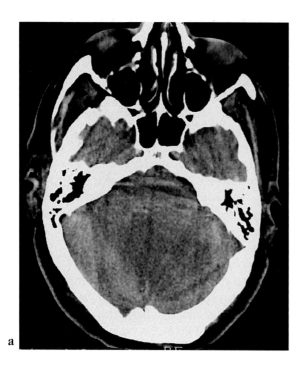

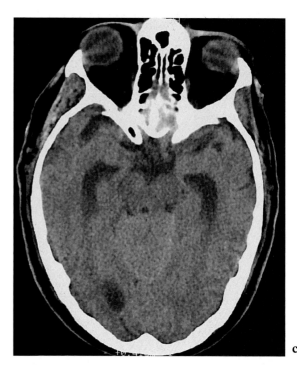

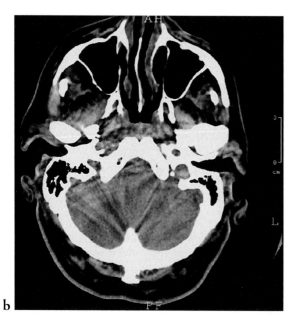

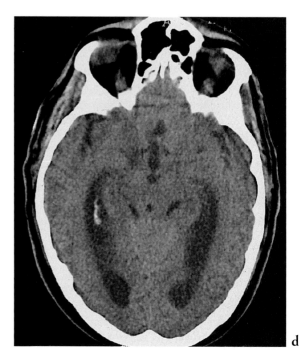

Fig. 4.16 - Acute infratentorial ischaemic swelling. Unenhanced cranial CT demonstrates a large area of hypodensity in the cerebellar vermis and hemispheres bilaterally. Note the evidence of ascending transtentorial herniation: the tentorial hiatus and the ambient cistern are both effaced. Also note the acute obstructive hydrocephalus with signs of transependymal extravasation of CSF from the lateral ventricular margins. [**a-e**) unenhanced axial CT].

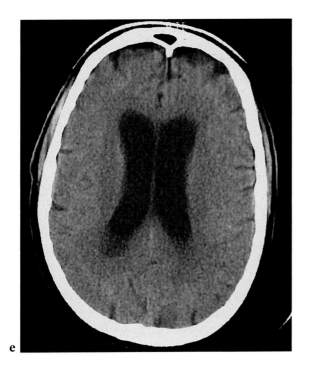

e

Fig. 4.16 (*cont.*).

tion or absence of the normally posteriorly directed convexity of the quadrigeminal plate/cistern. In the event of downward tonsillar herniation, special attention must be paid to the peribulbar CSF spaces and to the cisterna magna; with the progressive improvement in the quality of CT images, it is currently possible to observe clearly the downward displacement of the cerebellar tonsils into the foramen magnum.

Compression of the parenchyma of the brain stem can have very severe clinical consequences, especially if acute. However, the effect of the internal cerebral herniation upon the related blood vessels may also result in a considerable worsening of the neurological situation. This blood vessel involvement may result in venous stasis and ischaemia, itself engendering a further increase in cerebral swelling. This is the case, for example, in ischaemic infarction within the territory of the posterior cerebral artery consequent to its compression-occlusion in the perimesencephalic segment caused by the direct external mass effect of the descending uncal herniation (Fig. 4.15).

The pressure effects described can set in rapidly under the force of a large, rapidly growing haemorrhagic collection such as an epidural haematoma, however, more frequently these observations are the result of a combination of the primary mass lesion coupled with related phenomena such as oedema, complications of ischaemia or widespread brain swelling engendered by vasospasm. Changes in the mass effect and the formation of internal cerebral herniation follow very variable chronological patterns that often do not correspond to objective clinical neurological signs that might otherwise be useful in evaluating evolution of the overall process. Direct measurements of ICP and its patterns over time using subdural or subarachnoid catheters do provide one important objective parameter; however, this procedure is not always possible, and it is only available in specialized neurosurgery centres. This calls for frequent CT re-evaluations, properly integrated with other diagnostic techniques such as MRI or transcranial-echo colour Doppler, as required. Therefore, requests for frequent diagnostic imaging checks by resuscitation staff must not be considered superfluous on either a clinical basis or in order to justify difficult ICP measurements. The CT findings may in fact change dramatically in the course of just a few hours, in a crescendo that can only be controlled by swift implementation of appropriate treatment.

With regard to serial re-valuation of the evolution of intracranial findings in patients with coma, we must point out the significance of hydrocephalus associated with the primary pathology. In the case of diffuse brain swelling caused by a principal insult (e.g., trauma, haemorrhage with vasospasm, etc.), the onset of hydrocephalus can have dramatic consequences. Therefore, it is necessary to make a correct diagnosis early in its progress, before marked ventricular dilatation occurs. The earliest signs of hydrocephalus must be recognized, such as mild dilatation and outward rounding of the margins of the temporal horns of the lateral ventricles (Figs. 4.16, 4.17).

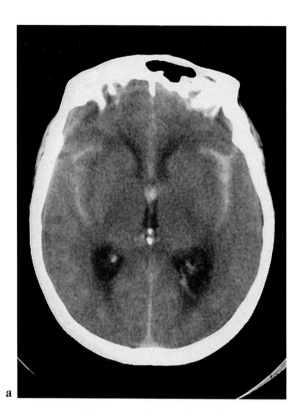

a

TECHNICAL CONSIDERATIONS

The technical approach adopted when treating patients in coma does not vary greatly from that generally applied in most cranial emergencies as has been described in the previous chapters. The general scheme uses CT as the initial examination technique, backed up by MRI and, less frequently, by other techniques that may prove useful in patients in critical condition.

CT is the preferred method of imaging in coma patients due to its very rapid examination acquisition speeds, with single or multiple slice scanning times faster than one second in latest generation appliances; in addition to its general diagnostic capabilities, it is also very sensitive in recognizing acute and hyperacute phase intracranial haemorrhages, in localizing the cranial compartment of the bleed (e.g., subdural/epidural, subarachnoid, intraparenchymal); finally it is almost universally available in the

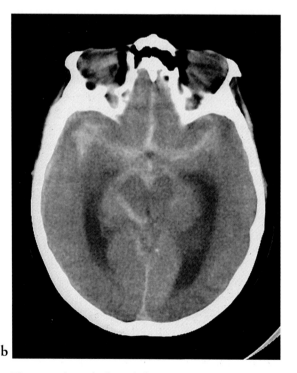

b

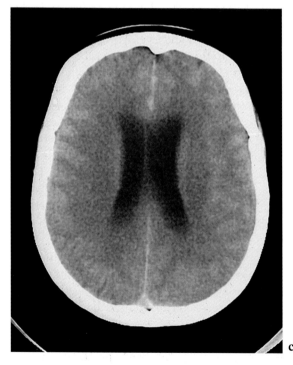

c

Fig. 4.17 - Acute hydrocephalus in a case of spontaneous subarachnoid haemorrhage. Unenhanced cranial CT shows an intraventricular blood clot at the level of the foramina of Monro and the symmetrical subarachnoid haemorrhage. Also note the dilatation of the lateral ventricles, including the temporal horns, as a consequence of the obstructive hydrocephalus. [a-c) unenhanced axial CT]

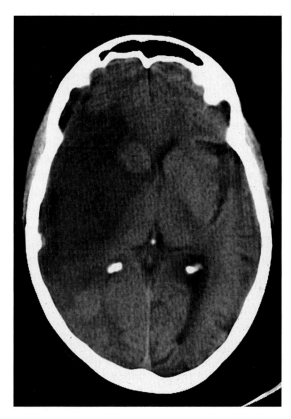

Fig. 4.18 - Subacute cerebral infarction within the right middle cerebral artery territory. Unenhanced cranial CT shows widespread cortical-subcortical hypodensity in the right temporoparietal region. Moderate mass effect is present, as a result of vasogenic oedema, represented by the effacement of the regional superficial subarachnoid spaces and the compression of the right lateral ventricle.

various communities of industrialized regions (Figs. 4.15, 4.17, 4.19).

MRI maintains a secondary role, in part because of its low sensitivity in demonstrating haemorrhages in the early phases of evolution, its rather long scan acquisition times making it unsuitable for use in non-cooperative patients and those in critical condition, and the still rather scarce availability of MRI appliances in some hospitals and healthcare centres.

Despite these limits, in the near future it is likely that MRI will be more frequently applied as scanning times are drastically reduced and as specific techniques for early detection of cerebral parenchymal haemorrhage become more readily available.

One example of this technological advancement is the recent introduction of diffusion techniques, which enable the very early detection of cerebral ischaemia and other pathological conditions characterized by cytotoxic/intracellular oedema utilizing very fast scanning times employing echo-planar acquisition sequences. Diffusion imaging makes it possible to detect parenchymal injury at a very early stage, when CT images are completely negative. In addition, diffusion imaging is equally sensitive in demonstrating posttraumatic diffuse axonal injury (Fig. 4.19) (4).

The rapid progress in MRI angiography and CT angiography (the latter especially since the recent introduction of multidetector appliances) has made it somewhat rare to have to resort to the use of invasive selective angiography in coma patients. Invasive angiographic techniques are currently primarily used following the CT or MR diagnosis of vascular malformations, where angiography remains important for the fine definition of the angioarchitecture of the documented malformation. While on the subject of vascular examinations it should be pointed out that when monitoring coma patients, especially in resuscitation centres, transcranial Doppler and transcranial echo-colour-Doppler may assume fundamental roles due to their ability to evaluate and quantify CBF (3, 5).

These techniques can also be used to evaluate reductions in cerebral perfusion pressure and vasoparalysis in order to rebalance CBF on the basis of ICP trends (1, 2).

ACUTE PRIMARY FOCAL CEREBRAL LESIONS

Haemorrhage

In the acute phase, freshly clotted blood has a density of approximately 70-80 H.U. It therefore appears hyperdense in comparison to the surrounding cerebral parenchyma; however, when fluid in consistency, newly extravasated blood can appear relatively isodense. Over time the CT density of the haematoma tends to decrease, with

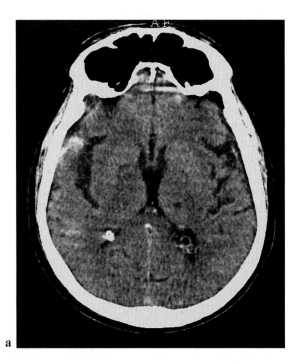

a

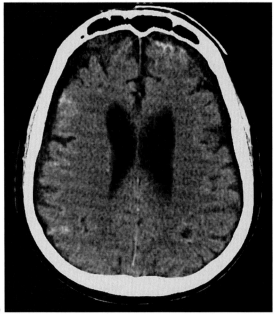

b

Fig. 4.19 - Diffuse axonal injury (damage). Unenhanced cranial CT shows the presence of multiple, small cortical-subcortical junction haemorrhagic foci. These haemorrhages are an expression of axonal shearing, some of which are not visible due to the absence of bleeding. The parenchymal, and therefore functional, damage is often greater than predicted on the basis of CT alone. [**a**, **b**) unenhanced axial CT].

an eventual evolution towards hypo- isodensity, a phenomenon that begins in the outside layers and moves inward towards the centre of the haematoma. The time required for the above-mentioned alterations depends on the size and site of the blood collection; in general, parenchymal haemorrhages remain hyperdense for many days and only appear frankly hypodense after several weeks. The evolution of mass effect follows a similar pattern: after a few hours, as oedema grows, the mass effect increases; in the absence of treatment, mass effect reaches a peak after 3-5 days, before gradually shrinking and disappearing, resulting in a loss of brain substance in late stages after many weeks or even months.

As mentioned previously, MRI at present is far less sensitive relative than CT in its ability to recognize the hyperacute phase haemorrhages: oxyhaemoglobin present a nearly or completely isointense signal in almost all image sequences (both T1- and T2-dependent sequences). With the subsequent transformation into methaemoglobin, MRI becomes more specific and sensitive than CT: initially the methaemoglobin that is contained within the non-lysed red cells presents a signal that is hyperintense on T1- and isointense on T2-weighted MR sequences, whereas subsequently, with the lysis of the red blood cells, extracellular methaemoglobin appears hyperintense on all sequences. Lastly, the subsequent evolution of the bleed into haemosiderin results in the haemorrhage becoming hypointense on T2-weighted sequences. This is especially apparent if the acquisitions (e.g., gradient recalled echo) are sensitive to the presence of paramagnetic substances (e.g., haemosiderin and ferritin) (11).

Cerebral ischaemia

In the hyperacute phase, the CT and MR manifestations of cerebral ischaemia consist mainly in cytotoxic oedema (Fig. 4.20); subsequently, from 12-24 hours later, vasogenic oedema appears, enlarges and becomes more readily visible, this in part due to mass effect (Fig. 4.16) (10, 13). Early CT signs of ischaemia are particularly evident in the lentiform nucleus (when the deep territory of

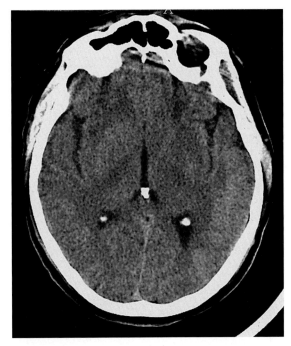

Fig. 4.20 - Cytotoxic oedema. Unenhanced cranial CT reveals a subtle absence of the normal hyperdensity of the left putamen as compared to the contralateral structure, indicating the presence of ischaemic cytotoxic oedema.

totoxic oedema. Cytotoxic oedema, an expression of cellular injury, principally involves the cerebral cortex and the basal nuclei of the cerebral hemispheres. Oedema generally shows a relative reduction in density on CT, a reduction in signal on T1-weighted MR and hyperintensity in T2-weighted sequences. Clinical practice has recently witnessed the introduction of T2-dependent FLAIR sequences (Fig. 4.22), on which abnormal signal alterations adjacent to the superficial and deep subarachnoid spaces are more immediately recognizable, thanks to the choice of parameters that cancel out the CSF signal; these sequences are currently the most sensitive in demonstrating oedema and pathological tissue in general in the acute phase of patient deterioration. Oedema can also be recognized by its mass effect, however, this may be very modest in the cytotoxic phase; in this early time period, the oedema may appear on CT not as hypodensity, but simply as a loss of the slight normal physi-

the middle cerebral artery is affected) due to the disappearance of its normal physiological hyperdensity. This finding, which can sometimes be very slight, is strengthened by any finding of clear hyperdensity (thrombosis, embolism) in the lumen of the first segment of the middle cerebral artery; in the same manner, this CT hyperdense signal can be observed in the basilar artery in cases of acute thrombosis/embolism.

Utilizing classic T1- and T2-weighted MR acquisitions in the initial phase of cerebral ischemia, findings and sensitivity are similar to those of CT. However, with new diffusion weighted sequences, both sensitivity and specificity are far greater relative to CT and enable, when appropriate, the prompt application of systemic or selective intraarterial antithrombotic treatment.

Cerebral oedema

Cerebral oedema is a non-specific phenomenon. Many events can cause intracellular cy-

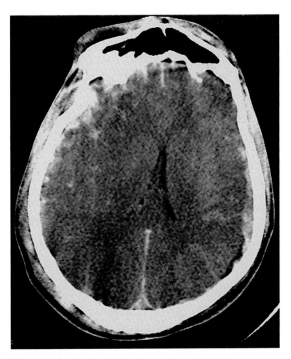

Fig. 4.21 - Brain death. Unenhanced cranial CT demonstrates bilateral subdural and subarachnoid blood collections. There is also diffuse brain swelling, with loss of the grey-white matter differentiation, and bilateral compression of the cerebral ventricular system due to parenchymal oedema.

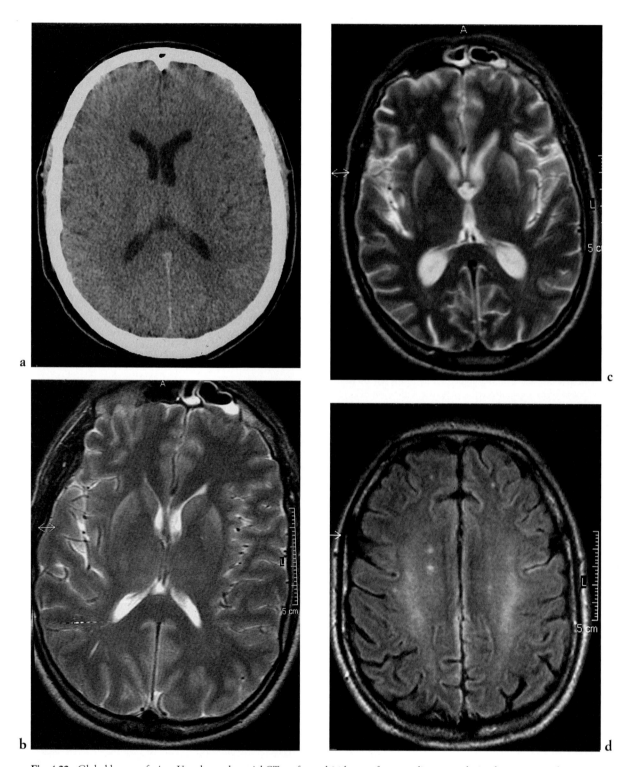

Fig. 4.22 - Global hypoperfusion. Unenhanced cranial CT performed 24 hours after a cardiac arrest during heart surgery documents relative isodensity of the lenticular nuclei bilaterally. Axial T2-weighted MRI 48 hours after the event reveals MRI signal hyperintensity within the lenticular nuclei. Axial T2-weighted and FLAIR MRI 3 weeks later demonstrates minor dilation of the ventricular system as a result of resolution of cerebral swelling, and an increase in the hyperintensity of the MRI signal of the lenticular nuclei. The FLAIR image at 3 weeks shows hyperintense cortical-subcortical MRI signal alterations. [**a**) initial axial CT; **b**) axial T2-weighted MRI at 48 hours; **c**) axial T2-weighted MRI at 3 weeks; **d**) axial FLAIR MRI at 3 weeks].

ological hyperdensity of grey matter in relation to the white matter (i.e., loss of grey-white matter differentiation).

Solid/cystic/mixed neoplastic lesions

Patients with solid/cystic/mixed neoplastic lesions may also present acutely, because of a sudden worsening in intracranial hypertension, due for instance to intratumoral haemorrhage (13), acute obstructive hydrocephalus or following a seizure precipitated by the tumor. The general CT/MRI findings will not be dealt with in this chapter, but once again the general rule applies that in such cases CT is suitable for the initial diagnosis and analysis in emergency situations, whereas MRI is better suited to more complete and definitive evaluation after the acute stage has passed.

WIDESPREAD INSULT/BRAIN SWELLING

The main clinical and radiological aspects appropriate to dealing with intracranial emergencies are dealt with in specific chapters, however, we will here examine a number of different conditions that may present with coma with varying aetiology. We will also demonstrate how, in addition to CT and MRI, important information can be gleaned from their integration with other imaging techniques.

Both conditions resulting in widespread brain swelling (especially of traumatic aetiology associated with DAI) and those associated with vasospasm (especially that caused by subarachnoid haemorrhage) have important consequences on CBF (6, 7, 17). These lead to diffuse ischaemic injury, with further brain swelling, greater increases in ICP and therefore a more marked reduction in CBF. In the case of DAI (13), the primary injury is accompanied by the exacerbating effect of compression of and damage to the hypothalamic substructure that in itself leads to a loss of vascular autoregulation.

Transcranial Doppler and transcranial echo colour-Doppler make it possible to monitor variations in the speed of flow in arterial segments undergoing vasospasm. In conditions of normal or slightly raised ICP, the increase in flow velocity (systolic or diastolic) represents compensation between the reduction in arterial calibre and the perfusion downstream from the arterial narrowing. In conditions of significant increases in ICP, a gradual increase in flow resistance occurs, with a drop in flow velocity (mainly diastolic) and a consequent reduction in overall peripheral perfusion. DAI can affect the substance of the thalamus and the brainstem, tissues that are responsible for cerebral vascular autoregulation, a physiological phenomenon that is aimed at maintaining CBF constant over a range of cerebral PP's between 60 and 150 mm Hg.

When cerebral PP drops below the minimum threshold in a brain trauma patient, cerebral hypoperfusion occurs as a result of progressively enlarging intracranial hypertension. Transcranial Doppler velocity measurements enable the identification of an increase or decrease in cerebral arterial flow speeds, which are generally in line with CBF alterations. CBF increases secondary to increased flow velocity caused by vasoparalysis are responsible for an increase in ICP and therefore the gradual, progressive decrease in CBF ultimately leading to the condition of cerebral vascular stasis (12, 17).

In recent years, establishing the diagnosis of brain death has gained particular importance because of the consonant importance in the harvesting of transplant organs from patients in irreversible coma. In addition to neurophysiological and metabolic tests, current regulations also require the certification of cerebral blood flow arrest (cerebral vascular stasis).

In such situations, angiography and transcranial ECD can be used for this purpose. Angiographic examinations document the stoppage of contrast medium progression within the internal carotid arteries and within the basilar artery, in the absence of delayed opacification of the cerebral arteries. Stasis of the arterial structures in the infratentorial compartment typically follows that of the supratentorial region (Fig. 4.21).

Another important clinicoradiological situation to consider is the condition consequent to widespread hypoperfusion (caused for instance by massive coronary infarction or prolonged severe systemic hypotension) or to global hypoxygenation (13) (for example following carbon monoxide inhalation). The most frequently affected areas are those with highest physiological oxygen demand, such as the basal nuclei of the cerebral hemispheres and the cerebral cortex. CT is usually negative immediately after the event, but may subsequently (Fig. 4.22) reveal the disappearance of the normal physiological hyperdensity of basal nuclei and the differential density between grey and white matter. On occasion, the only sign of such pathology is a non-specific observation of brain swelling. MRI performed on the 2nd-7th day following the inciting event documents with greater certainty the alteration in signal of the basal ganglia and later the typical cortical necrosis having a gyriform (laminar) distribution. Evolution towards a severe generalized atrophy of the affected regions can ensue rather quickly.

REFERENCES

1. Aaslid R, Lindegaard KF: Cerebral hemodynamics in transcranial doppler sonography. Aaslid R., Ed. Wien Springer-Verlag 60-85, 1986.

2. Aaslid R, Markwalder TM, Nornes H: Noninvasive transcranial doppler ultrasound of flow velocity in basal cerebral arteries. J Neurosurgery 57, 769-774, 1982.

3. Ahman PA, Carrigan TA, Carlton D et al: Brain death in children: characteristics common carotid arterial velocity patterns measured with pulsed doppler ultrasound. J. Pediatr. 110, 723-728, 1987.

4. Castillo M. et al: New techniques in MR neuroimaging. MRI Clinics of North America. Saunders 1998.

5. Chan CH, Dearden MN, Miller DJ et al: Transcranial doppler waveform differencies in hyperemic and nonhyperemic patients after severe head injury. Surg. Neur. 38, 433-436, 1992.

6. Gean M: Head trauma. Raven Press 1994.

7. Gentry LR: Current concepts in Imaging Cranio-facial trauma. Neuroimaging Clinics of North America. December 1991.

8. Grossmann RI, Younsem DM: Neuroradiology: the requisites. Mosby, St. Louis 1994.

9. Hachinskj V, Norris JW: Ictus. Athena editrice Roma 1988.

10. Masakuni Kameyama, Masanori Tomonaga, Tadashi Aiba: Cerebrovascular disease. Igaku-Shoin, Tokjo-New York 1988.

11. Hayman LA: Nontraumatic intracranial hemorrhage. Neuroimaging Clinic of North America 2:1, 1992.

12. Kassel NF, Sasaki T, Colohan Art et al: Cerebral vasospasm following aneurismal subarachnoid hemorrage. Stroke 16, 573-581, 1985.

13. Osborne A: Diagnostic neuroradiology. Mosby Year Book 1994.

14. Osborne A: Handbook of Neuroradiology. Mosby Year Book 1991.

15. Scarabino T, Cammisa M: Urgenze cranio-spinali: diagnostica per immagini. Ed. Liviana 1993.

16. Scotti G: Manuale di Neuroradiologia diagnostica e terapeutica. Masson 1993.

17. Seckhar L, Wechsler LR, Yonas H, et al: Value of TCD examination in the diagnosis of cerebral vasospasm after subarachnoid hemorrage. Neurosurg. 22, 813-821, 1988.

4.3

NUCLEAR MEDICINE IN NEUROLOGICAL EMERGENCIES

M.G. Bonetti, P. Ciritella, G. Valle, T. Scarabino

INTRODUCTION

The observation, clinical evaluation and prognosis of coma patients is always a demanding matter and one that requires reliable diagnostic instruments capable of providing answers in real time. This evaluation is further complicated by the varying aetiology of comas of acute onset. Some of the most frequent causes of coma include: head injuries, brain tumours, cerebrovascular lesions, meningitis, encephalitis and cerebral abscesses, epilepsy (postcritical coma), exogenous intoxication, endogenous intoxication (metabolic coma, severe hydroelectrolytic imbalances), respiratory insufficiency, and cardiocirculatory insufficiency. However, irrespective of the cause of the coma, the pathophysiology of functional brain damage rests on dynamic factors whose evolution must be recognized and monitored with care.

We believe that in neuroresuscitation, alongside the essential, accurate objective neurological examination and monitoring of cardiorespiratory and metabolic functions, diagnostic examinations with medical instruments are finding an increasingly important place. It is now possible to study the many aspects of cerebral pathophysiology using neurophysiological (e.g.: EEG, evoked potentials), morphological (e.g.: CT, MRI) and functional (e.g.: PET, SPECT) methods aimed at swiftly understanding events that alter the balance between the various components of the cranioencephalic system and cerebral perfusion.

Alterations in cerebral perfusion can be studied using two possible categories of analysis: invasive (e.g.: measuring ICP; measuring the jugular venous saturation of oxygen, $SvjO_2$; conventional selective angiography) and non-invasive (transcranial Doppler [TCD] and radionuclide scintigraphy of brain perfusion [SPECT]).

The introduction of SPECT into clinical neuroresuscitation practice has made it possible to obtain more rapid and accurate diagnoses and make more certain prognostic judgements. The most satisfactory results have been obtained in the examination of postanoxic coma, where perfusion parameters have proved reliable for guiding therapy, and in cases of suspected brain death, where SPECT is useful in dispelling doubts in either direction. In cases of posttraumatic coma or coma caused by stroke, brain perfusion as determined by SPECT has enabled a more certain prognostic prediction.

MEASURING CBF

The brain is the organ that more than any other requires a constant supply of oxygen and glucose transported by the blood (7). Measuring CBF makes it possible to visualize the haemodynamic and pathophysiological consequences of intracerebral pathology.

At the current time, there are no valid alternatives to the use of radionuclides to obtain quantitative flow measurements, especially in the posterior cerebral fossa and brainstem. The principal methods of the various techniques for studying CBF with gamma-emitting radioactive tracers are shown in Table 4.1. In our experience, we have used the repartition method utilizing hexamethyl propylene-amine-oxime (HMPAO) marked with 99mTc as a tracer.

The main steps of the technique we use are as follows (1, 3):

1. intravenous injection of a 99mTC HM-PAO;

2. when the fat-soluble HM-PAO molecules are taken by the blood to the brain, they pass through the blood-brain barrier, with a high extraction from the blood bed, and bond to the brain tissue;

3. as a consequence the distribution within the brain is proportionate to the regional cerebral blood flow (rCBF);

4. a bond between the HM-PAO molecule and the cerebral tissue forms and remains constant for at least one hour (sufficient time in which to perform the SPECT examination);

5. subsequent redistribution of the molecule in the white and grey matter.

The interpretation of the images obtained using brain SPECT with hexametazyme is based on visual criteria (through a comparison with chromatic scales correlated with the levels of radioactivity recorded in the various areas of the brain) and on the possibility of a semiquantitative study performed by comparing homologous areas with gamma-emission differences higher than 12-16%. In particular, in all those cases in which a cerebral hemisphere, or part of it, is significantly differently perfused than the contralateral, it is possible to calculate a perfusion ratio using the following expression (2):

$$\text{Perfusion ratio} = \frac{\text{Counts/pixel affected side x 100}}{\text{Counts/pixel healthy side}}$$

The resulting value constitutes a measurement of the asymmetry between the two hemispheres.

SPECT also makes it possible to make a more accurate prognostic evaluation of the underlying problem, which is usually simply classified into a favourable or unfavourable prognosis (Table 4.1).

Method	Radiotracer	Advantages/Disadvantages
Vascular Clearance	133Xe	A: quantitative (if intracarotid injection) D: invasive
Dilution	99mTcO$_4$ 99mTc-albumin 99mTc-DTPA	A: simple, easily available radiotracer D: not quantitative
Repartition	99mTc-HM-PAO 123I-IMP	A: steady state D: unknown uptake process

Tab. 4.1 - Prognostic evaluation of cerebral lesions by SPECT.

Good prognosis	Bad prognosis
Meningeal lesions	Focal lesions
Not focal lesions	Many lesions
Small lesions	Large lesions
Few lesions	Parietal lesions
Occipital lesions	Brainstem lesions
Frontal lesions	Cerebellar lesions
	Temporal lesions

Tab. 4.2 - Prognostic evaluation of brain lesion using SPECT.

In our practice we use a rotating gammacamera with a single dedicated head (GE 400 AC, Milwaukee, Wisconsin, USA) a few minutes after an intravenous injection of freshly prepared 950 MBq of 99mTc -HM-PAO (Ceretec, Amersham-Sorin, Saluggia, Italy).The following acquisition parameters are used: 64 planar images with a 1.6x zoom, 64 x 64 pixel matrix, radius of rotation = 15 cm (on average), 20% symmetric window on photopeak of 140 keV of the 99mTc, acquisition time 25-30 minutes and a general purpose parallel hole collimator.

During the examination the patient is ventilated using a portable automatic respirator (Puritan Bennet Companion 2801, USA), monitoring blood pressure with a portable electronic modulus (Propaq 102, Protocol System Inc. Oregon, USA); ECG and the arterial saturation of O_2 of the haemoglobin is determined with a peripheral digital detector.

CLINICAL USAGE OF HM-PAO SPECT

The study of brain perfusion in coma patients has come to be part of routine clinical practice in our Resuscitation Centre in all those cases in which conventional neurophysiological and radiological techniques are inadequate in providing a reliable prognostic estimate. The findings from a number of coma patients are summarized in the text below. For comparative purposes, Fig. 4.23 shows a SPECT image for a normal brain.

Posttraumatic coma

SPECT's superiority over CT in studying head injuries that do not demonstrate focal le-

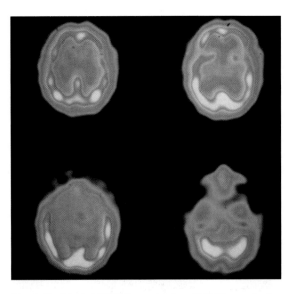

Fig. 4.23 - Normal SPECT examination. SPECT examination of the brain utilising 99mTC HM-PAO in a healthy subject for comparison.

sions consists mainly in its ability to detect pathophysiological cerebral perfusion alterations before the appearance of gross injuries that CT can detect (8).

Cerebral ischaemia can be a consequence of vasospasm occurring immediately after a trauma or following episodes of cardiocirculatory instability. This situation calls for serial studies of cerebral flow in order to detect either increases or decreases in perfusion. CBF also correlated with the final clinical outcome: persistently low CBF values have an unfavourable prognosis, whereas patients whose CBF rapidly returns to normal levels will typically have a better recovery.

Another important aspect of CBF measurements is that SPECT highlights a reduction in flow that may be directly proportionate to the degree of cerebral oedema. For example, an increase in cerebral oedema can reduce or even completely interrupt CBF.

Clinical Case

PATIENT	T.R.
AGE	25 years
DIAGNOSIS	head injury
GCS on admission	5
SAPS (Simplified acute Physiology Score)	8

The CT examination (Fig. 4.24) was negative for focal lesions; the BAEP's determination (Brainstem Auditory Evoked Potentials) was normal. The scintigraphic study of cerebral perfusion in this patient showed (Fig. 4.25) multiple small perfusion defects in both cerebral hemispheres, with good perfusion of the cerebral cortex. The patient came out of coma approximately one month from the injury. He was subsequently referred to a functional rehabilitation centre in order to complete the recovery of neuromuscular activity.

Acute cerebrovascular pathology

To reiterate, in studies of rCBF in cerebrovascular disease, SPECT is able to document flow alterations at an early stage, within a few hours after the trauma. This is observed before CT becomes positive, which in this stage occurs in less than 1 case every 5. Serial rCBF studies have considerable prognostic importance: patients with limited perfusion defects subsequently generally show complete or near complete recovery, whereas almost 50% of pa-

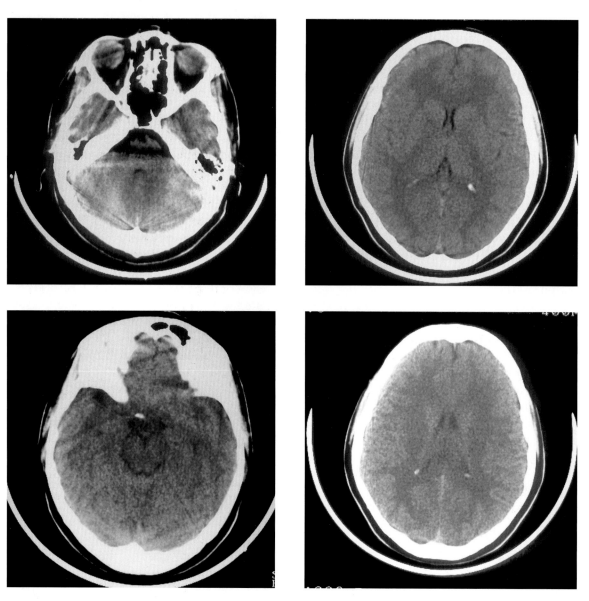

Fig. 4.24 - Post-traumatic coma. Unenhanced CT shows no abnormality.

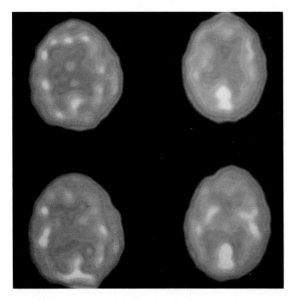

Fig. 4.25 - Same case as in Fig. 4.24. Left hand images: SPECT images reveal multiple small perfusion defects. Right hand images: Another normal case is shown on the right for comparison.

tients with diffuse areas of hypoperfusion, or especially a complete absence of perfusion (4,5), have an unfavourable outcome as is shown in the following case.

Clinical Case

PATIENT	A. G.
AGE	75 years
DIAGNOSIS	right temporoparietal haemorrhage
GCS on admission	6
SAPS	14

CT documented the presence of an extensive right temporoparietal haemorrhagic focus with lateral ventricular compression and midline shift (Fig. 4.26). SPECT demonstrated a large area of perfusion absence involving the upper portion of the right parietal lobe that extended more caudally, frontally, medially and posteriorly, thereby including the right subcortical grey matter structures. Overall, the remaining cerebral cortical and subcortical structures appeared to be well perfused. Crossed cerebellar diaschisis was also present (Fig. 4.27).

A subsequent SPECT examination performed approximately one month from the first study documented (Fig. 4.28): discreet improvement of the perfusion in a right posterior-frontal region, immediately in front of the haemorrhagic area; marked recovery of perfusion at the right temporal level, substantial normalization of the crossed cerebellum diaschisis. Overall, the picture showed a more or less complete recovery of perfusion within the areas of ischaemic penumbra surrounding the haemorrhage. Nevertheless, the patient, who died approximately 6 months after the stroke due to the extent of the original focus, was unable to recover beyond the level of coma.

Postanoxic coma

The cerebral consequences of cardiocirculatory arrest often determine the vital prognosis regardless of the success of the initial cardiopulmonary resuscitation. In fact, only 15-30% of patients with cardiopulmonary arrest survive either with or without neurological sequelae (6).

Two separate clinical conditions precipitated by cardiopulmonary arrest can be identified: global cerebral hypoxia and incomplete cerebral ischaemia. The former is due to diminished arterial oxygen content together with an increase in cerebral blood flow requirement that occur in acute respiratory insufficiency; the second is due to a reduction in the blood supply to the brain with normal arterial oxygen content that occurs in cases of shock and in intracranial hypertension (6).

The relationship between cerebral blood flow, O_2 transport (DO_2) and cerebral oxygen consumption (VO_2) are shown in Table 4.3. Fortunately, there is a margin of safety that the brain has in hypoxia or anoxia, because the quantity of O_2 transported by the blood is equal to 2 or 3 times cerebral VO_2. Cerebral perfusion SPECT in postanoxic coma therefore shows impoverished cerebral blood flow, or if this is normal, depressed neuronal function, thus enabling the neuroresuscitator to construct a prognostic judgement while guiding him in the implementation of a specific therapeutic protocol.

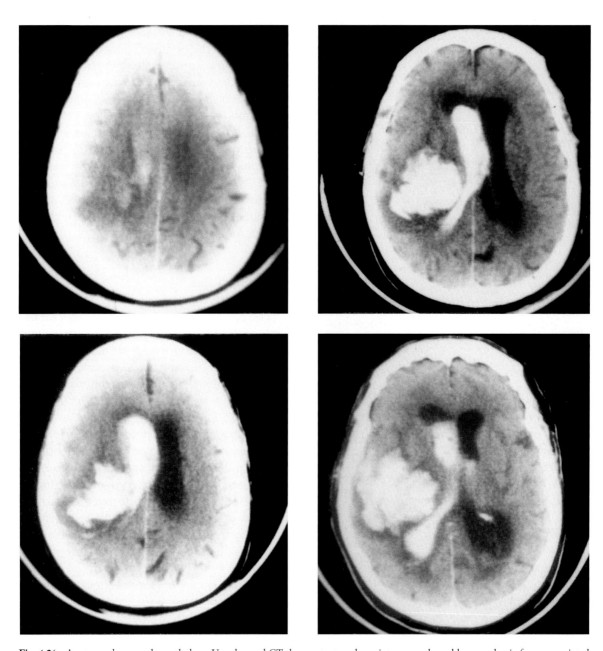

Fig. 4.26 - Acute cerebrovascular pathology. Unenhanced CT demonstrates a large intraparenchymal haemorrhagic focus associated with rupture into the ventricular system and ventricular dilatation.

CBF x CaO_2 = DO_2
    CBF=5Oml/min/ 100 g
    CaO_2 = 20 ml / 100 ml
    DO_2 = 10 ml / min / 100 g
    VO_2 = 3-5 ml / min / 100 g

CaO_2 = arterial oxygen concentration

Tab. 4.3 - Relationship between CBF, O_2 transport (DO_2) and cerebral oxygen consumption (VO_2).

Clinical case
PATIENT   T.A
AGE   49 years
DIAGNOSIS   postanoxic coma
GCS on admission 7
SAPS   14

The first scintigraphic study in this patient documented a marked reduction in blood sup-

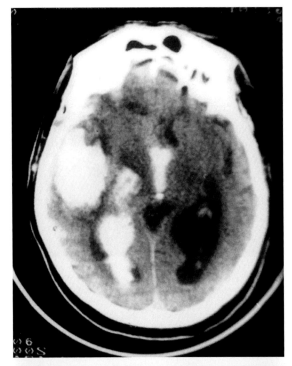

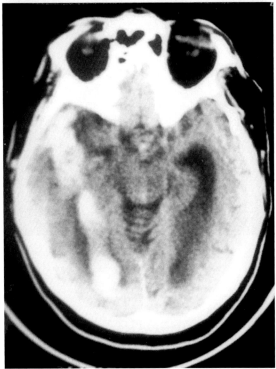

Fig. 4.26 - (*Contd.*).

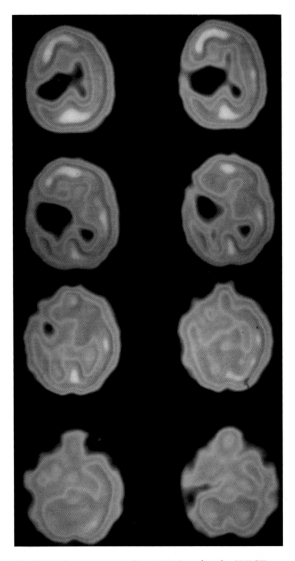

Fig. 4.27 - Same case as in Fig. 4.26. Note that the SPECT images reveal extensive perfusion defects and evidence of cerebellar diaschisis.

ply throughout the cerebral cortex and in the subcortical grey matter structures, without demonstrating focal deficits. Cerebellum and brainstem perfusion were generally well conserved (Fig. 4.29). A subsequent study (Fig. 4.30) highlights the asymmetry of the peripheral blood flow distribution between the two cerebral hemispheres with global hypoperfusion of the left hemisphere.

Finally, the third examination (Fig. 4.31) performed 15 days from the first, documented good overall cortical perfusion within both cerebral hemispheres and the disappearance of lateralized flow asymmetries. The improvement in brain perfusion documented by SPECT correctly predicted the patient's gradual recovery from coma.

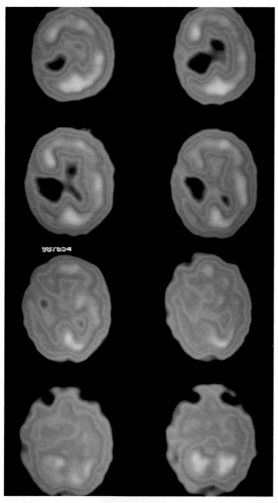

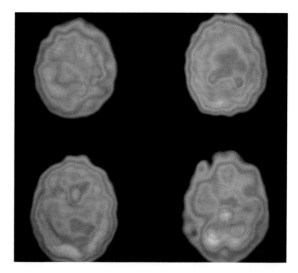

Fig. 4.30 - Same case as in Fig. 4.29. A SPECT follow up examination conducted seven days later shows that the global hypoperfusion of the left cerebral hemisphere persists. The CT study in this patient was negative (not shown).

Fig. 4.28 - Same case as in Figs. 4.26 and 4.27. The follow up SPECT examination shows an improvement in brain perfusion.

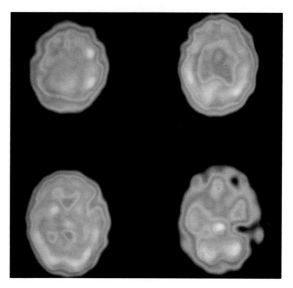

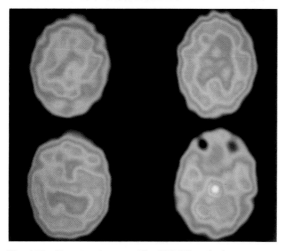

Fig. 4.31 - Same case as in Figs. 4.29 and 4.30. Two weeks after the first examination, the SPECT images show good cerebral perfusion recovery.

Fig. 4.29 - Post-anoxic coma. The SPECT study demonstrates diffuse, bilateral marked reduction in perfusion of the cerebral cortex.

REFERENCES

1. Avogaro F, Zamperetti N, Pellizzari A: Studio del flusso ematico cerebrale. In: Trattato Enciclopedico di Anestesiologia, Rianimazione e Terapia Intensiva, pp. 51-76. Piccin ed., Padova. 1991.

2. Choksey MS, Costa DC, Iannotti F et al: 99mTc-HM-PAO SPECT stuclies in traumatic intracerebral haematoma. J. Neurol. Neurosurg. Psych. 54: 6-11, 1991.

3. Costa DC, Ell PJ, Cullum ID et al: The in vivo distribution of 99mTcHM-PAO in normal man. Nucl. Med. Com. 7: 647-652, 1986.

4. Fayad PB, Brass LM: Single Photon Emission Computed Tomography in cerebrovascular disease. Stroke 26: 950-954, 1991.

5. Giubilei F, Lenzi GL, Di Piero V et al: Predictive value of brain perfusion single-photon emission computed tomography in acute ischemic stroke. Stroke 21: 895-900,1990.

6. Haberer JR, Hottier E: Encéphalopathies postanoxiques. Ann. Fr. Anesth. Réan. 9: 212-219, 1990.

7. Manni C, Della Corte F, Rossi R et al: La perfusione cerebrale in Anestesia e Rianimazione. Atti XLV Congr. Naz.le SIAARTI, pp. 1117-1127, Milano 8-12 ottobre 1991.

8. Obrist WD, Gennarelli TA, Segawa H et al: Relation of CBF to neurological status and outcome in head injured patients. J. Neurosurg. 51: 292-297, 1979.

4.4

DIAGNOSING BRAIN DEATH

M.G. Bonetti, F. Menichelli, T. Scarabino, U. Salvolini

INTRODUCTION

Throughout mankind's history, the concept of death has changed constantly in parallel with the scientific, cultural and social evolution of the various eras. Until the nineteenfifties, the interruption of the heart beat or breathing marked the point in time in which an individual was deemed to be dead. With the introduction and dissemination of resuscitation techniques as well as with the availability of total artificial respiratory and cardiocirculatory support, it is no longer sensible to equate the time of death with the time of cardiorespiratory arrest. In fact, externally controlled respiratory and cardiocirculatory techniques have made it possible to consider that a patient who is no longer able to breath autonomously is nevertheless alive.

However, these cardiopulmonary resuscitation techniques may also allow a patient to continue to be well oxygenated and maintain sufficient haemodynamic stability for limited periods even when all cerebral functions have been completely and irreversibly lost. It therefore follows that the confirmation of death cannot be based on the observation or conservation of autonomous cardiopulmonary activity alone.

Over the past thirty years this observation has led to the introduction of the concept of "brain death", intended as a definitive and complete loss of all functions of the CNS. In the 1960's the French school of medicine proposed the term *coma depassée* to describe this condition, however from a semantic point of view the term is inaccurate because, as it indicates a state of brain death, it is no longer possible to speak of coma. Coma in fact implies that brain activity is still present, albeit compromised to a greater or lesser extent. It is therefore preferable to avoid such expressions as "irreversible coma" but instead use the term "brain death" (BD) to indicate a subject whose cerebrum is no longer vital but whose cardiopulmonary function is still present.

By BD, we therefore signify the irreversible arrest of all brain function, including that of the brainstem, which is precisely the structure whose loss of function is required for the verification of brain death (14).

PATHOPHYSIOLOGY

The skull, a rigid and inelastic container, contains: brain substance, interstitial fluid, arterial and venous blood and the cerebrospinal fluid (CSF). Any variation in the volume of one or more of these components must necessarily be compensated for by a variation in one of the other components in order to maintain total intracranial volume and pressure constant.

With progressive increases in volume, within certain limits, a slight and equally gradual increase in intracranial pressure (ICP) takes place. A part of this compensation takes place as a consequence of the cranial CSF being displaced into the subarachnoid space of the spinal canal (14). If the increases in volume are sufficiently large to exceed so-called cerebral compliance, intracranial hypertension sets in, which if not treated can be life threatening.

The close relationship that exists between ICP and cerebral blood flow (CBF) means that any increase in intracranial pressure must correspond to an increase in venous and arterial pressure. This mechanism serves to prevent a collapse of the cerebral blood vessels and therefore makes it possible to maintain adequate cerebral perfusion pressure (CPP).

There are cases in which this compensation mechanism is inadequate and in such instances the ICP increases beyond the limit required to ensure adequate CPP. This occurs when nonspecific cerebral mass effect is not controlled or controllable using therapy, resulting in an increase in brain volume within the rigid skull. This in turn causes a consequent compression of the intracranial vascular structures in order to gain additional intracranial space. In an attempt to compensate for this situation, a vicious circle is established whereby CBF rapidly increases, contributing to further increases ICP and, ultimately, to further reductions in CPP.

At this point ICP, which can increase beyond 40 mm Hg, prevents adequate CPP with consequent anoxia and death of the brain within a very few minutes. The compressive effect of high ICP upon the cerebral vessels with eventual arrest of the blood flow correlates with studies showing an absence of cerebral perfusion.

DIAGNOSIS

The diagnosis of BD is first and foremost a clinical one, the main signs being clinical coma, together with the absence of brainstem reflexes and apnea. The main pathogenic factor leading to BD is a severe state of brain swelling with a progressive reduction and eventual complete interruption of intracranial blood flow.

The further clinical criteria (16) for the diagnosis of BD are the absence of spontaneous somatic movements, total areflexia and an absence of activity on the EEG as well as on the brainstem auditory evoked potentials (BAEP). However, such findings can be mimicked by various causes such as intoxication from medicines, hypothermia and technical problems with the recording equipment (14). For this reason the Italian law (Law n. 578 of 29/12/93; Italian Ministry of Health Decree n. 582 of 22/8/94) establishes that complementary investigations aimed at highlighting the absence of cerebral blood flow need to be performed in order to prove BD (15, 18). However, ancillary examinations used for the confirmation of BD are only conducted if the usual clinical criteria are unable to provide an unquestionable diagnosis.

Transcranial Doppler (TCD) examinations can be performed with ease at the patient's bedside and can demonstrate the interruption of arterial flow with a sensitivity that varies from 90% to 99%, and with a specificity that approaches 100%. In order to confirm a TCD diagnosis of vascular stasis, it is recommended that the examination be repeated 30 minutes following the first determination.

TCD can be used to diagnose BD (3, 8) (although it remains decidedly operator-dependent) on condition that the examination is carried out with both a supra- and subtentorial approach while checks of systemic systolic blood pressure insure that the recorded values do not drop below 70 mmHg.

In cases of brain death, in addition to revealing the potential presence of focal lesions, *computed tomography* (CT) enables the detection (21) of cytotoxic oedema secondary to ischaemia- related diffuse cellular necrosis. This is responsible for the predominant hypodensity of the grey matter, with the disappearance of the grey-white grey matter differentiation. This is also accompanied by a reduction and eventu-

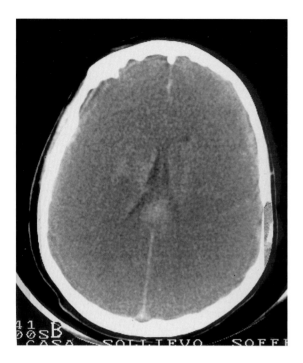

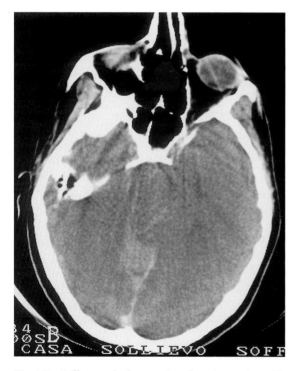

Fig. 4.32 - Diffuse cerebral cytotoxic oedema in a patient with subarachnoid haemorrhage. Unenhanced CT shows swelling of the brain with compression of the ventricular and subarachnoid spaces of the supratentorial compartment and posterior fossa. Note also the disappearance of the grey-white matter differentiation indicating diffuse cytotoxic oedema.

al disappearance of sulcal, pericerebral and ventricular CSF spaces due to cerebral swelling (Fig. 4.32).

However, CT alone does not allow an unquestionable distinction between diffuse parenchymal insult and frank brain death. The use of *spiral CT* has been proposed as a method that may overcome this limitation. A demonstration of the absence of cerebral blood flow (4), as required for the diagnosis of BD, is performed by means of the acquisition of images in the arterial and venous phases after the administration of intravenous contrast medium utilizing a rapid bolus injection. This technique enables the measurement of blood flow, blood volume, mean transit times and flow peak times of the cerebrum corresponding to the territories of the main arterial vessels, including the anterior, middle and posterior cerebral arteries (13).

CBF measurements can also be obtained by evaluating the distribution of inhaled xenon, which diffuses into the brain to form a variation in tissue density (10, 17).

It is also possible to visualize the arterial vessels directly by using the angio-CT technique. The administration of a bolus of intravenous contrast medium is followed by a high spatial resolution volumetric acquisition, with results that are similar to those obtained by conventional selective angiographic catheterization.

However, all the various possibilities of establishing BD diagnosis by CT described above have yet to be validated for use for forensic purposes.

Cerebral angiography by means of selective arterial catheterization (Fig. 4.33), preferably utilizing digital imaging equipment, has limitations in that it is invasive and cannot be performed in all centres (20). In the past this technique has repeatedly been proposed as a method for diagnosing BD. If this method is utilised, we suggest tailoring the examination to include a study of the supraaortic vessels and the intracranial circulation by a simple catheterization of the ascending aorta, with injection of contrast medium at this point using the automatic injector. In order to certify BD, one must be able to demonstrate the absence of filling of the internal carotid arteries and the

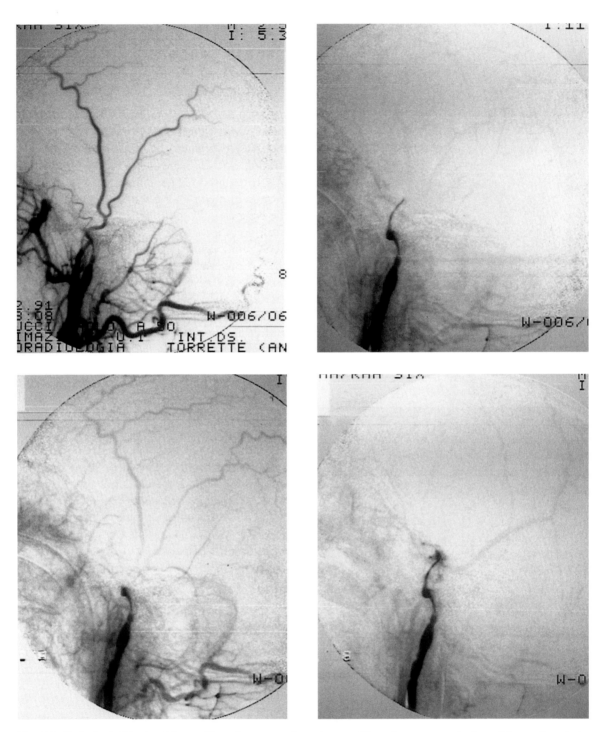

Fig. 4.33 - Brain death. Selective right carotid arteriogram reveals an absence of flow of contrast past the base of the cranium via the internal carotid artery. Similar findings were observed in the left carotid and vertebral arteries (not shown).

vertebral arteries at the point where they enter the skull together with normal filling of the external carotid arteries (2, 5, 9). Being an inva-

sive technique, and given the known potential for the toxic effect of the contrast medium on organs suitable for transplantation, certain

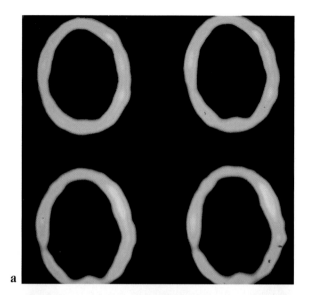

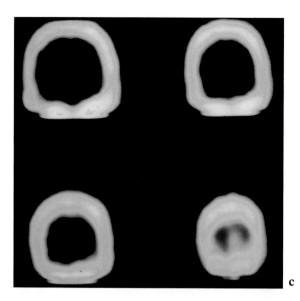

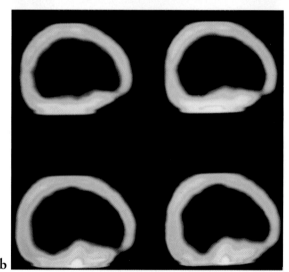

Fig. 4.34 - Brain death. SPECT scans reveal a complete absence of cerebral and cerebellar perfusion. [**a**) axial **a**), sagittal **b**) and **c**) coronal SPECT].

doubts have been voiced concerning the use of conventional cerebral angiography for verifying BD (20).

Magnetic resonance imaging (MRI) easily demonstrates diffuse cerebral oedema, even at an early stage, using T2-weighted or diffusion-weighted imaging sequences; MR spectroscopy can directly show the presence of lactic acid, an early indication of cellular necrosis; MR angiography can indicate the presence or absence of flow in the cerebral veins and arteries. De-

spite the fact that MRI does present certain difficulties in execution and has some clear limitations, the initial results would suggest further future investigation into its potential medico-legal use in the evaluation of BD (11, 12).

With regard to *nuclear medicine methods*, the study of cerebral perfusion with 133-Xenon, which is not readily available, does not enable evaluation of the deep brain structures and is hindered by artefacts caused by increased extracranial flow (19). In addition, cerebral angioscintigraphy can be difficult to interpret, and importantly, it is unable to study the vascular structures of the posterior fossa (7, 19).

On the other hand, in our experience and that of others, SPECT with HM-PAO has proved to be simple to perform and interpret (1, 6). Additionally, it has made it possible to diagnose brain death at an early stage.

Using SPECT, the diagnosis of brain death is made by demonstrating an absence of perfusion throughout the brain. One example of this finding is shown in Fig. 4.34: absence of detection of the radionuclide in the brain; detection of radionuclide in the subcutaneous muscular and bony tissues of the skull. In the same case CT demonstrated the presence of a deep intraparencymal haematoma (Fig. 4.35). In another patient (scintigraphic planar scans in AP: Fig. 4.36; SPECT: Fig. 4.37), CT and MRI studies (Figs. 4.38-4.42) demonstrated the presence of an intraparenchymal haema-

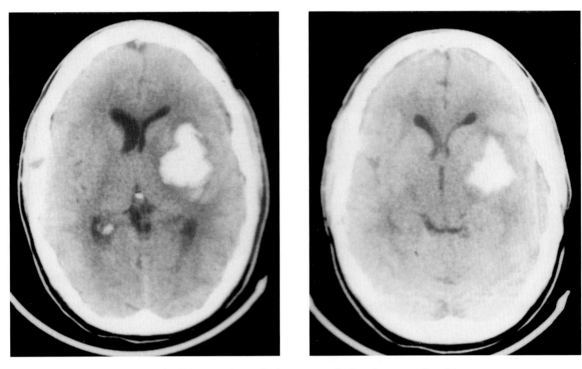

Fig. 4.35 - Same case as Fig. 4.34. The CT images show only the presence of a deep intraparenchymal haematoma.

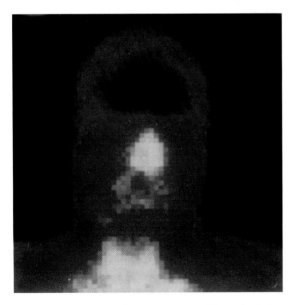

Fig. 4.36 - SPECT, CT and MRI comparison of brain death. See text.

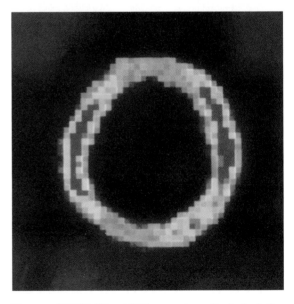

Fig. 4.37 - SPECT, CT and MRI comparison of brain death. See text.

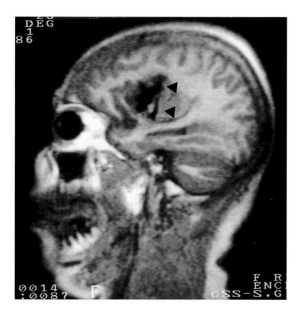

Fig. 4.38 - SPECT, CT and MRI comparison of brain death. See text.

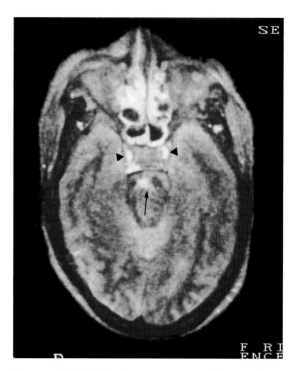

Fig. 4.40 - SPECT, CT and MRI comparison of brain death. See text.

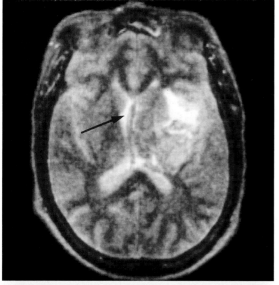

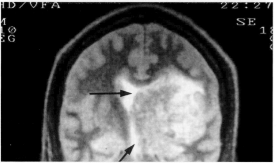

Fig. 4.39 - SPECT, CT and MRI comparison of brain death. See text.

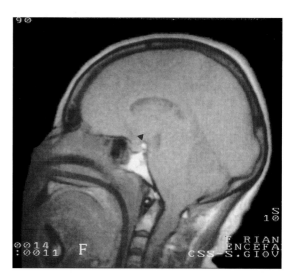

Fig. 4.41 - SPECT, CT and MRI comparison of brain death. See text.

toma, intraventricular and midbrain haemorrhage and brain swelling. MRI also demostrated a loss of grey-white matter differentiation and the absence of blood flow in the main intracranial vessels, suggested by a high intravascular MR signal intensity.

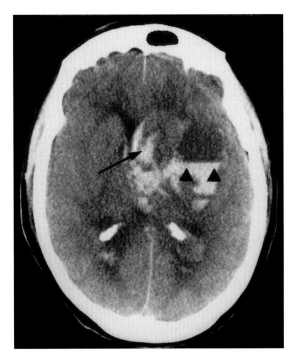

Fig. 4.42 - SPECT, CT and MRI comparison of brain death. See text.

Whichever methodology is embraced, it is recommended that explicitly approved protocols are adopted in all hospitals were BD certification is performed taking into account local situations and conditions.

REFERENCES

1. Bonetti MG, Ciritella P, Valle G et al: 99mTc HM-PAO brain perfusion SPECT in brain death. Neuroradiology 37: 365-369, 1995.
2. Bradac GB, Simon RS: Angiography in brain death. Neuroradiology 7: 25-28, 1974.
3. Ducrocq X, Braun M, Debouverie M et al: Brain death and transcranial Doppler: experience in 130 cases of brain death patients. J. Neurol. Sci. 160: 41 -46, 1998.
4. Dupas B, Gayet-Delacroix M, Villers D et al: Diagnosis of brain death using two-phase spiral CT. Am. J. Neuroradiol. 19: 641-647, 1998.
5. Eelco FM, Wijdicks MD: The diagnosi of brain death. N. Engl. J. Med. Vol. 344, 16: 1215-1221, 2001.
6. Facco E, Zucchetta P, Munari M et al: 99mTc-HMPAO SPECT in the diagnosis of brain death.death. Intensive Care Med. 24: 911-917, 1998.
7. Flowers WM Jr., Patel BR: Radionuclide angiography as a confirmatory test for brain death: a review of 229 studies in 219 patients. South Med. J. 90: 1091-1096, 1997.
8. Hadani M, Bruk B, Ram Z et al: Application of transcranial doppler ultrasonographv for the diagnosis of brain death. Intensive Care Med. 25: 822-828, 1999.
9. Heiskanen O: Cerebral circulatory arrest caused by acute increase of intracranial pressure. Acta Neurol. Scand. 40: 7-59, 1964.
10. Johnson DW, Warren AS, et al.: Stable Xenon CT Cerebral Blood Flow Imaging: Rationale for and Role in Clinical Decision Making. Am. J. Neuroradiol. 12: 201-213, 1991.
11. Karantanas AH, Hadjigeorgion GM, Paterakis K: Contribution of MRI and MR angiography in early diagnosis of brain death. Eur. Radiol. 12 (11): 1210-6, 2002.
12. Kendall MJ, Patrick PB: MR diagnosis of Brain Death. Am. J. Neuradiol. 13: 65-66, 1992.
13. Kornig M, Kraus M, et al.: Quantitative Assessment of the Ischemic Brain by means of Perfusion-Related Parameters Derived from Perfusion CT. Stroke 32: 431-437, 2001.
14. McL. Black P: Brain Death. N. Eng. J. Med. 299: 338-344, 393-401, 1978.
15. Norme per l'accertamento e la certificazione di morte. Legge 29 dicembre 1993. n. 578. Gazzetta Ufficiale della Repubblica Italiana, Serie generale - n. 5, of 8/1/94, pp. 4-5.
16. Pellizzari A, Digito A, Pellegrin C et al: Accertainento di morte cerebrale: aspetti clinici. In Atti del 19° Corso Nazionale di Aggiornamento in Rianimazione e Terapia Intensiva, pp. 11-26. Piccin ed., Padova, 1990.
17. Pistoia F, Johnson DW, et al.: The role of Xenon CT measurements of cerebral blood flow in the clinical determination of brain death. Am. J. Neuroradiol. 12: 97-103, 1991.
18. Regolamento recante le modalità per l'accertamento e la certificazione di morte. Decreto del Ministero della Sanità 22 agosto 1994, n. 582. Gazzetta Ufficiale della Repubblica Italiana, Serie generale - n. 245, of 19/10/94, pp. 4-7.
19. Reid RH, Gulenchyn KY, Ballinger JR: Clinical use of Technetium- 99m I IM-PAO for Determination of Brain Death. J. Nucl. Med. 30: 1621-1626, 1989.
20. Salvolini U, Montesi A: Diagnostica angiografica di morte cerebrale. Annali Italiani di Chirurgia XLVII: 88-98, 1971-72.
21. Yoshikai T, Tahara T, Kuroiwa T et al: Plain CT findings of brain death confirmed by hollow skull sign in brain perfusion SPECT. Radiat. Med. 15: 419-424, 1997.

4.5

POSTSURGICAL CRANIOSPINAL EMERGENCIES

T. Popolizio, A. Ceddia, V. D'Angelo, F. Nemore, N. Maggialetti, A. Maggialetti, T. Scarabino

INTRODUCTION

Postsurgical craniospinal emergencies constitute an important aspect of neuroradiology because early, accurate diagnosis forms the basis for rapid, optimally undertaken treatment and potentially improved patient outcomes. The correct interpretation of cranial and spinal imaging studies requires an extensive knowledge of the underlying pathology as well as the specific operative techniques used, making a close cooperation between neuroradiologist and neurosurgeon imperative. The imaging findings in postsurgical emergencies depend on the site of the operation, the surgical technique and the clinical status of the patient.

As a general rule, the choice of the neuroradiological modality for the study of such pathology depends primarily on specific clinical indicators. For acute phase evaluations of the skull, CT remains the diagnostic technique of choice. This is both because there are no contraindications to the use of CT in patients with metal cerebral aneurysm clips or in the presence of patient support devices (as with MRI), as well as for the very short time period required for performing the examination.

This being said, MRI is the most sensitive technique for use in spinal cord evaluation, in particular for the evaluation of haemorrhage, oedema and ischaemia. Nevertheless, CT and traditional radiography still play an important role in the evaluation of the spinal column itself, such as the investigation of suspected postsurgical vertebral collapse or signs and symptoms linked to the malpositioning or movement of implanted surgical spinal appliances.

It should be highlighted that the diagnostic sensitivity of both CT and MR in evaluating the skull and, especially, the spinal cord, is substantially reduced by the presence of artefacts caused by the ferromagnetic materials used or implanted during surgical procedures (e.g., clips, shunt catheters, plates, screws, rods and metal residues from drilling and bone resection). In order to minimize this phenomenon, fast spin echo sequences (44-46, 54) are used in MRI; because these acquisitions are less sensitive to magnetic susceptibility than are conventional sequences, there is a consequent reduction in the artefacts induced by the ferromagnetic material. Moreover, these sequences are particularly useful for studying the spinal subarachnoid spaces and the meningeal nerve root sheaths.

In this chapter, we will outline the most common postsurgical neuroradiological emergencies, discussing both those following cranial surgery and those subsequent to spinal operative procedures; emergencies secondary to hypophyseal surgery will be dealt with separately.

CRANIAL EMERGENCIES

The surgical approach to the cranium involves a surgical route of choice that does not have a substantial impact on the possible complications that may ensue. Simplistically speaking, the operative techniques used are craniotomy and craniectomy. In the former, the resected bony operculum is repositioned after the operation, while in the latter it is removed from the skull.

Within a few hours after the operation, several things occur in the surgical site that do not cause concern from a clinical point of view. For example, small haematomas, extraaxial fluid or air collections and swelling of the extracranial soft tissues (Fig. 4.43). These findings tend to resolve spontaneously within a few days of the surgical procedure.

Haemorrhages

On certain occasions, the postsurgical outcome may be seriously complicated by acute events that significantly compromise the patient's clinical situation. Acute oedema and haemorrhage are the most commonly observed emergencies, followed by hydrocephalus, infections and infarct (39).

Haemorrhage occurring immediately after surgery is not rare, although the progress made in surgical techniques and postsurgical management have minimized the frequency of this complication (7, 18, 52, 58). CT is undoubtedly the technique of choice for the evaluation of postoperative haemorrhage, although tiny bleeds, such as those adjacent to the vertex or base of the skull, may prove difficult to visualize (7). Haematoma density depends on the packed cell volume as well as duration, and on blood concentration as well as protein content. In severely anaemic patients, for example, it may be possible to encounter

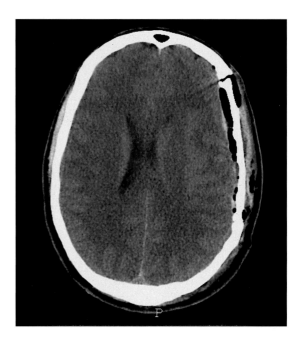

Fig. 4.43 - Craniotomy alterations. Unenhanced axial CT shows expected alterations of a recent prior craniotomy procedure to remove a left temporoparietal neoplasm.

only very slightly hyperdense or even isodense haematomas, which are difficult to diagnose on the basis of CT. On the other hand, clotting disorders and other causes of repeated haemorrhages may also profoundly alter the appearance of haematomas (6, 59).

Intraaxial haemorrhages

A large number of pathogenic mechanisms may be responsible for postsurgical intraaxial haemorrhage (Fig. 4.44). These haemorrhages may be secondary to surgical procedures or to systemic causes; in the case of the former, causes may include inadequate haemostasis, subtotal removal of hypervascular neoplasia, direct vascular trauma, postsurgical venous thrombosis, and rapid decompression in cases of intracranial hypertension (20). Systemic causes (18, 59) may include systemic perisurgical hypertension and clotting disorders (e.g., anticoagulation therapy, kidney and liver disease and disseminated intravascular coagulation) (Fig. 4.45). The removal of cerebral AVM's may cause intraaxial haemorrhage; in such cases

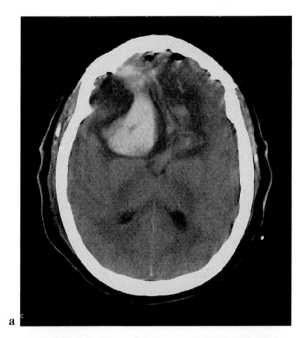

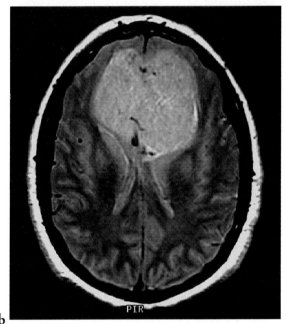

Fig. 4.44 - Postoperative intra-axial haemorrhage. Axial CT (**a**) shows extensive intraparenchymal haematoma in patient recently operated on for large frontal meningioma (**b**). [**a** postoperative unenhanced axial CT; **b**) preoperative T2-weighted MRI].

bleeding develops because of a loss of a low impedence vascular bed in favour of normal capillary circulation. One may also observe the breakthrough phenomenon, indicating the presence of congestion of the cortical capillary circulation with consequent vasogenic oedema due to a breakdown of the blood-brain barrier (34, 51).

Although less frequently observed, postsurgical haemorrhages may also present at a distance removed from the surgical site (32, 37, 38, 48). In fact, cases of cerebellar haemorrhage have been observed following supratentorial operations. In this case, the supine position could favour the stretching of the upper vermian veins and their tributaries, with the resulting laceration of the wall; this process could be facilitated by CSF overdrainage or by the intracranial influx of air through the postoperative drainage tube (59).

Extraaxial haemorrhage

Extraaxial haemorrhage may occur in the form of subgaleal, epidural and subdural haematomas. The pathogenic mechanism most commonly underlying subgaleal haematomas is inadequate haemostasis during the reconstruction phase of the muscular and subcutaneous planes, which results in a blood collection below the surgical flap.

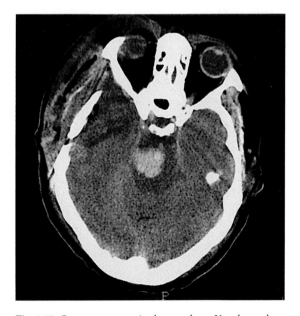

Fig. 4.45 - Spontaneous pontine haemorrhage. Unenhanced axial CT demonstrates an acute pontine haematoma in a patient with plasmacytopenia following the surgical removal of a neoplastic metastatic deposit in the right temporal region.

Epidural haematomas, on the other hand, are typically caused by a failure to treat haemostasis of the dural mater. Less frequently epidural bleeding may be precipitated by extended exposure of the dura mater with resultant injury to this meningeal tissue ultimately leading to delayed haemorrhage (Fig. 4.46).

Subdural haemorrhagic collections are usually a consequence of a sudden reduction in CSF volume that causes a negative pressure over the cerebral hemispheres. This in turn results in the stretching and then laceration of the bridging cortical veins (25, 30, 57). These haematomas may occur following seemingly straightforward surgical procedures such as the positioning of a ventricular shunt for non-specific hydrocephalus or as a consequence of sudden decompression of obstructive hydrocephalus during a posterior fossa mass resection.

Cerebral oedema

Cerebral oedema may be caused by a number of factors, such as surgical manipulations

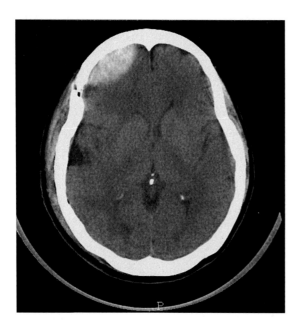

Fig. 4.46 - Postoperative extra-axial haemorrhage. Unenhanced axial CT reveals an acute epidural haematoma over the frontal convexity in patient following surgery for ipsilateral temporoparietal meningioma.

that result in direct tissue trauma, vascular spasm, various alterations of venous drainage and fluid-electrolyte imbalances in the postoperative period. Brain swelling usually begins within a few hours after the operation and lasts up to 3 to 4 days, before slowly spontaneously resolving (39).

The hypodensity and mass effect of oedema as detected on CT scans may affect the area closely associated with the surgical procedure, or the entire hemisphere in which the operation was performed. In certain circumstances, external herniation of cerebral tissue through the craniectomy site may occur. In other cases of more massive swelling, internal herniation of cerebral tissue may occur, such as in downward transtentorial or transfalcian herniations (8). In cases of complicated surgery in the posterior fossa, cerebellar oedema may result in downward internal herniation of the cerebellar tonsils through the foramen magnum (11, 28, 61).

Infections

Postsurgical infections may involve the surgical flap alone or may spread to the adjacent cerebral parenchyma (39). The infection of the surgical site represents a potentially very serious complication (5). The first sign of an infectious process on imaging is the progressive thickening of the meningogaleal complex with intense enhancement of the inflamed dura mater (Fig. 4.47). Generally speaking, MRI is more sensitive to these changes than is CT (14, 23, 24).

Sterile inflammation within the first 24 hours of the operation will cause benign, non-infectious dural enhancement as well as similar enhancement of the entire mengingogaleal complex on MRI after the IV administration of gadolinium (43). On CT, this type of postsurgical enhancement usually will only be seen at the end of the first week after surgery. This normal postsurgical enhancement may persist for a number of months or even years on enhanced MRI examinations, but does not typically endure for more than six months on enhanced CT studies (27).

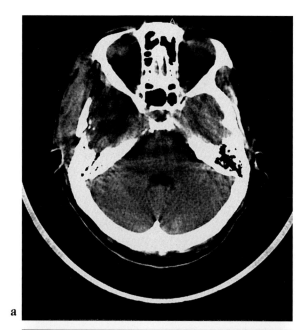

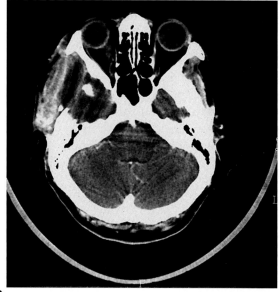

Fig. 4.47 - Infection of the surgical site in patient previously operated on for intracranial meningioma. Axial CT after contrast medium administration shows extensive swelling and enhancement of the superficial soft tissues overlying the temporal surgical site which ultimately proved to be active infection.

Following craniotomy, the bone flap is devascularized and therefore devitalized. For this reason, bacterial proliferation and consequently bony infection is facilitated (16). Standard treatment of bone flap infection involves the removal of the infected bone and the drainage of any associated suppurative collec-

tion that may have formed. In a similar manner to haemorrhages, infectious collections may be subgaleal, epidural or subdural in location.

Intraparenchymal postsurgical infection occurs in a subacute phase following the operative procedure. In such cases, physical signs of intracranial hypertension or fever can represent a clinical and neuroradiological emergency.

Cerebritis represents the initial stage of a purulent brain infection, which if not treated may evolve into a purulent abscess. Both cerebritis and abscess are associated with oedema and mass effect. On CT it is usually impossible to distinguish cerebritis from a sterile postsurgical reaction, infarction or benign oedema. However, after the administration of contrast medium, early cerebritis will reveal minor degrees of enhancement within the first few days following the operation. If not treated, this area will develop a necrotic core, which will show rim-shaped contrast enhancement on imaging. On delayed images (60-90 minutes), enhancement may fill the centre of the abscess cavity (53).

Hydrocephalus

Postsurgical hydrocephalus may occur in up to 33% of patients subjected to craniotomy (28). In this case there is a slow, steady increase in intracranial pressure resulting in neurological signs and symptoms more typical of normotensive hydrocephalus than of acute intracranial hypertension (30, 34).

On the other hand, repeated (42) and excessive ventricular shunt drainage in cases of treated hydrocephalus can generate the so-called "slit ventricle syndrome". This is an acute-subacute syndrome characterized clinically by vomiting, headache and alterations of consciousness. On imaging, the lateral ventricles in such cases are collapsed, thus giving the appearance of slit-like ventricles (12, 17, 21).

Infarction

Causes of a postsurgical cerebral infarction can be found in factors closely linked to the operation itself (Fig. 4.48). The most frequent surgical causes of infarction are the accidental occlusion of arteries associated with cerebral aneurysms or with clips on the components of cerebral AVM's. The total or partial occlusion of an artery may also be caused by the use of a bipolar coagulator during the removal of a brain tumour.

The ischaemic area can be adjacent to the site of the operation, or alternatively can occur at a distance. In the latter case, the pathogenic mechanism may be laceration of the bridging meningeal veins due to rapid decompression of cases of non-specific raised intracranial pressure, cerebral retraction or compression during surgery, marked systemic hypertension or prolonged hypoxia during the operation (2, 3 15, 39).

HYPOPHYSIS

Postsurgical emergencies following operations on the hypophysis by the transsphenoid approach are somewhat rare; most cases are due to haemorrhage (intracerebral, subarachnoid and intraventricular), hydrocephalus, meningitis, marked pneumocephalus and cerebrospinal fluid fistula formation. Alterations of vision have also been observed following prolonged surgical compression or direct surgical trauma to the optic chiasm, tracts or nerves. Operations requiring surgical dissection that extends to the level of the cavernous venous sinus may injure the adjacent cranial nerves. A rare complication of transsphenoid surgery is the laceration or rupture of the cavernous segment of the internal carotid artery, which may be rapidly fatal (36).

SPINAL EMERGENCIES

Postsurgical spinal emergencies can be divided into lesions of the neurological, bony or soft tissues. In addition, spinal implant dysfunction can also lead to clinical emergencies. This section has been divided into several parts

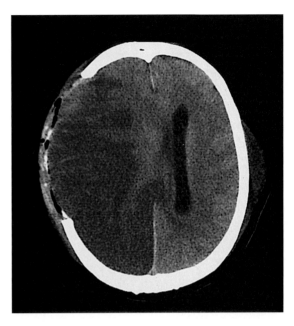

Fig. 4.48 - Postoperative cerebral infarction. Unenhanced axial CT shows an extensive right hemisphere infarction associated with mass effect in patient recently operated on for aneurysm of the right internal carotid artery.

dedicated respectively to the upper cervical spine (skull base-C2), the lower cervical spine (C3-C7), the thoracolumbar spine and the lumbosacral spine. The type of operation and the type of surgical approach commonly adopted (anterior, anterolateral, posterior) are discussed in each subsection (55, 56).

The upper cervical spine (skull base-C2)

Due to the particular mechanics of the atlanto-occipital articulation, techniques for fixing and fusing the upper cervical spine are different from those used in the lower areas of the spine (10, 19). The anterior approach can be broken down into transoral, anterior retropharyngeal and anterolateral retropharyngeal. Each of these techniques presents surgical risks that may potentially result in a clinical emergency (55).

The transoral approach has been reported to result in infection in up to 59% of cases (40). Another complication is the creation of a pharyngeal fistula due to the dehiscence of the surgical incision.

Complications affecting the spinal tissues include CSF fistulae with associated anterior pseudo-meningocele formation. The latter is due to a dural tear. Pseudo-meningoceles on imaging appear as well-defined fluid collections that extend along the intraspinal surgical tract into the soft paraspinal tissues. Although on MRI it commonly demonstrates the same intensity as CSF, in certain cases it is possible to observe fluid-fluid levels with the relative differences in signal intensity being caused by the presence of blood and other products (55).

In emergencies secondary to the malpositioning of vertebral screws, there can be direct injury to the neural structures adjacent to the surgical site as well as to regional vascular structures such as the vertebral arteries (22, 26).

Being extramucosal, the other approaches to surgery in the upper cervical spine have lower rates of postsurgical infections. However, given the close relationship that the surgical route has with major vascular structures (e.g., anterior vertebral arteries, ascending anterior pharyngeal arteries, upper costo- thyrocervical branches), this still constitutes a relative risk. For example, retropharyngeal or lateral cervical haematomas may be observed, as well as the formation of pseudo-aneurysms secondary to subacute vascular ruptures due to the weakening of the wall of an overdistracted-compressed vessel during surgery (4).

The posterior approach is generally used for the reduction and subsequent fusion of the atlanto-occipital articulation in order to correct atlantoaxial subluxation associated with instability. This surgical route enables access to the foramen magnum, the posterior arch of the atlas, the spinous process of C2 and the laminae and articular facets of C1-C2 (9).

Generally speaking, surgical emergencies are principally linked to pathology involving the nerves or the spinal cord. In such situations it is possible to observe, preferably by MRI, fluid collections, posterior pseudo-meningocele formation or the encroachment upon neurological tissue by bony or soft tissue abnormalities.

Complications from implanted surgical appliances include incorrect positioning of the screws within the lateral masses of C1-C2 adversely affecting the nearby spinal nerves or the vertebral arteries. Moreover, in the event of posterior C1-C2 stabilization procedures, the collapse of the prosthetic implant or of the bone graft may result in varying degrees of central spinal canal stenosis with spinal cord compression.

In such cases, the diagnostic imaging technique of choice is conventional radiography first, to evaluate the bony spine and the spinal implant, followed by MRI and then complemented by CT myelography in extraordinary cases in which the first two examinations do not answer the clinical questions (41).

The lower cervical spine (C3-C7)

Surgery performed upon the lower part of the cervical spine also includes anterior, anterolateral and posterior approaches. Overall, the anterior and posterior routes are far more commonly utilized than the anterolateral one, and we will therefore focus our analysis of potential surgical complications on these (19).

In operations involving the anterior approach, it is possible although rare to observe arterial (e.g., carotid, vertebral, superior thyroid arteries) and venous (e.g., internal jugular vein) lacerations, spinal cord injury and oesophageal and tracheal trauma. Overall, temporary or permanent injury to the recurrent laryngeal nerve has been described as the most common postsurgical complication of anterior approach cervical spine surgery (31, 60).

Acute postsurgical infections of the cervical spine are rare. In such cases prominent epidural enhancement may be observed associated with mass effect and, if severe, spinal cord compression. In some instances, the intravenously administered contrast medium may penetrate into the intervertebral disk spaces at the levels of surgery. It is important to note that neither disk space enhancement nor hyperintensity of the intervertebral disk on T2-weighted images of the operated region are to be considered absolute indicators of spinal infection in the immediate postsurgical period. Such observations may only be due to expected postoperative oedema or the presence of blood at the surgical site. Related to these observations, within days of the surgery MRI may reveal areas of altered signal at and near the operative site; such alterations, characterized by low MRI signal on T1-weighted images and high signal on T2-weighted acquisitions, indicate the presence of oedema and haemorrhage that may only be a physiological response to the normal trauma of surgery (19, 41).

Acute complications of anterior cervical discectomy principally centre on the type of the surgical implant utilized, including the malpositioning of the fixation screws, due either to their being too long or to the accidental extension of the screws into the spinal neural foramina. An emergency observed in the chronic phase relates to the fracture of the implanted spinal appliances (Fig. 4.49) associated with the collapse of the surgical construct (26).

In cases of anterior fusion utilizing bone grafts, the following neuroradiological emergencies may occur: collapse of the native bone graft, collapse of a synthetic bone graft, over-distraction of the spine causing straightening or even kyphosis of the cervical spinal curvature as observed in the sagittal plane, and subsidence of the synthetic bone graft into the supra- and subjacent vertebral body marrow spaces (Fig. 4.50).

Finally, we should point out the neuroradiological emergencies related to extrusions of prosthetic materials, such as in the case of expulsion of interbody bone grafts with compression of the oesophagus and trachea. In such cases, both MR and conventional radiography are ideal imaging modalities for demonstrating the problem (13).

The posterior surgical approach is the most common technique for the decompression of the cervical spinal canal. This surgical route is also typically used to stabilize complex fractures. Postsurgical emergencies commonly observed related to the posterior surgical approach are characterized by injuries to the spinal or cervical spinal cord.

CSF leaks with pseudo-meningocele formation are also observed at this level of the spine

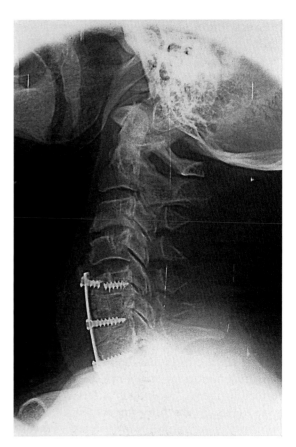

Fig. 4.49 - Fracture of surgical spinal appliance. A lateral radiograph of the cervical spine shows a fracture of the upper vertebral body screw in a patient with cervical myelopathy operated on for spinal cord decompression and anterior fusion.

in cases where the meninges are inadvertently breached. Finally, especially in cases of coagulation disorders, the formation of epidural blood collections can present as clinical emergencies.

Other neuroradiological emergencies concern the surgical technique used in posterior decompression. In cases of cervical laminectomy, the extent of the removal of the vertebral laminae can be insufficient, thus causing a possible stenosis upstream and downstream from the bone decompression.

Lastly, in relation to cervical laminoplasty (with widening of the cervical canal leaving the plates in place), the stabilization systems used (plates and screws, bone grafts, metal wires) can recreate a condition of canal stenosis with subsequent worsening of the clinical situation.

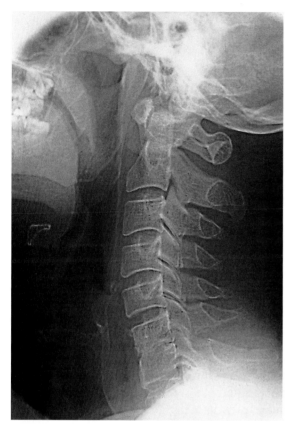

Fig. 4.50 - Collapse of spinal interbody bone graft in patient undergoing for diskectomy and spinal fusion. A lateral radiograph of the cervical spine shows postoperative intervertebral disc space collapse at the C6-7 level following diskectomy and attempted bone graft placement.

Emergencies linked to posterior instrumentation include the malpositioning of transarticular screws and those screws placed into the lateral masses of the cervical vertebral bodies, fractures of the posterior spinal facet joints, direct surgical injuries of the vertebral arteries and impingement on the exiting spinal nerves and nerve roots.

The thoracic spine

As in other levels of the spine, clinical emergencies of the thoracic spine (19) depend on the type of surgery performed and the surgical technique used.

The anterior surgical approach to the thoracic spine is best suited to the treatment of neoplastic and infectious disease, and for the management of complex problems such as scoliosis. Potential complications that may require emergency medical imaging studies include lung and pleural trauma, haemorrhage from injuries of the intercostal arteries or the azygos vein and complications arising from injury of the lymphatic trunk. In such cases, the diagnostic modality of choice is spiral CT performed either with or without the use of intravenous contrast media.

Accidental penetration of the spinal meninges resulting in CSF leakage may cause fluid collections in a pleural, extrapleural, posterior spinal soft tissue or retroperitoneal location. In rare cases, haematomyelia may occur from direct trauma of the spinal cord (47).

The posterior approach to spinal surgery is utilized for laminotomy and/or laminectomy used for the treatment of spinal fractures, decompression of spinal stenosis and neoplastic lesions (13). In addition, the posterior route is classically used for the correction of skeletal deformities, such as scoliosis.

The posterior surgical approach is also most commonly used for the stabilization of the thoracic spinal column. With regard to spinal surgical instrumentation, the same complications may occur in the thoracolum-

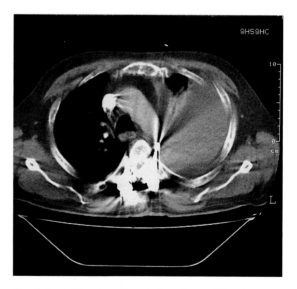

Fig. 4.51 - Dislocation of surgical appliances following vertebral collapse in patient with multiple myeloma operated on for posterior stabilisation. [axial CT].

bar spine as those outlined for the cervical spine.

The most common radiological emergencies are related to malpositioning of surgical implants. In such cases, poorly positioned transpedicular fixation screws can injure the vascular and neural structures adjacent to the vertebral pedicles or anterior to the vertebral bodies. Injuries to the thoracic or abdominal aorta (Fig. 4.52), the intercostal arteries, the inferior vena cava, the azygos vein, the thoracic spinal nerves and the thecal sack may occur. With malpositioning of translaminar surgical hooks, the most commonly recognized complication involves the compression of the adjacent neural structures to include the spinal nerves and spinal cord.

Finally, dorsal epidural haematomas may be encountered, especially following decompressive laminectomies in patients with vertebral neoplasia or in those having coagulation disorders.

The lumbosacral spine

Anterior surgical procedures on the lumbosacral spine, carried out via the retroperitoneal or transperitoneal route are performed for the removal of vertebral neoplasia, the treatment of spinal column infections and for anterior stabilization procedures in cases of spinal trauma and degenerative disease.

Perhaps the most frequently encountered clinical emergency is the formation of a retroperitoneal haematoma that may result in circulatory system shock. Other clinical emergencies not infrequently involve injuries of the regional soft tissues. In particular, trauma to the large retroperitoneal vessels (e.g., common iliac arteries, common iliac veins) may be seen (33, 35). Lesions of the ureter can also be observed, as can perforations of the intestinal viscera and urinary bladder (34, 36, 47). Surgical neurological injuries and those linked to prosthetic malpositioning are identical to those mentioned for the thoracic spine (49, 50).

With regard to complications linked to the posterior surgical approach, the same observations made previously in the cervical and tho-

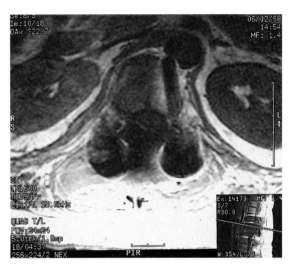

Fig. 4.52 - Over insertion of transpedicular screw with impingement upon the aorta. Axial T1-weighted MRI shows penetration of the transpedicular screw on the left side through the anterior cortex of the vertebral body associated with impingement upon the abdominal aorta.

racic spine sections apply in the lumbosacral spine concerning injuries of the lumbosacral roots and those of the thecal sack (e.g., CSF fistulae, pseudo-meningocele formation) (1, 29).

REFERENCES

1. Barron JT: Lumbar pseudomeningocele. Orthopedics 13:608-609, 1990.
2. Bejjani GK, Duong DH, Kalamarides M et al: Cerebral vasospasm after tumor resection. A case report. Neurochirurgie 43 (3):164-8, 1997.
3. Bejjani GK, Sekhar LN, Yost AM et al: Vasospasm after cranial base tumor resection:pathogenesis, diagnosis and therapy. Surg Neurol 52(6):577-84, 1999.
4. Bell GR: The anterior approach to the cervical spine. In Ross J,ed. Neuroimaging Clinics of North America: Philadelphia: WB Saunders 465-480, 1995.
5. Blomstedt GC: Craniotomy infections. Neurosurg Clin North Am 3:375-385, 1992.
6. Bradley WG: MR appearance of hemorrhage in the brain. Radiology 189:15-26, 1993.
7. Brant-Zawadzki M, Pitts LH: The role of CT in evaluation of head trauma. In: Federle MP, Brant-Zawadzki M, eds. Computed Tomography in the evaluation of trauma. Baltimora: Williams e Wilkins 1-82, 1982.
8. Bruce DA, Alavi A, Bilaniuk L et al: Diffuse cerebral swelling following head injuries in children: The syndrome of malignant brain edema: J Neurosurg 65:170-178, 1981.
9. Castel E, Lazennec JY, Chiras J et al: Acute spinal cord compression due to intraspinal bleeding from a vertebral hemangioma:2 case-report. Eur Spine 8(3):244-8, 1999.
10. Connolly PJ, Yuan HA: Anterior instrumentation of the cervical spine. In: White AH,ed. Spine Care. Baltimore: Mosby 1428-1436, 1995.

11. De La Paz RL, Davis KR: Postoperative imaging of the posterior fossa.In: Taveras JM, Ferrucci JT,eds.Radiology diagnosis imaging intervention,vol. 3. Neuroradiology and radiology of the head and neck(Cpt 75). Philadelphia: JB Lippincott 1-11, 1988.

12. Di Rocco C: Is the slit ventricle syndrome always a slit ventricle syndrome? Child's Nerv Syst 10:49-58, 1994.

13. Djukic S, Lang P, Morris J et al: The postoperative spine: Magnetic resonance imaging. Orthop Clin North Am 28: 341-360, 1990.

14. Elster AD, Di Persio DA: Cranial postoperative site: assestment with contrast-enhanced MR imaging. Radiology 174:93-98, 1990.

15. Enevoldsen EM, Torfing T, Kjeldsen MJ, et al: Cerebral infart following carotid endarterectomy. Frequency clinical and hemodynamic significance evaluated by MRI and TCD. Acta Neurol Scand 100(2):106-10, Aug 1999.

16. Enzmann DR, Britt RH, Yeager AS: Experimental brain abscess evaluation: computed tomographic and neuropathologic correlation. Radiology 133:113-122, 1979.

17. Epstein F, Lapras C, Wisoff JH: Slit ventricle syndrome: etiology and treatment.Pediatr Neurosc 14(1):5-10, 1988.

18. Franke CL, dJonge J, van Swieten JP et al: Intracerebral hematomas during anticoagulant treatment. Stroke 21:726-730, 1990.

19. Heller JG, Whitecloud TS, Butler JC: Complications of spinal surgery. In: Herkowitz HN,Garfin SR Baldeston RA et al, (eds.): The Spine,3rd ed.Philadelphia: WB Saunders 385-400, 1995.

20. Hyman LA, Pagani JJ, Kirkpatrick JB et al: Pathophysiology of acute intracerebral and subarachnoid hemorrhage: applications to MR imaging: Am J Neuroradiol 10:457-461, 1989.

21. Ide T, Aoki N, Miki Y: Slit ventricle syndrome successfully treated by a lumboperitoneal shunt. Neurol Res 17(6):440-2, Dec 1995.

22. Ito H, Shimizu A, Miyamoto T et al: Fracture of the axis after dome-like cervical laminoplasty. Arch Orthop Trauma Surg 118 (1-2):106-8, 1998.

23. Jeffries BF, Kishore PRS, Simgh KS et al: Postoperative computed tomographic changes in the brain. An experimental study. Radiology 135:751-753, 1980.

24. Jeffries BF, Kishore PRS, Singh KS et al: Contrast enhancement in the postoperative brain. Radiology 139:409-413, 1981.

25. Kadson DL, Magruder MR,Stevens EA et al: Bilateral interhemispheric subdural hematomas. Neurosurgery 5:57-59, 1979.

26. Karasick D: Anterior cervical spine fusion:struts,plugs,and plates.Skel Radiol 22:85-94, 1993.

27. Knauth M, Aras N, Wirtz CR et al: Surgical induced intracranial contrast enhancement:potential source of diagnostic error in intraoperative MR imaging.AJNR 20(8):1547-53, Sep 1999.

28. Lanzieri CF, Lakins M, Mancall A et al: Cranial postoperative site: MR imaging appearance. Am J Neuroradiol 9:27-34, 1988.

29. Lee KS, Hardy IM: Postlamynectomy lumbar pseudomeningocele: report of four cases. Neurosurg 30:111-114, 1992.

30. Manninen PH, Raman SK, Boyle K et al: Early postoperative complications following neurosurgical procedures. Can J Anaesth 46 (1): 7-14, Jan 1999.

31. Manski TJ, Wood MD, Dunsker SB: Bilateral vocal cord paralysis following anterior cervical discectomy and fusion. Case report. J Neurosurg 89(5):839-43, 1998.

32. McLelland H, Couillard P: Postoperative heamatoma distant from the surgical site. A case report and review of the literature. Neurochirurgie 43(5):322-4, 1997.

33. Mercier P, Donnez MC, Papon X et al: Vascular complications during surgery of lumbar disk herniation. Apropos of 3 personal cases and 37 cases from a national investigation. Neurochirurgie 42(4-5):202-8, 1996.

34. Miller JD, Stanek A, Langfitt TW: Concepts of cerebral perfusion pressure and vascular compression during intracranial hypertension. Pro Brain Rse 35:411-32, 1972.

35. Pillet JC, Pillet MC, Braesco J et al: Vascular complications of lumbar disk surgery.Report of two cases and review of the literature on 122 cases. J Mal Vasc 20(3):219-23, 1995.

36. Rajaraman V, Schulder M: Postoperative MRI appearance after transsphenoidal pituitary tumor resection. Surg Neurol 52(6):598-9, 1999.

37. Rao CVGK, Kishore PRS, Barlett J: Computed tomography in the postoperative patient. Neuroradiology 19:257-263, 1980.

38. Rapana A, Lamaida E, Pizza V et al: Multiple postoperative intracerebral haematomas from the site of craniotomy.Br J Neurosurg 12(4):364-8, Aug 1998.

39. Rastogi H, Baazan III C, da Costa Leite C et al: The posttherapeutic cranium. In: Randy Jinkins J edt. Posththerapeutic neurodiagnostic imaging. Philadelphia: JB Lippincott 3-39, 1997.

40. Richardson WJ, Spinner RJ: Surgical approaches to the cervical spine. In: White AH, ed. Spine Care. Baltimore: Mosby 1335-1350, 1995.

41. Ross JS, Masaryk TJ, Schrader M et al: MR imaging of the postoperative lumbar spine: assesment with gadapentate dimeglumine. Am J Roentgenol 155:867-872, 1990.

42. Samii C, Mobius E, Weber W et al: Pseudo Chiari type I malformation secondary to cerebrospinal fluid leakage. J Neurol 246(3):162-4, Mar 1999.

43. Sato N, Bronen RA, Sze G et al: Postoperative changes in the brain:MR imaging findings in patients without neoplasms. Radiology 204(3):839-46, Sep 1997.

44. Scarabino T, Giannatempo GM, Perfetto F et al: Mielogrfia con Risonanza Magnetica con sequenze Fast Spin Echo. La Radiol Med 91:202-206, 1996.

45. Scarabino T, Perfetto F, Giannatempo GM et al: Riduzione degli artefatti ferromagnetici mediante sequenza Fast Spin Echo nella valutazione post-operatoria delle malattie degenerative del rachide cervicale. La Radiol Med 91:174-176, 1996.

46. Scarabino T, Poponara G, Perfetto F et al: Studio RM fast Spin Echo dei traumi midollari acuti. La Radiol Med 9:565-571, 1996.

47. Shafaie FF, Bundschuh C, Jinkins R: The posttherapeutic Lumbar spine. In: Randy Jinkins J edt. Posththerapeutic Neurodiagnostic imaging. Philadelphia: JB Lippincott 223-243, 1997.

48. Shimizu S, Tachibana S, Maezawa H et al: Lumbar spinal subdural hematoma following craniotomy: case report. Neurol Med Chir Takio 39(4):299-301, Apr 1999.

49. Slone MR, MacMillan M, Montgomery WJ et al: Spinal fixation: Part 2. Fixation techniques and hardware for the thoracic and lombosacral spine. Radiographics 13:521-543, 1993.

50. Slone MR, MacMillan M, Montgomery WJ et al: Spinal fixation: Part 3. Complications of spinal instrumentation. Radiographics 13:797-816, 1993.

51. Spetzler RF, Wilson CB, Weinstein P et al: Normal perfusion pressure breakthough theory. Clin Neurosurg 25:651-72, 1978.

52. Taber KH, Ford JJ, Hayman LA: Magnetic resonance imaging appearance of hemarrhage:sources of imaging contrast. Neuro Clin North Am 2:61-741, 1992.

53. Takahashi M, Korogi Y: Sovratentorial neoplasm: postopertive changes. In: Taveras JM, Ferrucci JT, (eds.): Radiology Diagnosis, Imaging, Intervention, vol. 3. Neuroradiology and Radiology of the Head and neck (Cpt 56). Philadelphia: JB Lippincott 1-10, 1988.

54. Tartaglino LM, Flanders AE, Vinitski S et al: Metallic artifacts on the MR images of the postoperative spine: reduction with fast spin echo techniques. Radiology 190:565-569, 1994.

55. TeplicK JG, Haskin MR: Intravenous contrast-enhanced CT of the postoperative lumbar spine: improved identification of recurrent disc herniation, scar arachnoiditis and disckitis: Am J Roent 143:845-855, 1984.

56. Thompson J, Smith M, Castillo M et al: The posttherapeutic cervicothoracic spine. In: Randy Jinkins J edt. Posthterapeutic Neurodiagnostic imaging. Philadelphia: JB Lippincott 193-221, 1997.

57. Tjan TG, Aarts NJM: Bifrontal epidural haematoma after shunt operation and posterior fossa exploration. Report of a case with survival. Neuroradiology 19:51-53, 1980.

58. van Calembergh F, Goffin J, Plets C: cerebellar hemorrhage complicating supratentorial craniotomy: report of two cases: Surg Neurol 40:336-338, 1993.

59. Walenga JM, Mamon JF: Coagulophaties associated with intracranial haemorrhage. Neuroimag Clin North Am 2:137-152, 1992.

60. Winslow CP, Meyers AD: Otolaryngologic complications of the anterior approach to the cervical spine. Am J Otolaryngol 20(1):16-27, Jan-Feb 1999.

61. Zimmerman RA, Bilaniuk LT, Dolinskas C et al: Computed tomography of pediatric head trauma: Acute general swelling. Radiology 126:403-408, 1978.

V

SPINAL EMERGENCIES

5.1

CLINICAL AND DIAGNOSTIC SUMMARY

T. Scarabino, M.G. Bonetti, M. Cammisa

Given the variety of potential types of pathology and their varied clinical presentations, spinal emergencies are considered among the most challenging of all neuroradiological investigations. Spinal emergencies can be divided into traumatic and non-traumatic causes and can involve the spinal column itself and its related bony, ligamentous and muscular tissues, as well as the intraspinal contents to include the meninges, spinal roots/nerves and spinal cord.

Non-traumatic spinal emergencies can originate from a vast number of causes. These non-injury lesions of the spine are classified as benign/malignant neoplastic (primary or metastatic, including haematological malignancies) or infectious-degenerative. Lesions of the spinal contents may be extradural (e.g., haematoma, infection), intradural-extramedullary (e.g., primary or secondary neoplasia) or intramedullary (e.g., infarction, haemorrhage, demyelinating plaque formation) in location.

NEURORADIOLOGICAL PROTOCOLS

From a clinical point of view, the most important crisis whatever the cause is the presentation of a patient with signs and symptoms suggesting compression of the spinal cord and the spinal nerve roots. In this case, the neuro-radiologist's role is to identify the cause of the clinical presentation quickly so that decompression of the compromised neurological tissue can be undertaken in a timely manner: the earlier the diagnosis, the greater is the probability of functional recovery following therapy. For this purpose a number of imaging methods can be used, depending upon the specific clinical situation.

Conventional radiography is still considered the first technique of choice in spinal emergencies, despite the fact that it is not always conclusive, especially in the more complex cases of spinal pathology. Considering its low cost, universal patient access and its rapidity and simplicity of execution, conventional radiography provides a general diagnostic evaluation, revealing the majority of pathological spinal conditions responsible for the compression of the spinal cord and the nerve roots.

The subsequent diagnostic imaging modality chosen varies depending on the presence and nature of the neurological signs and symptoms indicating direct involvement of neural structures. In cases where neurological symptoms are present, MRI is preferable to CT where it is available (1, 3-5, 9-11). By combining multiplanar capabilities and high sensitivity to subtle tissue abnormalities, MR provides a very thorough analysis of the spinal column, its contents and the perivertebral soft tissues. In general, MRI provides information non-invasively that it currently unobtainable using other imaging techniques.

Given its high sensitivity, MRI is capable of visualizing bone marrow abnormalities earlier than other imaging techniques. In addition to limited access in some areas, there may also be practical drawbacks to the use of MRI, especially in patients with acute vertebral collapse and spinal cord compression. Life support devices in such patients, for example, may preclude the use of MRI.

If MRI is unavailable or it is not technically possible, CT can provide useful information regarding bony morphology, the central spinal canal and the perispinal soft tissues (2, 4, 8). However, CT provides little data concerning the contents of the central spinal canal. Nevertheless, intervertebral disk herniations and vertebral compressions/burst fractures of traumatic origin are well visualized (7). In such instances the examination can be performed quickly, without having to immobilize the patient. In addition, CT investigations can be extended to include other organs and regions in polytrauma patients, providing results that are unquestionably superior to and more informative in most cases than those obtained with conventional radiography. Of course, in order to avoid excessive irradiation the CT examination should be focused on limited levels of the spine by the preliminary identification of problem areas by means of x-ray or MRI, or on the basis of specific localizing clinical signs and symptoms.

It is not always possible to clearly define the location of the pathology responsible for the clinical presentation. In such cases, MR is once again the most reliable examination technique,

as it clearly defines the spinal pathology responsible for the neural compromise, analysing at once the epidural space, the intradural-extramedullary space and the spinal cord (16). To repeat, CT's principal drawback in this regard is its inability to visualize the intradural structures (7).

In conclusion, MRI currently represents an indispensable instrument in spinal diagnosis. In certain cases it enables a complete diagnostic evaluation even when used alone. In other cases it can be combined profitably with other conventional neuroradiological techniques to facilitate a definitive diagnosis.

REFERENCES

1. Baleriaux DL: Spinal cord tumors. Eur Radiol 9(7):1252-1258,1999.
2. Brant-Zawadzki M, Miller EM, Federle MP: CT in the evaluation of spinal trauma. AJR 136:369-375, 1981.
3. Han JS, Kaufman B, El Youse SJ et al: NMR imaging of the spine. AJNR 4:1151-1159, 1983.
4. Kaiser JA, Holland BA: Imaging of the cervical spine. Spine 23(24):2701-712, 1998.
5. Keiper MD, Zimmerman RA, Bilaniuk LT: MRI on the assessment of the supportive soft tissue of the cervical spine in acute trauma in children. Neuroradiology 40(6):359-363, 1998.
6. Klein GR, Vaccaro AR, Albert TJ: Efficacy of magnetic resonance imaging in the evaluation of posterior cervical spine fractures. Spine 24(8):771-774, 1999.
7. Kretzschmar K: Degenerative disease of the spine: the role of myelography and myelo-CT. Eur J Radiol 27(3):229-234, 1998.
8. Lee CP, Kazam E, Newman AD: Computed tomography of the spine and spinal cord. Radiology 128:95-102, 1978.
9. Modic MT, Weinstein MA, Paulicek W et al: MRI of the spine. Radiology 148:757-762, 1983.
10. Paleologos TS, Fratzoglou MM, Papadopoulos SS et al: Posttraumatic spinal cord lesions without skeletal or discal and ligamentous abnormalities: the role of MR imaging. J Spinal Disord 11(4):346-349, 1998.
11. Wilmink JT: MR imaging of the spine: trauma and degenerative disease. Eur Radiol 9(7):1259-1266, 1999.

5.2

CT IN SPINAL TRAUMA EMERGENCIES

S. Perugini, S. Ghirlanda, R. Rossi, M.G. Bonetti, U. Salvolini

INTRODUCTION

The frequency of spinal trauma, which in developed countries affects 70% of cases under the age of 40, has gradually increased over the last 50 years. Typical causes of spinal trauma include road traffic accidents (50%), sports activities (25%), occupational accidents (20%) and accidental falls (5%) (19).

Neurological injuries occur in 10-14% of cases of spinal trauma; 85% of these cases present at the time of the trauma, between 5-10% originate shortly afterwards, and between 5-10% become evident at a later time (9). Diagnostic and therapeutic advancements have increased patient survival rates; however, little can be done to reverse frank spinal cord injury. Improvements in survival rates have led to a parallel increase in the number of younger invalids. It is in part for this reason that prevention, rapid diagnosis and proper patient management are of paramount importance in minimizing neurological patient deficit (16).

Timely radiological diagnosis is fundamental in the modern management of patients with spinal trauma. Mastery of this includes a thorough knowledge of the anatomy and biomechanics of the spine, an understanding of the mechanism of the trauma, experience in the correct execution of radiological examinations, knowledge of the indications and limitations of the individual imaging techniques under consideration and a correct appreciation of the importance of the correlation between the imaging findings and the clinical signs and symptoms.

Practically speaking, the spinal column has two functions: to facilitate stability and movement, and to protect the spinal cord and spinal nerves. Consequently, we have two separate yet closely connected considerations when evaluating the patient with spinal trauma: the spinal column itself and the underlying neural and meningeal structures. At the level of the present state of the art, medical imaging techniques make it possible to glean information concerning all components of the spine, including its contents and the perivertebral tissues. Conventional radiology, CT and MRI are the techniques currently available, although the most advanced techniques do not necessarily represent the best ones in every case (2, 12, 15).

Fundamental diagnostic information is provided by conventional x-rays which, when complemented by conventional tomography, are the best choice for evaluating acute trauma of the spinal column itself. Radiographic analysis also makes it possible to perform the examination in a number of projections without moving the patient. In addition, the entire spine as well as other body parts can be examined at the same time. According to the literature, 43% of patients with burst spinal fractures may have other spinal injuries. Associated both distal and proximal traumatic spinal lesions are present in 10-17% of patients. For example, in patients with cervical injuries, 12% also have thoracic fractures and 3% reveal lumbar fractures.

With regard to conventional radiography, particular attention should be paid to evaluating the following parameters in the patient with spinal trauma:

Vertebral alignment abnormalities:
– reversal of normal spinal curvature
– abrupt increase in the spinal curvature
– alignment of the articular processes, laminae, spinous processes, transverse processes and vertebral bodies
– widening of the interspinous/interlaminar spaces

Abnormalities of the perivertebral soft tissues:
– enlargement of the retropharyngeal and retrotracheal spaces
– enlargement of the thoracic and lumbar paraspinal spaces

Disk/Articular abnormalities:
– abnormalities of the intervertebral disk space
– abnormalities of the posterior spinal articular facet processes (zygapophyses).

It is also necessary to evaluate spinal stability in patients with spinal trauma. The term instability in this context indicates a posttraumatic state of intersegmental hypermobility that may require surgical restabilization. In order to properly discuss and study the spinal column for possible instability, the spine has been divided into three columns (6, 7): anterior column, middle column and posterior column. Practically speaking, the involvement of a single column does not necessarily entail instability, however, the involvement of two adjacent columns usually does.

Recent studies (5) have identified five radiological signs of spinal instability associated with spinal injuries. These five signs can be summarized as follows:
1) anterior or posterior vertebral subluxation greater than 2 mm
2) enlargement in the interlaminar space of more than 2 mm
3) enlargement in the joint space between the articular facet processes; malalignment of the same a loss of contact between contiguous facets
4) fracture involving the posterior cortex of the vertebral bodies
5) enlargement in the lateral dimension of the central spinal canal of more than 2 mm as measured by the interpedicular distance between adjacent vertebrae.

It is also essential to know the mechanism of the trauma as well as the biomechanics of the spine, which make it possible to identify the areas most at risk of injury. The highest risk areas are those sites at which a greater degree of mobility exists, such as the cervical and lumbar spinal segments, or where a junction exists between a relatively mobile segment and one that is less so or not at all (e.g., the cervico-thoracic junction, the thoraco-lumbar junction, the lumbo-sacral junction).

On the basis of the dynamics of trauma, it is possible to recognize injuries caused by: simple flexion, flexion-distraction, flexion dislocation, flexion and compression, simple extension, extension-distraction, extension-dislocation, "shearing" forces, and rotation. Although there is overlap between the various types, each of these traumatic mechanisms may cause a particular type of fracture.

To summarize, when investigating traumatic lesions of the spine one must: understand the mechanism of the trauma; ensure that the patient is only moved once it has been determined that it is possible to do so with safety by expert personnel and preferably under medical guidance; remember that patients with spine trauma not infrequently have polytrauma and that neurological injuries can conceal involvement of internal organs (e.g., the spleen); perform a preliminary medical imaging investigation that will focus clinical attention to relevant areas and survey the areas at highest risk; interrupt the diagnostic evaluation if a lesion requiring emergency treatment is detected; demand that a specialist interpret the medical images and that a radiologist be present when these examinations are carried out.

TECHNIQUES

Although one must consider a technique's limits and advantages (18), only thorough investigations provide reliable diagnostic information. Naturally the imaging modality chosen and the parameters selected will vary according to the type of injury and the imaging equipment available.

The CT investigation technique initially involves a lateral scanogram in the cervical, thoracic and lumbar areas in order to centre the axial sections of the spine and an anteroposterior scanogram in the thoracic spine in order to number the vertebrae. Axial sections are then angled to the direction of the intervertebral disk. A second set of stacked axial images are then obtained using relatively thin section width and without space between the sections (this will enable multiplanar reconstructions to be performed). For the cervical spine it is advisable to use a slice thickness of 2 mm, whereas at the thoracic and lumbar levels it is possible to use slice thicknesses of up to 5 mm. Thicker slices will not reveal fractures or other types of injury due to the partial volume effect. The use of thin (2 mm) slices makes it possible to obtain more reliable electronic reconstructions on the coronal, lateral and oblique planes. The acquisition field of view (FOV) must be wide enough to cover the entire volume being examined (e.g., cervical spine: 25 cm; cervicothoracic: 35 or 50 cm; lumbar: 35 or 50 cm). The data postprocessing FOV must be of 15 or 18 cm in order to be able to visualize the spinal column as well as the perivertebral structures. Larger postprocessing FOV's are used for studying the surrounding tissues (e.g., lung, liver, kidney and spleen), especially when the clin-

ical situation or trauma dynamics suggest injuries of these organs.

The introduction of spiral and multislice CT into clinical practice has considerably expanded the diagnostic possibilities of CT. A major advantage of this technique is the ability of acquiring volume data rapidly, enabling subsequent processing in multiple planes.

As a result, motion artefacts are reduced and one can obtain reconstructed images of excellent quality. These advantages make spiral CT particularly well suited to studying acute trauma patients (17).

Conventional radiography, as compared to CT, has a sensitivity of 60%, a specificity of 100% and positive and negative predictive values of 100% and 85%, respectively (13). Spiral CT on the other hand has a sensitivity of 90%, a 100% specificity and positive and negative predictive values of 100% and 95%, respectively (1, 11).

The spinal segment most at risk of injury in trauma patients is C1-2. A spiral CT of this spinal segment is preferably performed at the same time as the cranial CT (4, 20). Another high risk level is the cervico-thoracic junction, one that is often inadequately visualized with conventional x-rays (22). The CT screening of this level is also considered valid from an economic point of view (21). Overall, high resolution spiral CT examinations offer a detailed analysis of the spine, generating information that sometimes is of decisive importance in treatment planning (8, 10, 11).

An optimized spiral CT technique of the cervical spine includes: for routine imaging, a slice thickness of 3 mm (pitch 1) is used with section reconstructions acquired at 1.5 mm intervals; for higher resolution imaging, a slice thickness of 1 mm with 1.5 mm intervals (pitch 1.5) is recommended with section reconstructions acquired at 0.75 mm intervals. At the thoracic and/or lumbar levels the spiral technique suggested is: for routine imaging, a slice thickness of 5 mm with 5 mm intervals (pitch 1), with reconstructions acquired at 2.5 mm intervals; for more detailed examinations, the same protocol is used as for the cervical spine.

However, CT principally focuses upon the bony structures. Obviously, the spinal cord is generally poorly visualized. When studying the CT images, the data must always be viewed with windows suited to both bony structures as well as the soft tissues. The investigation must be complemented by electronic reconstructions in the sagittal, coronal and oblique planes. If possible, three-dimensional reconstructions are also performed.

INDICATIONS

Correct diagnostic medical imaging of the patient with spinal trauma demands that the spine be examined in the sagittal and coronal planes. Axial imaging alone is inadequate. It should also be pointed out that the clinical status of spine trauma patients varies greatly as do the clinical and diagnostic priorities. Four different clinical situations can be encountered: severe polytrauma patient in a coma, patient with spinal cord damage not in a coma, patient with radicular signs/symptoms, and patient without neurological deficits but with clinical suspicion of spine damage.

1) *Severe polytrauma patient in a coma*

In this case, and until proven otherwise, the patient must be considered to have spine injury. The cranial trauma and the state of coma require CT scanogram(s) extending from the top of the skull through the cervical spine in the lateral projection. With certain types of CT equipment, it is possible to obtain oblique projection scanograms. The current state of scanography only permits the determination of gross vertebral alignment alterations in the frontal, lateral and oblique projections; in the latter projection it is sometimes possible to see dislocations of the posterior spinal facet joints. The scanogram can also be used to evaluate the thoracolumbar spine, analysing the same injuries as in the cervical spine.

Therefore, while at the current time the scanogram does not replace conventional radiography, it nevertheless can constitute the initial examination in the spine trauma patient.

2) *Patient with spinal cord injury not in a coma*

In this case the CT should be performed in patients when it is essential for emergency surgical planning and in patients where MRI is not possible. Importantly, the CT examination makes it possible to discover if traumatic bony encroachment into the central spinal canal is present (7).

3) *Patient without neurological deficit*

CT should be performed in spinal areas where conventional x-rays are inconclusive or in order to better define the extent of an injury detected using x-rays.

4) *Patient with radicular symptoms*

The CT examination should focus on the spinal level indicated by the clinical examination in order to search for a traumatic abnormality giving rise to radicular compression (e.g., traumatic disk herniation, bony fracture fragment, vertebral subluxation).

SEMEIOTICS

CT provides an excellent analysis of the bony spinal structures. However, while fractures along the coronal and sagittal planes are well visualized, fractures in the axial plane are poorly identified. Dislocations in the axial plane can also be difficult to determine from the axial images. Nevertheless, multiplanar reconstructions when of high resolution quality can visualize these abnormalities in the axial plane, and lessens this limitation of CT. Finally, posttraumatic swelling of the paravertebral soft tissues is well seen on CT examinations.

Radiography and CT

For descriptive purposes, vertebral column trauma can be divided into: trauma of the proximal cervical spine (from the occipital condyles to C2) (case nos. 1, 2, 3, respectively, Figs. 5.1, 5.2, 5.3); trauma of the mid-distal cervical spine (from C3 to C7) (case nos. 3, 4, 5, respectively, Figs. 5.3, 5.4, 5.5); trauma of the thoracolum-

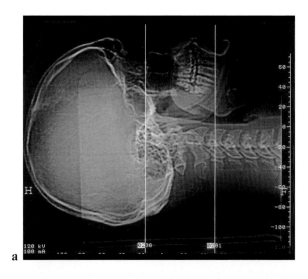

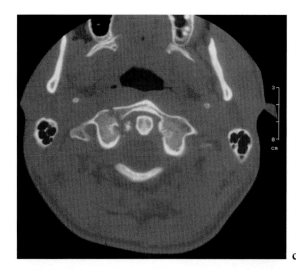

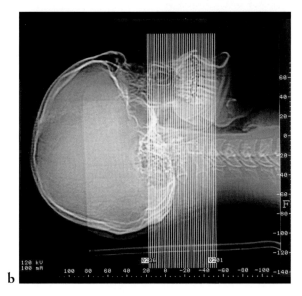

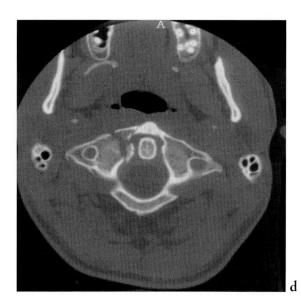

Fig. 5.1 - Acute cervical spine trauma. **a**), **b**) Axial CT of the cervical region includes the distance extending from the entire thickness of the skull base to at least the bottom of C2, scanned with 2mm thickness or less slices. **c**), **d**) Contiguous axial sections show a comminuted fracture of the anterior arch of the C1 with associated involvement of a lateral mass. The posterior arch of C1 is intact.

bar spine (case nos. 6 and 7, respectively, Figs. 5.6, 5.7).

Proximal (craniad) cervical trauma

Fractures of the occipital condyle are rare and are typically caused by vertical compression; they are examined very well with thin slice CT; *atlanto-occipital dislocation* is usually fatal and therefore rarely observed on radiography. In non-fatal cases, lateral projection x-rays show marked thickening of the perivertebral soft tissues associated with atlanto-occipital dislocation.

C1 fractures can involve the anterior or posterior arch, and because C1 constitutes a bony ring, they are almost always seen in combination. The mechanisms of trauma are essentially hyperextension (i.e., whiplash) or vertical com-

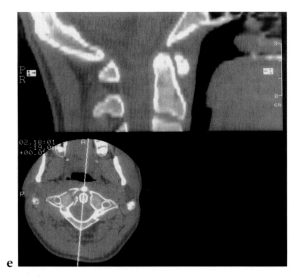

e

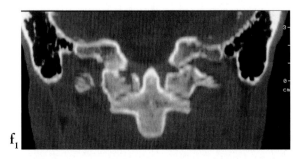

f₁

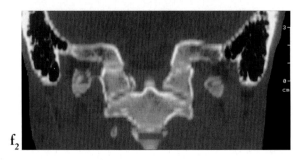

f₂

Fig. 5.1 - (*Cont.*) **e**) A reconstructed sagittal section demonstrates the relationship between the anterior arch of the C1 and the odontoid process. **f₁**), **f₂**) Reconstructed coronal sections show the normal relationship between the occipital condyles (**f₂**) and the lateral masses of C2 (**f₁**); there is no lateral dislocation of the lateral articular masses of C2.

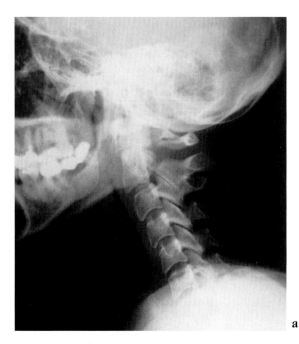

a

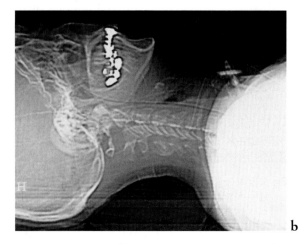

b

Fig. 5.2 - Acute cervical hyperextension trauma. **a**) Lateral x-ray of the cervical spine shows a hangman fracture associated with anterior subluxation of C2 and bilateral fractures of the posterior arch of C1. **b**) Lateral scanogram and **c**) **d**) axial CT confirms the x-ray findings of the C1 and C2 fractures.

pression. Each of these causes a different type of fracture: hyperextension trauma results in a fracture of the posterior arch of C1, compression trauma causes a fracture of both the anterior and posterior arches of C1. Posterior arch

fractures are clearly visible on both x-rays and CT images.

Fractures of the anterior and posterior arch of C1, or Jefferson's fractures, also result in the dislocation of the articular facets of C1 in rela-

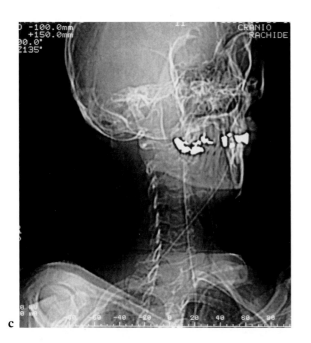

c

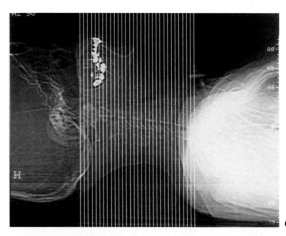

e

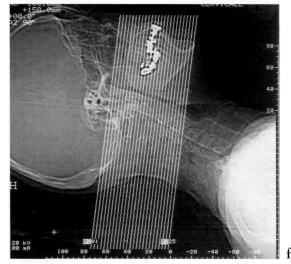

f

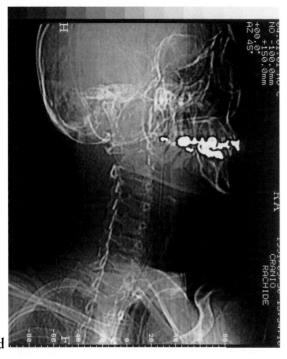

d

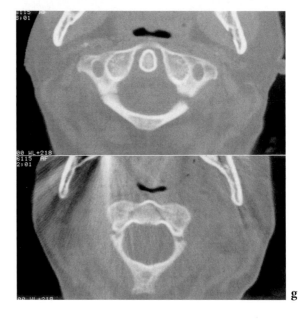

g

Fig. 5.2 (*cont.*) - **c**), **d**) oblique scanograms highlight the distal portion of the cervical spine at the cervicothoracic junction. **e**), **f**) Axial CT is performed initially with no angulation utilising 4 mm thick slices covering the entire cervical spine; this is then followed by a second set of axial CT scans utilising thinner slices (2 mm or less) extending from C1 to C3, angled generally to the cross-sectional plane of the longitudinal axis of the cervical spine. **g**) 2 mm-thick axial CT scans demonstrate the C1 and C2 fractures.

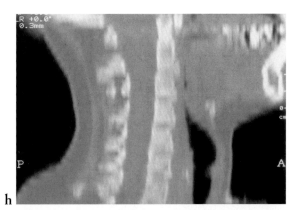

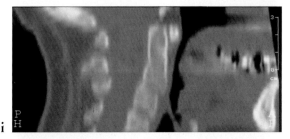

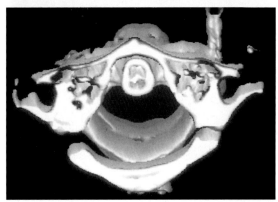

Fig. 5.2 (*cont.*) - **h**), **i**) Sagittal reconstructions of the 4 m (**h**) and the 2 mm (**i**) thick slides. Note the relative difference in spatial definition. **j**) A three-dimensional reconstruction clearly shows the bilateral fractures of the posterior arch of C1 and confirms the integrity of the anterior arch.

tion to those of C2. This alteration is clearly visible on the open mouth anteroposterior projection radiograph that is principally used for studying the odontoid process. This projection also makes it possible to measure the degree of lateral dislocation of the articular facets which, if greater than 7 mm, suggests a rupture of the transverse atlantal ligament. Axial CT makes it possible to visualize the fractures, however the examination must be performed using thin contiguous slices complemented by reconstruc-

tions in the sagittal and coronal planes in order to show the subluxation of the articular facet processes.

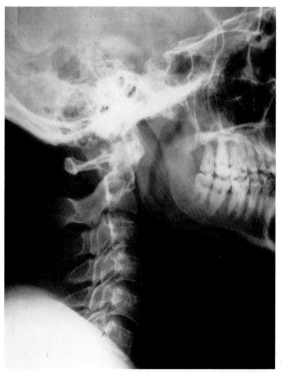

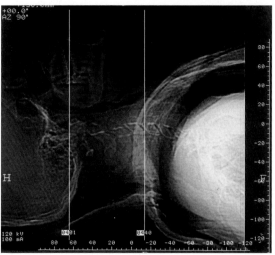

Fig. 5.3 - Acute cervical spine trauma. **a**) Lateral x-ray of the cervical spine shows a fracture of the anterior-inferior corner of C3 associated with a very minor retrolisthesis of C3 on C4. There is also a malalignment of the body of C2 with relationship to C1. **b**) Lateral CT scanogram proscribed to acquire axial images extending from C1 to C4.

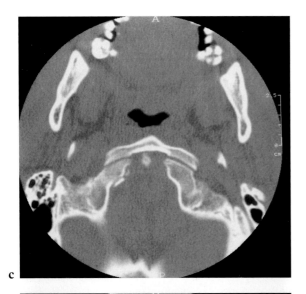

c

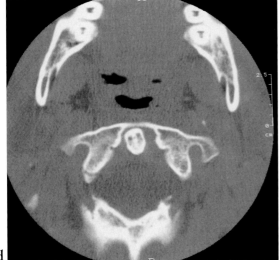

d

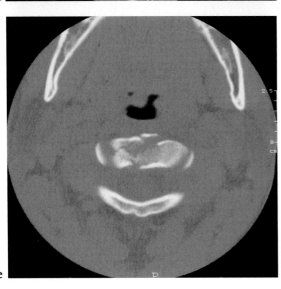

e

Dislocations between C1 and C2 in the sagittal plane are rare because the transverse ligament is both strong and resilient. However, rotary subluxations between C1 and C2 associated with injuries of the articular capsule in the face of an intact transverse ligament may be encountered. Such rotary dislocations result in a traumatic-acquired form of torticollis. CT makes it possible to clearly identify the degree of rotation between C1 and C2.

C1 fractures are often associated with *C2 fractures* and these in turn are seen in combination with fractures of the C7 spinous process. C2 fractures can involve the posterior arch, the odontoid process and the vertebral body. Frac-

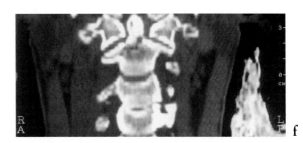

f

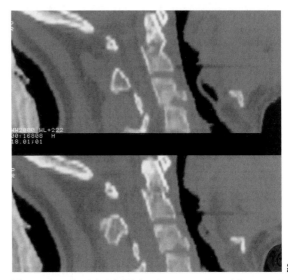

g

Fig. 5.3 (*cont.*) - **c**) Axial CT showing a comminuted fracture of the right occipital condyle, **d**) rotation of the odontoid process with relationship to C1 and **e**) a comminuted fracture of C2 at the base of the odontoid process. **f**) Coronal CT reconstruction poorly demonstrates the fracture at the base of the odontoid process. **g**) Sagittal CT reconstructions show the fracture at the odontoid base of C2 and the posterior dislocation of the C3 vertebral body on that of C4.

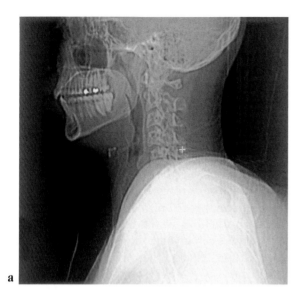

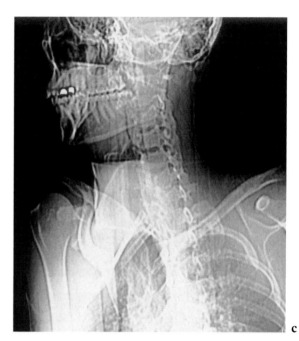

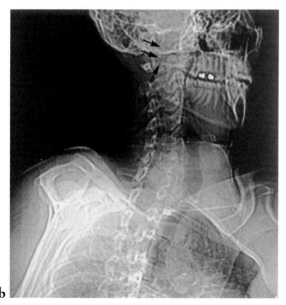

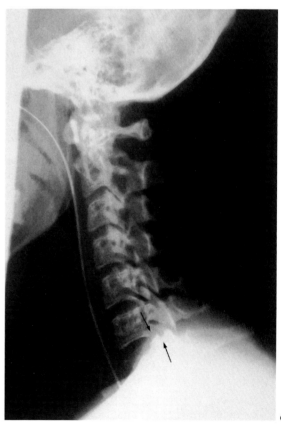

Fig. 5.4 - Acute cervical spine trauma. **a)** Lateral cervical CT scanogram suggests the presence of rotation-subluxation in the mid cervical spine. **b)** Right anterior-oblique scanogram showing the malalignment of the posterior aspect of the C6-7 vertebrae (arrows). **c)** Left anterior-oblique scanogram shows normal alignment of the bony structures. **d)** Lateral x-ray confirms the finding of rotation of the distal cervical spine and shows the presence of a fracture of the anterior-superior corner of C7 and retrolisthesis of C6 on C7.

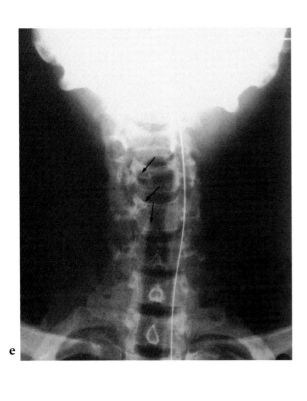

e

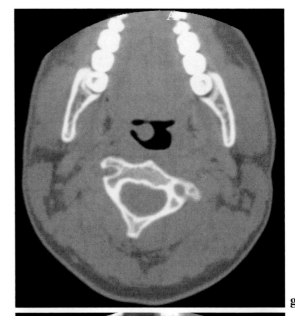

g

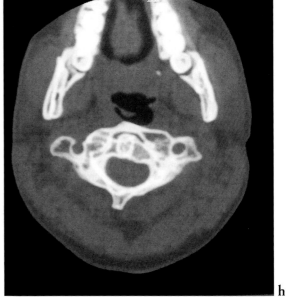

h

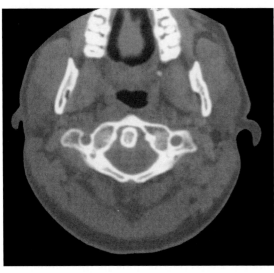

f

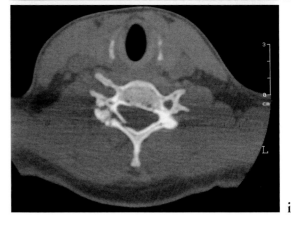

i

Fig. 5.4 (*cont.*) - **e**) Anterior-posterior x-ray shows an abrupt deviation of the spinous processes of C6 and higher to the right in relationship to the spinous processes of C7 and below. **f**), **g**) High resolution axial CT of the cervico-occipital shows a deviation to the right of the C2 spinous process in the absence of a fracture. **h**) A digital summation of the C1 and C2 images (**f** + **g** = **h**) show a degree of atlanto-axial rotation, which nevertheless may within physiological limits. **i**) Fracture of the right C6 lamina and the right posterior articular spinal facet processes of C6-7.

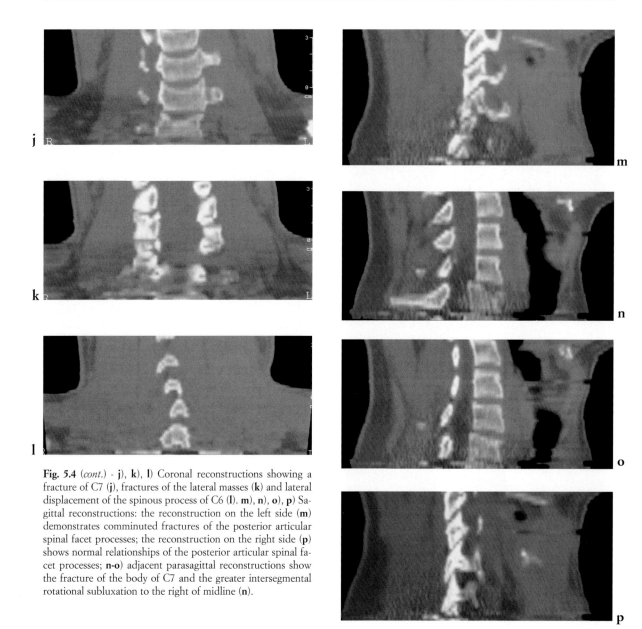

Fig. 5.4 (*cont.*) - **j**), **k**), **l**) Coronal reconstructions showing a fracture of C7 (**j**), fractures of the lateral masses (**k**) and lateral displacement of the spinous process of C6 (**l**). **m**), **n**), **o**), **p**) Sagittal reconstructions: the reconstruction on the left side (**m**) demonstrates comminuted fractures of the posterior articular spinal facet processes; the reconstruction on the right side (**p**) shows normal relationships of the posterior articular spinal facet processes; **n-o**) adjacent parasagittal reconstructions show the fracture of the body of C7 and the greater intersegmental rotational subluxation to the right of midline (**n**).

tures of the body, caused by various types of traumatic forces, are classified as three different types, depending upon the site of the injury. C2 fractures are associated with neurological injuries in 20% of cases (2, 3).

Hyperextension C2 fractures, or hangman's fractures, affect the pedicles bilaterally either symmetrically or asymmetrically and can be associated with fractures of the inferior-anterior corner of the vertebral body itself; there is often a related subluxation of C2 on C3. Radiography in such cases will clearly demonstrate these

fracture-dislocations. CT must be performed using thin slices, extending from the foramen magnum through C4 and must be complemented by reconstructions in the sagittal and coronal planes. CT is necessary when the patient feels pain in the upper neck, when cervical spine x-rays are negative or when radiography shows thickening of the perivertebral soft tissues.

Limitations of CT include the often poor visualization of linear fractures that develop along the axial plane of section. In this case it is

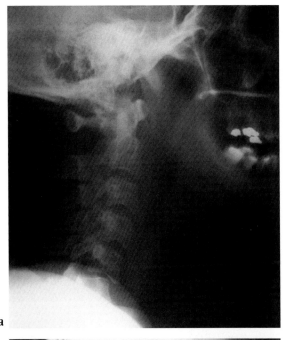

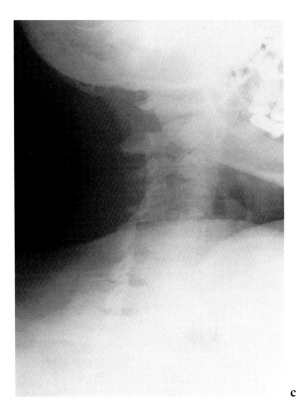

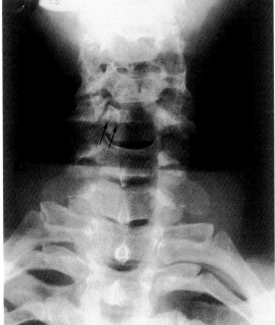

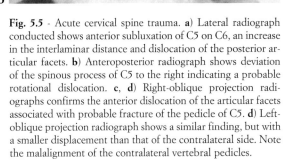

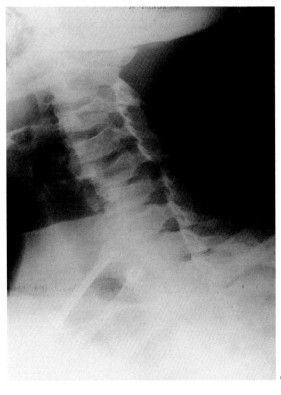

Fig. 5.5 - Acute cervical spine trauma. **a)** Lateral radiograph conducted shows anterior subluxation of C5 on C6, an increase in the interlaminar distance and dislocation of the posterior articular facets. **b)** Anteroposterior radiograph shows deviation of the spinous process of C5 to the right indicating a probable rotational dislocation. **c, d)** Right-oblique projection radiographs confirms the anterior dislocation of the articular facets associated with probable fracture of the pedicle of C5. **d)** Left-oblique projection radiograph shows a similar finding, but with a smaller displacement than that of the contralateral side. Note the malalignment of the contralateral vertebral pedicles.

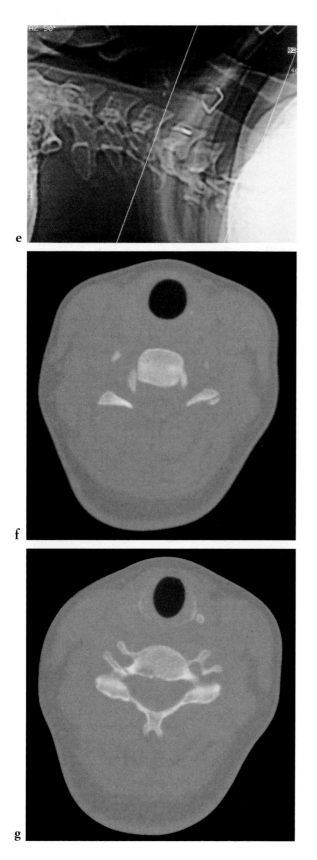

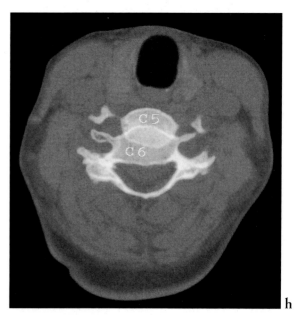

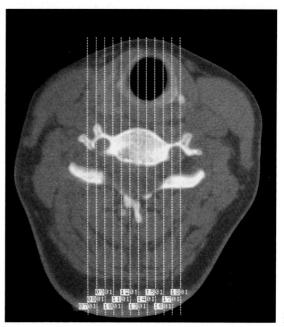

Fig. 5.5 (*cont.*) - **e**) Lateral CT scanogram . **f**) Axial CT shows asymmetric dislocation of the body of C5 with relationship to C6. **g**) Axial CT shows a fracture of the right pedicle of C5. **h**) Image summation technique including the bodies of C5 and C6 showing the C5-6 anterior subluxation. **i**) Oblique-sagittal reconstruction method from preceding axial image set.

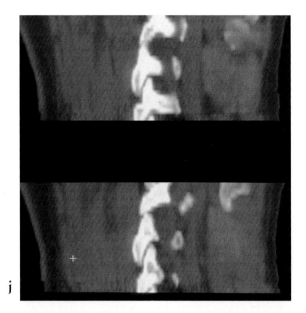

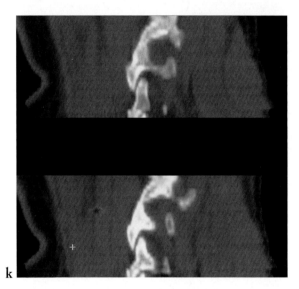

Fig. 5.5 (*cont.*) - **j**), **k**) Parasagittal right and left reconstructions that show the asymmetric dislocation of posterior articular spinal facets.

essential to supplement the examination with high resolution multiplanar reconstructions and with conventional tomography.

Mid-distal (caudal) cervical spine trauma

Cervical spine trauma associated with minor spinal fractures does not in general result in neural tissue injury, with the exception of cases in which there is underlying congenital-acquired stenosis of the central spinal canal.

In adults the mid-distal cervical region is the level of the spine that is most frequently affected in cases of trauma. This is especially common at the C5-C7 level (81% according to Berquist) (2, 3). Distal cervical spine traumatic injuries are categorized according to the mechanism of the trauma: hyperflexion, hyperextension and axial compression.

Hyperflexion trauma: the forces that obtain in hyperflexion involve a distraction of the posterior ligamentous structures and a compression of the anterior structures. Posterior distraction injuries can alter the spine's stability even in the absence of visible bony fractures. In such cases the spine radiographs only reveal an increase in the interlaminar and interspinous spaces at one or more levels. This type of injury may be associated with fractures of the articular facets. These facet process fractures can be well documented in oblique radiographic projections or lateral conventional tomographic examinations. The combination of such fractures with posterior ligamentous injury results in spinal instability.

X-rays are therefore fundamental to this diagnosis, although CT can add important supplemental information, especially when there are diagnostic doubts. As elsewhere in the spine, CT should always be performed using thin sections, complemented with reconstructions in the sagittal, coronal and oblique planes.

In hyperflexion trauma, fractures of the upper-superior corner of the involved vertebra are often observed. Should the flexion forces obtain with the neck in rotation, it can be possible to have the same or similar fracture injury, but there may be an asymmetric subluxation. Orthogonal x-ray studies must therefore be supplemented with oblique projections.

Another type of flexion fracture that may affect the cervical spine is the so-called "teardrop fracture" in which all three columns of the spine are involved in a characteristic triangular fracture of the vertebral body often associated with stenosis of the central spinal canal due to retropulsion of fracture fragments. This type of

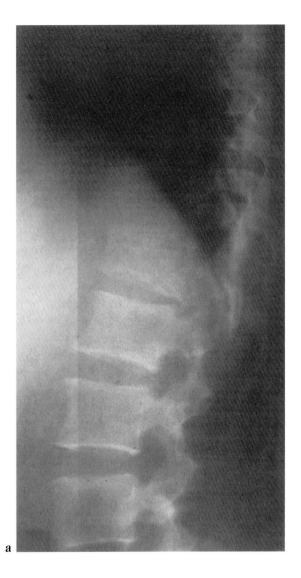

a

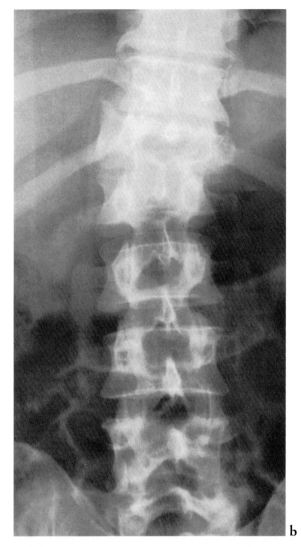

b

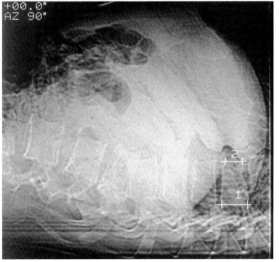

c

Fig. 5.6 - Acute thoracic spine compression trauma. **a**) Lateral radiograph of the thoracolumbar junction shows compression of T12 with poor definition of the T11-12 disc space. **b**) Anteroposterior radiograph showing an increase in the interpedicular distance of T12 as compared to the vertebrae above and below; this indicates the presence of a *burst* fracture of T12. **c**) Lateral CT scanogram confirms the fracture of T12 and shows the anterior wedging of T8. .

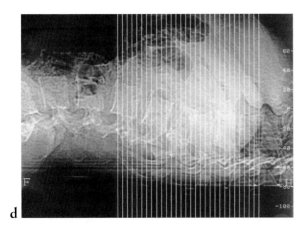

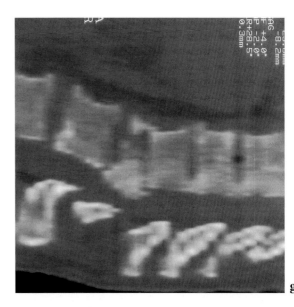

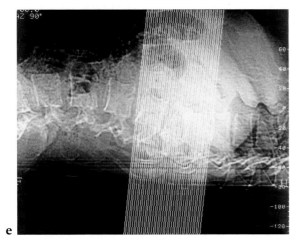

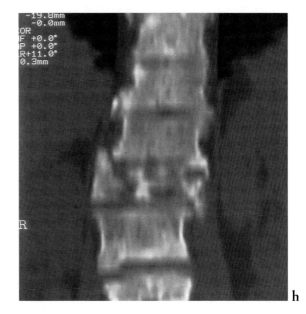

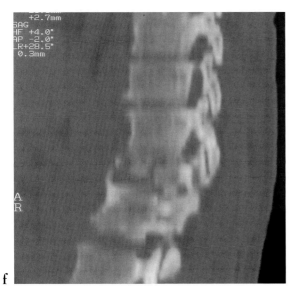

Fig. 5.6 (*cont.*) - **d**) Lateral scanogram annotating 5mm and **e**) lateral scanogram annotating 2 mm (**e**) slices. **f**), **g**) Sagittal midline (**f**) and paramedian (**g**) reconstructions using the 5mm axial sections show a reduction in the sagittal dimension of the central spinal canal caused by retropulsed bony fragments. **h**) Coronal reconstructions again show the vertebral burst fracture and the left lateral subluxation of the spine.

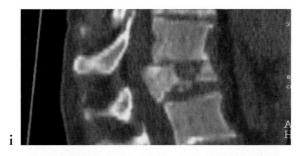

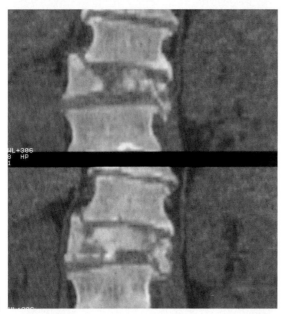

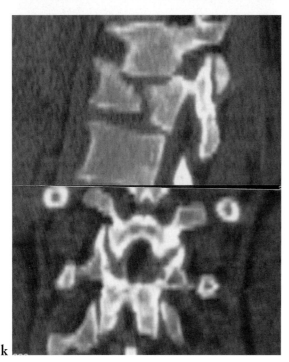

fracture should be differentiated from *burst fractures* that may be stable. CT enables the differentiation between these two types of fracture by showing the characteristic involvement of the three pillars in teardrop fractures.

Spinal cord injury in hyperflexion fractures is common when there is a vertebral dislocation associated with a subluxation of the posterior articular facets bilaterally, and in cases of teardrop fractures. Cervical spinal nerve injuries are more commonly observed in unilateral fracture-dislocations.

Hyperextension trauma tends to injure the posterior spinal elements in a compressive manner, whereas the anterior elements are affected by distraction with avulsion of a fragment of the inferior-anterior corner of a vertebral body associated with rupture of the anterior longitudinal ligament. This traumatic mechanism can also result in vertebral subluxation which in turn is often linked with spinal cord injury. Unlike hyperflexion injuries, hyperextension trauma can be associated with fractures of the posterior bony elements of the spine.

Generally speaking, fracture-dislocations are unstable. A precise diagnosis of posttraumatic spinal instability is important for surgical planning (14). Extension and rotation forces can injure both an articular mass as well as a lamina. This injury, which is difficult to document using conventional radiography, is clearly visualized on CT. CT also makes it possible to determine if any bone fragments have been displaced into the neural foramina.

Axial compression trauma of a severe degree results in burst fractures of the vertebral body. Fractures of the pedicles may also be seen. CT is excellent for demonstrating retropulsion of bony fragments into the central spinal canal. Generally speaking, neurological injury is caused

Fig. 5.6 (*cont.*) - **i**), **j**), **k**) Multiplanar reconstructions using the 2mm axial sections. The increase in spatial definition facilitates the demonstration of both the traumatic findings of the anterior spinal bony structures as well as the injury to the posterior bony elements and their three dimensional relationships.

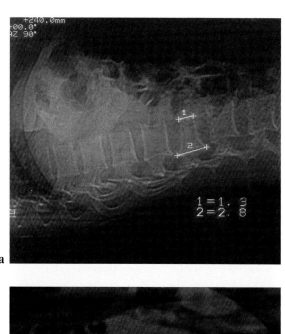

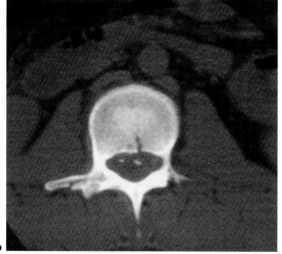

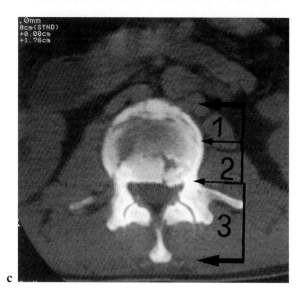

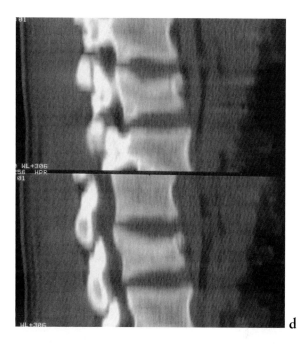

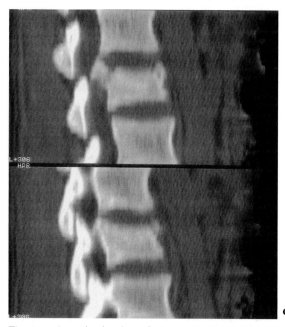

Fig. 5.7 - Acute lumbar hyperflexion trauma. **a)** Lateral CT scanogram shows a wedge fracture of L1. **b, c)** Axial CT sections demonstrating a comminuted fracture of L1 and some retropulsion of bony fragments into the central spinal canal indicating a burst fracture. (1: anterior column; 2: middle column; 3 posterior column) **d, e)** Sagittal reconstructions show the posteriorly displaced fragment (**e**).

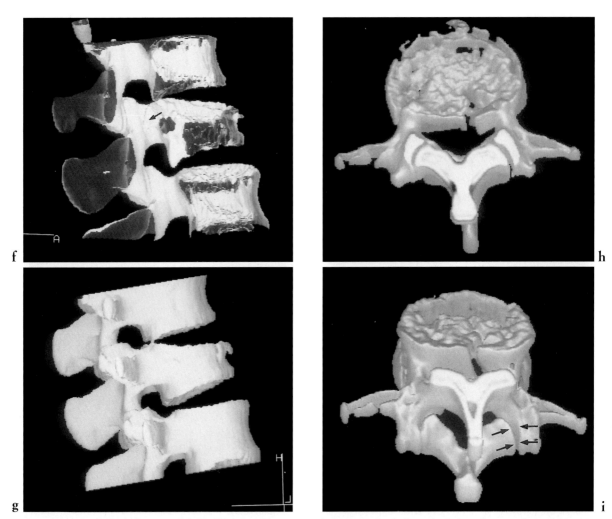

Fig. 5.7 (*cont.*) - **f)** Three-dimensional (3-D) CT sagittal plane sectional reconstruction in the sagittal plane shows a relative increase in the density of the vertebral marrow in three adjacent vertebrae (darker vertebral body shading), indicating that there is marrow compression and concentration of bony trabeculae. **g)** 3-D CT reconstruction demonstrating a superficial overview of the vertebral trauma. **h), i)** 3-D CT reconstruction of L1 shows the posterior vertebral body fracture, the central spinal canal stenosis and the widening of the posterior spinal facet joint articular space on the left side (arrows).

by this posterior displacement of bone with direct trauma to the spinal nerves/roots and spinal cord.

CT may also prove essential in differentiating between certain types of fractures, for example in distinguishing between teardrop and burst fractures. CT must be performed using thin slices, examining the vertebrae above and below the focus of the trauma. It is of vital importance to supplement the examination with image reconstructions in the sagittal and coronal planes in order to better demonstrate the three dimensional relationships of the spinal trauma.

Trauma of the thoracic and lumbar segments of the spinal column

Most thoracolumbar spinal trauma (3, 5) occurs at and near the thoraco-lumbar junction, between T12 and L2. In this area there is an anatomical change in the orientation of the posterior articular spinal facet joints and a transition from a relatively hypomobile spinal segment to one with greater mobility.

The mechanisms of trauma are the same as those described for the cervical spine, although the majority of thoracolumbar injuries occur in hyperflexion.

Flexion trauma entails a compression of the anterior structures and a distraction of the posterior spinal-perispinal tissues. Anterior compression results in wedge-shaped compression fractures of the vertebral body, burst fractures, fracture-dislocations and distraction-fractures, depending in part upon the forces applied. Distraction-fractures may affect the articular facet processes or laminae.

Anteroposterior and lateral x-rays make it possible to identify the vertebral compression as well as burst fractures. In some cases, the relevant alterations can be quite minor, such as a slight curve of the anterior margin of the vertebral body or condensation of the bony trabeculae. Multiple, adjacent compression fractures are common. In compression fractures, a loss of structural integrity of the posterior vertebral cortical surface can be suspected when the anterior height of the vertebral body is reduced by more than one-half that of the rear.

CT demonstrates the posterior retropulsion of bony fragments in cases of burst fractures, the dimensions of the central spinal canal and neural foramina, and documents fractures of the posterior bony elements.

Fractures caused by flexion forces can result in intersegmental subluxation, especially at the thoraco-lumbar junction. When there is an involvement of the posterior and middle columns at the lumbar level, the fracture-dislocation is unstable. However, such instability is only rarely observed in the thoracic spine due to the strong paravertebral muscles, the connected ribs and the orientation of the posterior spinal facet joints.

Vertical compression trauma resulting in burst fractures is most commonly observed at the thoraco-lumbar junction. Using conventional x-rays it is possible to show the compression and fragmentation of the vertebral body, including disruptions of the posterior vertebral cortical margin. However, CT shows the involvement of the posterior vertebral cortex better than conventional x-rays and makes it possible to visualize any migration of fragments into the central spinal canal. CT also makes it possible to highlight fractures of the posterior bony spinal elements that can indicate spinal instability.

Single burst fractures of vertebral bodies are associated with fractures at other levels that may or may not be contiguous in up to 43% of cases. An imaging survey of the entire spinal column is therefore imperative once a burst fracture is identified.

Hyperextension trauma is not commonly encountered in the thoracolumbar spine. When this is the mechanism of the trauma, isolated fractures of the spinous and transverse processes may be encountered. In the lumbar spine the latter can be associated with renal trauma.

In cases of *torsion trauma* CT reveals even small fractures of the articular facet processes, on the condition that thin contiguous sections are used.

CONCLUSIONS

In cases of spinal trauma, CT provides additional information to that obtained by conventional x-rays, thus permitting a more sensitive examination of the bony structures of the spinal column. Nevertheless, CT investigations are only carried out after x-rays have shown or suggested an injury. Contiguous, thin, stacked CT sections must be acquired in order to obtain optimal sagittal, coronal and oblique plane reconstructions. CT also reveals traumatic lesions of the adjacent soft tissue structures, however these abnormalities are typically gross; subtle injuries will be overlooked on CT.

REFERENCES

1. Berne JD, Velmahos GC, El-Tawil Q et al: Value of complete cervical helical computed tomographic scanning in identifying cervical spine injury in the unevaluable blunt trauma patient with multiple injuries: a prospective study. J Trauma, 47(5):896-902, 1999.
2. Berquist TH: Spinal trauma. Da: Trauma Radiology. Edited by Mc Cort – Churchill Livingstone: 31-74, 1990.
3. Berquist TH, Cabanella ME: The spine. Da: Imaging of the orthopedic trauma. Edited by TH Berquist – Raven Press: 93-206, 1992.
4. Cusmano F, Ferrozzi F, Uccelli M et al: Upper cervical spine fracture: sources of misdiagnosis. Radiol Med, 98(4):230-235, 1999.

5. Daffner RH, Deeb ZL, Goldeberg AL et al: The radiological assessment of post-traumatic vertebral stability. Skeletal Radiol, 19:103-108, 1990.

6. Denis F: The three column spine and its significance in the classification of the acute thoraco-lumbar spinal injuries. Spine, 8:817-831, 1983.

7. Denis F: Spinal instability as defined by three-column spine concept in acute spinal trauma. Clin Orthop, 189:65-73, 1984.

8. El-Khoury GY, Kathol MH, Daniel WW: Imaging of acute injuries of the cervical spine: value of plain radiography, CT, and MR imaging. AJR, 164(1):43-50, 1995.

9. Guareschi B: Le lesioni traumatiche vertebrali. Da A.P.C.: Rivisitiamo la radiologia tradizionale. L'urgenza radiologica, pp. 39-50.

10. Katz MA, Beredjiklian PK, Vresilovic EJ et al: Computed tomographic scanning of cervical spine fractures: does it influence treatment? J Orthop Trauma, 13(5):338-343, 1999.

11. LeBlang SD, Nunez DB Jr: Helical CT of cervical spine and soft tissue injuries of the neck. Radiol Clin North Am, 37(3):512-532, 1999.

12. Leite CC, Escobar BE, Bazan C 3rd et al: MRI of cervical facet dislocation. Neuroradiology, 39(8):583-588, 1997.

13. Mace SE: Emergency evaluation of cervical spine injuries: CT versus plain radiographs. Ann Emerg Med, 14(10):973-975, 1985.

14. Monti C, Malaguti MC, Bettini N et al: La TC nei traumi acuti del rachide. Da: La diagnostica per immagini nelle "urgenze", a cura di Romagnoli e Del Vecchio, Idelson, Napoli: 191-198, 1991.

15. Murphey MD, Batnitzky S, Bramble JM: Diagnostic imaging of spinal trauma. Radiol Clin North Am, 27:855-873, 1989.

16. Narayan RK: Emergency room management of the head-injured patient. Da: Textbook of head injury. Edited by DP Beker and SK Gaudeman, W.B. Saunders: 23-66, 1989.

17. Nuñez DB Jr, Quencer RM: The role of helical CT in the assessment of cervical spine injuries. AJR, 171:951-957, 1998.

18. Olsen WL, Chakeres DW, Berry I et al: Traumatismes du rachis et de la moelle. Da: Imagerie du rachis et de la moelle, Scanner, IRM, Ultrasons. Edited by C Manelfe, Vigot:387-426, 1989.

19. Pistolesi GF, Bergamo Andreis IA: L'imaging diagnostico del rachide. Edizione Libreria Cortina, Verona: 637-706, 1987.

20. Schmieder K, Hentsch A, Engelhardt M et al: Results of spiral CT in patients with fractures of the craniocervical junction suspected on conventional radiographs. Eur Radiol, 9(5):1008, 1999.

21. Tan E, Schweitzer ME, Vaccaro L et al: Is computed tomography of nonvisualized C7-T1 cost-effective?. J Spinal Disord, 12(6):472-476, 1999.

22. Tehranzadeh J, Bonk RT, Ansari A et al: Efficacy of limited CT for nonvisualized lower cervical spine in patients with blunt trauma. Skeletal Radiol, 23(5):349-352, 1994.

5.3

MRI IN EMERGENCY SPINAL TRAUMA CASES

A. Carella, A. Tarantino, P. D'Aprile

INTRODUCTION

Spinal trauma is a frequent cause of permanent disability which can often be severe. The social and financial costs involved in treatment and rehabilitation are substantial, especially when one considers the young age of many of those affected. The typical causes of such spinal trauma include motor vehicle accidents, falls, acts of violence and sports.

Spine traumas warrant early diagnosis in order to prevent or restrict spinal marrow damage. Conventional radiography, computed tomography and magnetic resonance imaging are all useful diagnostic instruments and are often complementary in trauma emergencies.

Conventional x-rays, which generally constitute the initial diagnostic modality utilized, may show the presence of vertebral fractures and/or subluxations, thereby identifying specific levels of abnormality allowing a more focused subsequent analysis. CT enables a particularly detailed evaluation of the bony structures under examination. MRI, however, plays a fundamental diagnostic role as it is the only investigation that is able to detect spinal cord injury and provide information on the osteoarticular structures, while covering large spinal segments or even the entire spine. One restriction of MRI,

in addition to the usual contraindications (e.g., metal clips, pacemakers, etc.), are life support and vital function monitoring devices used in trauma patients.

PATHOGENESIS

Osteoarticular trauma

The occurrence of vertebral trauma derives from the sum of both internal and external factors. On the one hand, traumatic forces are applied, and on the other there is resistance to these forces by the bony, muscular and ligamentous tissues of the spinal column. Internal variables include the individual's anatomy, the presence of underlying pathology that reduces osteoarticular resistance to trauma (e.g., osteoporosis, spondyloarthrosis, malformations, etc.) and the relative stance of the vertebral column at the moment of the trauma.

The frequency of vertebral trauma varies considerably depending upon the segment of the spine in question, this in turn being dependent in part on the biomechanical characteristics of that level. The more mobile segments of the spine (lumbar, cervical) are more frequently the sites of trauma, especially in the transition levels between spinal segments with differing mobility (e.g., thoraco-lumbar, cervico-thoracic, and cranio-cervical junctions). The thoracic spine is affected to a lesser degree, being more rigid and supported by the rib cage (2, 11).

Once the above factors have been taken into account, the type of vertebral trauma depends principally on the manner in which the traumatic force is applied (11, 37). On the basis of the vectors of the traumatic force, four main mechanisms of trauma can be recognized, which are usually seen in combination: compression, flexion, extension, rotation. Spinal column trauma can then affect any or all of the bony, articular, ligamentous and muscular tissues of the spine.

On an anatomical and pathological basis, vertebral fractures can be categorised as follows (11, 37):

Fractures of the upper (craniad) cervical spine:
– fracture of the posterior arch of C1, often along the sulcus of the vertebral artery
– fractures of the anterior and posterior arches of C1 (i.e., Jefferson's fracture)
– fracture of the odontoid process
– bilateral fractures of the pedicles of C2 (i.e., hangman fracture)

Fractures of the lower (caudal) cervical spine:
– anterior compression fractures
– fractures of the posterior bony elements
– burst fractures

Fractures of the thoracic and lumbar spinal segments:
– anterior compression fractures
– fractures of the posterior bony elements
– burst fractures

These bony fractures can also be associated with trauma to the spinal and perispinal soft tissues (e.g., spinal ligaments, articular capsules of the posterior spinal facet joints, intervertebral disks, intrinsic spinal muscles). Spinal ligaments can be subject to rupture, avulsions or stretching. The intervertebral disks can rupture, resulting in protrusions, herniations and

extrusions with disk fragment migration, the posterior spinal facet joints can rupture their capsules and the intrinsic spinal muscles can undergo rupture or avulsion.

Intersegmental subluxation can be observed with only very minor underlying bony injury and in some cases without bony trauma. The most common mechanism of such dislocations is "whiplash", consisting of two parts: rapid hyperextension followed by rapid hyperflexion. Types of subluxation include atlanto-axial rotary dislocation, anterior/posterior/lateral spondylolisthesis, and complete vertebral dislocation.

Trauma of the central spinal canal contents

Posttraumatic lesions of the contents of the central spinal canal can affect the spinal cord, spinal nerves/roots, thecal sac and epi- intradural arteries and veins. Spinal cord injuries represent the most severe form of spinal trauma. Cord damage may be from direct or secondary effects of the trauma (16). Direct traumatic lesions are derived from the sudden impact of the bone or protruded/extruded intervertebral disk material against the spinal cord. In the acute phase, secondary effects such as oedema, lympho-granulocytic infiltration, ischaemic alterations, formation and accumulation of free radicals, extracellular calcium, amino acids, arachidonic acid derivatives will have damaging effects upon the underlying cord tissue (17, 19, 23, 25, 34).

Within the first minutes following the traumatic incident it is possible to observe dramatic neuronal alterations and even frank necrosis of neural tissue, and micro- macrohaemorrhages. Although rare, gross haematomyelia may develop (21).

Posttraumatic repair processes include the reabsorption of necrotic tissue and haemoglobin breakdown products, reactive gliosis and residual cavity formation, processes that can take 2-3 years or more (13). Terminal events typically are spinal cord atrophy and cystic myelomalacia (12), a type of focal cavity that can evolve into extensive syringomyelia formation (5, 13). In the case of particularly extensive trauma, intramedullary gliosis and extramedullary fibrous scarring may develop, with the formation of subarachnoid adhesions (13).

In addition, the spinal nerves and roots can become traumatized. The most common occurrence is radicular compression, which may result from bone or intervertebral disk material. Radicular avulsions are usually caused by the violent hyperextension of a limb. Most avulsions involve the cervical nerve roots, usually as a consequence of the forced adduction of the shoulder and arm in motorcycle accidents (2, 18). Pseudo-meningocele formation is associated with such avulsions as the meninges are torn together with the neural tissue.

Finally, epidural haematomas result from the traumatic rupture of the epidural venous plexi. Because the spinal dura mater is not firmly adherent to the vertebral surface, extensive haematomas traversing multiple levels can develop.

SEMEIOTICS

MR investigations in cases of spinal trauma begin with the acquisition of sagittal images that yield an overview with which to select and orient subsequent axial imaging sequences focused on the areas of abnormality. A coronal plane study may also prove to be useful.

A combination of sequences must then be acquired directed toward critically examining all of the spinal tissues. These include the acquisition of sagittal T1-weighted spin-echo (SE) images that provide accurate anatomical-morphological information. This acquisition is followed by T2-weighted fast spin echo (FSE) sequences providing good detail and MR signal characteristics of the spinal cord and nerve roots (14, 20, 27, 31, 33). One limitation of T2-FSE sequences is the relative absence of fatty tissue suppression with persistence of the bright bone marrow fat signal, which can conceal the presence of oedema. This limitation can be overcome by using fat signal suppression techniques (35). Finally, it is imperative to

acquire T2*-weighted gradient recalled echo (GRE) images that are sensitive to the effects of magnetic susceptibility and which thereby reveal the presence of certain haemorrhagic products (3, 13, 31). Specifically the GRE sequences are sensitive to small areas of acute haemorrhage (e.g., deoxyhaemoglobin), and in the chronic phase in detecting haemosiderin.

Imaging of the container of the central spinal canal

To some degree, MRI makes it possible to visualize gross bony fractures, disk herniations/extrusions, intersegmental subluxation and certain ligamentous injuries (Figs. 5.8, 5.9). However, subtle fractures, especially those that are not distracted and those of the posterior bony elements of the spine, are poorly seen on MRI (3, 4, 13, 24, 32) (Fig. 5.10). Thin fracture lines are better visualized with T2/T2*- weighted sequences (Fig. 5.11). In addition, the detection of small bony fragments has also been partly overcome by the use of T2*-weighted GRE sequences.

It should be pointed out that MRI is unique in its ability to identify compression fractures of the vertebral bodies without gross evidence of fracture on conventional radiography. In such cases, the detection of MRI signal hyperintensity on T2-weighted images and consonant hypointensity on T1-weighted sequences indicates oedema of the marrow and microfractures of the trabecular structure of the vertebrae (Fig. 5.12).

One frequently encountered problem is that of the differentiation between benign posttraumatic fractures and pathological fractures resulting from underlying metastatic neoplastic disease. Unfortunately, it must be stated that there are no absolute differential diagnostic criteria that unquestionably confirm metastatic neoplasia on a first imaging study in an individual patient. Sequential follow-up imaging studies may be the only recourse in such cases.

Posttraumatic herniations are similar or identical to non-traumatic forms (Fig. 5.13). In fact it is usually impossible to distinguish the

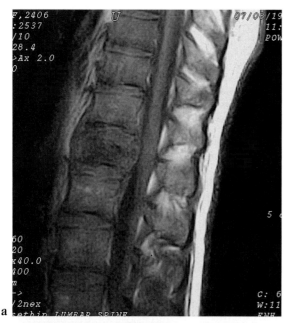

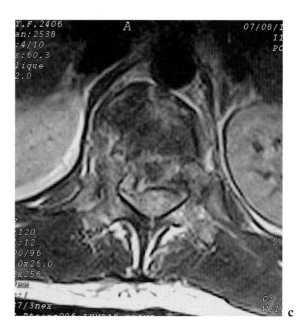

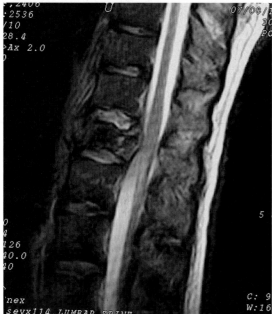

Fig. 5.8 - Acute thoracic spine trauma. The MRI images show a burst fracture of the T12 vertebral body, with posterior displacement of bony fragments into the central spinal canal and resulting stenosis. There are no visible signal alterations of the spinal cord. [**a**) Sagittal T1-weighted MRI; **b**, sagittal T2-weighted MRI; **c**) axial T2-weighted MRI].

posttraumatic degenerative disk herniations. Generally speaking, the presence of other associated posttraumatic injuries at the same level suggests the diagnosis of traumatic disk herniation (7, 13, 15).

Ligamentous trauma can be detected directly or indirectly on medical imaging studies. However, while MRI is capable of visualizing the spinal ligaments, it may not be able to differentiate between ruptured ligaments and adjacent tissue injury, all of which may be hypointense.

Serious vertebral trauma demands an evaluation of the stability of the spine. This type of assessment is aimed at recognizing those conditions that may require surgical stabilization in order to prevent secondary damage to the neural structures. Of the various methods employed to evaluate spinal stability, the simplest is that of Denis which identifies three functional columns of the spine (9, 10): the anterior column (the anterior longitudinal ligament and the anterior 2/3 of the vertebral body); the middle column (the posterior 1/3 of the vertebral body and the posterior longitudinal ligament); and the posterior column (the bony and ligamentous structures behind the posterior longitudinal ligament). According to this model, vertebral instability occurs with the loss of integrity of at least two contiguous columns.

A more recent method identifies five separate signs of spinal instability (6): intersegmental vertebral subluxation of more than 2mm; increase in the interlaminar space of more than

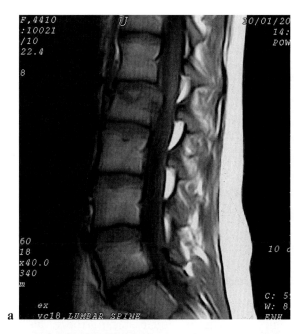

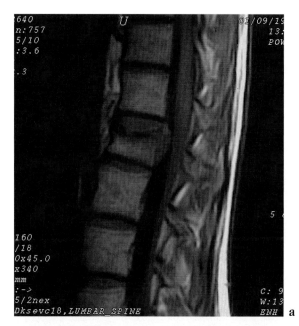

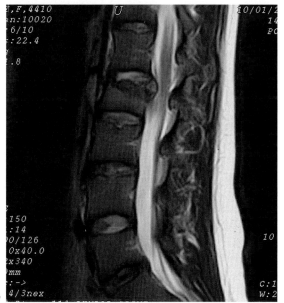

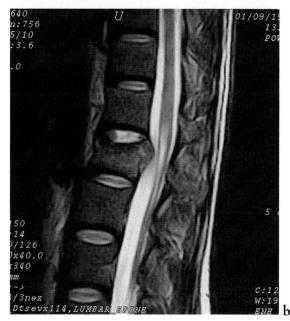

Fig. 5.9 - Acute lumbar spine trauma. The MRI reveals an L2 burst fracture with posterior displacement of the upper portion of the vertebral body into the central spinal canal and consequent canal stenosis. [**a**) sagittal T1-weighted MRI; **b**) sagittal T2-weighted MRI].

2 mm in relation to the adjacent levels; widening of the joint space of one or more posterior spinal facet joints; interruption of the posterior cortical margin of a vertebral body; and increase in the interpedicular distance of more than 2 mm between adjacent vertebrae.

Fig. 5.10 - Acute lumbar spine trauma. The MRI images show a burst fracture of the L1 vertebral body with anterior epidural tissue within the central spinal canal. The vertebral bone marrow of L1 is hypointense on T1-weighted acquisitions and hyperintense on T2-weighted images indicating posttraumatic oedema/haemorrhage. The axial MRI T1-weighted image shows compression of the thecal sac by indeterminate tissue. The supplemental CT examination better demonstrates an interruption of the bony cortex of the right posterolateral surface of the L1 vertebral body and better characterises the bone fragment that is displaced into the central spinal canal. [**a**, **d**) sagittal T1-weighted MRI; **b**, **c**) sagittal, coronal T2-weighted MRI; **e**) axial CT].

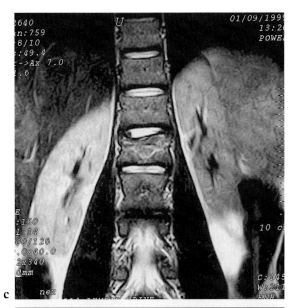

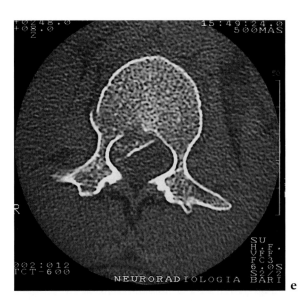

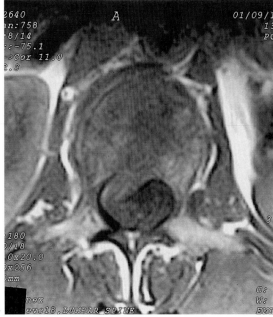

Fig. 5.10 (cont.).

Imaging of the spinal cord

Unquestionably, MRI is the imaging examination technique of choice in the evaluation of spinal cord injury (1, 2). In the acute phase, this facilitates the identification of those conditions that may benefit from emergency surgical treatment, while also enabling an immediate prognostic judgement to be made. MR examinations should aim in particular to detect oedema, contusions, intramedullary haemorrhage, and spinal cord transection, in addition to determining if cord compression is present (Figs. 5.14, 5.15, 5.16).

The study involves the acquisition of sagittal T1-weighted SE and T2-weighted FSE or T2*-GRE images; the acquisition of axial images, preferably utilizing T2*-GRE. FLAIR (fluid attenuated inversion recovery) sequences can also provide useful information regarding spinal cord injury, due to the high contrast definition between the lesion, normal tissue and CSF (26).

In the acute phase, the spinal cord may appear swollen due to the presence of oedema and haemorrhage. Spinal cord swelling is easily shown on T1-weighted sequences. This swelling is hyperintense on T2-weighted sequences in relation to the normal cord tissue, an expression of intramedullary oedema (1, 3, 4, 6) (Fig. 5.17).

This is defined by several authors as medullary contusion (16, 22) (Fig. 5.18). The presence of haemorrhagic products in the spinal cord injury is termed haemorrhagic contusion (Fig. 5.19). As mentioned above, frank intramedullary haemorrhage (i.e., haematomyelia) may be encountered. In any case, the MR appearance of haemorrhagic products varies depending upon the time that has elapsed since the traumatic event, the modifications undergone by the haemoglobin molecules

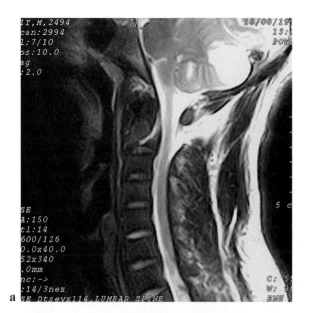

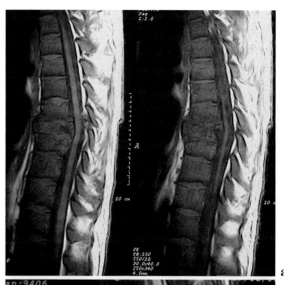

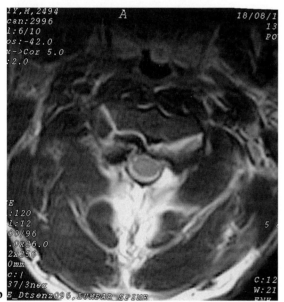

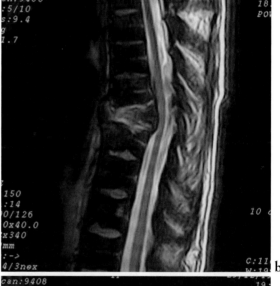

Fig. 5.11 - Acute cervical spine trauma. MRI in a patient with bilateral C2 pedicle fractures (Hangman fracture). **a**), **b**) Sagittal, axial T2-weighted MRI.

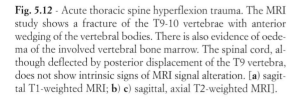

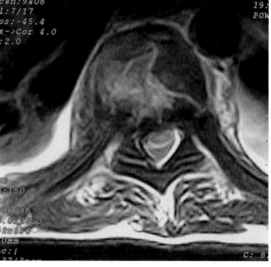

Fig. 5.12 - Acute thoracic spine hyperflexion trauma. The MRI study shows a fracture of the T9-10 vertebrae with anterior wedging of the vertebral bodies. There is also evidence of oedema of the involved vertebral bone marrow. The spinal cord, although deflected by posterior displacement of the T9 vertebra, does not show intrinsic signs of MRI signal alteration. [**a**) sagittal T1-weighted MRI; **b**) **c**) sagittal, axial T2-weighted MRI].

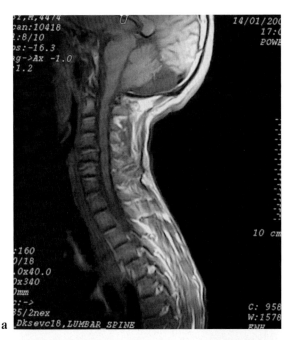

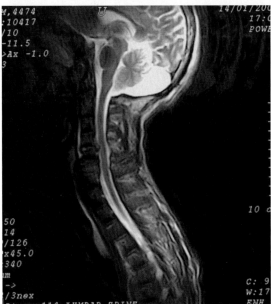

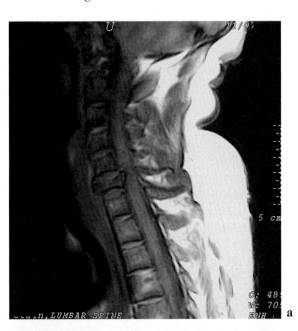

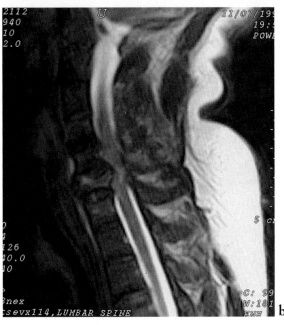

the deoxyhaemoglobin into methaemoglobin changes the signal to hyperintense on T1- and T2-weighted acquisitions. It should be noted that the evolution times of the various species of the haemoglobin molecule are slower than in

Fig. 5.13 - Acute cervical spine trauma. The images show a posttraumatic C4-C5 disk herniation and anterior subluxation of C4 on C5, with minor impingement upon the anterior surface of the cervical spinal cord. A minor C4 compression fracture is also noted. **a)** Sagittal T1-weighted MRI; **b)** sagittal T2-weighted MRI.

present, and the strength of the magnetic field. In the acute phase, deoxyhaemoglobin yields a hypointense signal on T2-, and even more strongly, on T2*-GRE sequences. A week or more after the trauma, the transformation of

Fig. 5.14 - Acute cervical spine trauma. Identified is a burst fracture of C6 and with associated narrowing of the central spinal canal and cervical spinal cord compression. Note the hyperintensity of the spinal cord on the T2-weighted images indicating contusion. [**a)** sagittal T1-weighted MRI; **b)** sagittal T2-weighted MRI].

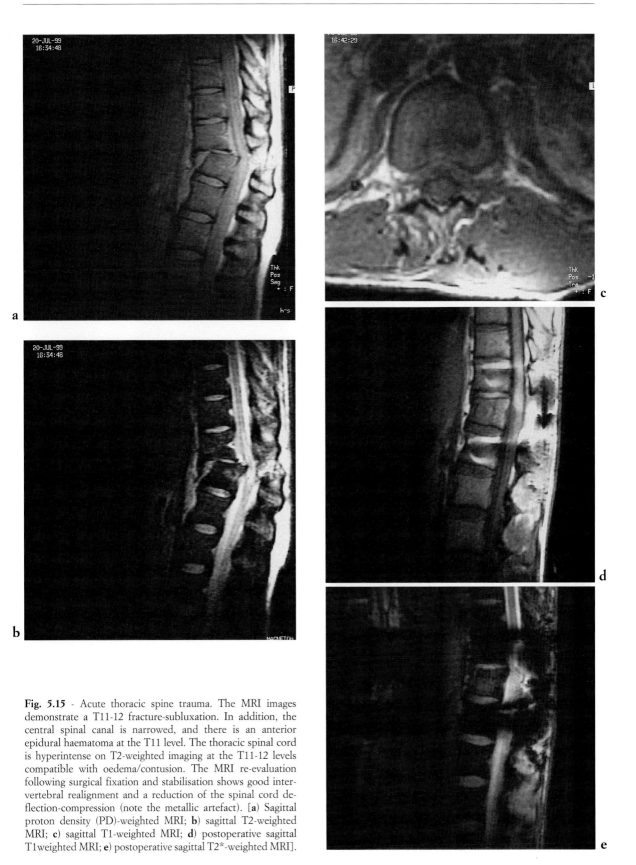

Fig. 5.15 - Acute thoracic spine trauma. The MRI images demonstrate a T11-12 fracture-subluxation. In addition, the central spinal canal is narrowed, and there is an anterior epidural haematoma at the T11 level. The thoracic spinal cord is hyperintense on T2-weighted imaging at the T11-12 levels compatible with oedema/contusion. The MRI re-evaluation following surgical fixation and stabilisation shows good intervertebral realignment and a reduction of the spinal cord deflection-compression (note the metallic artefact). [**a**) Sagittal proton density (PD)-weighted MRI; **b**) sagittal T2-weighted MRI; **c**) sagittal T1-weighted MRI; **d**) postoperative sagittal T1weighted MRI; **e**) postoperative sagittal T2*-weighted MRI].

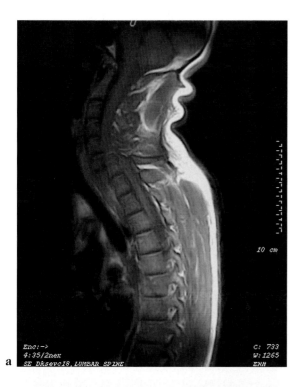

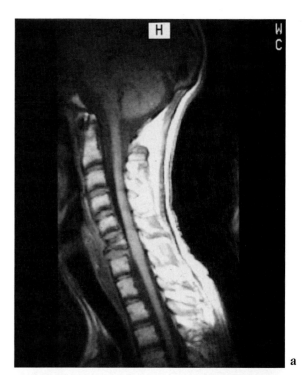

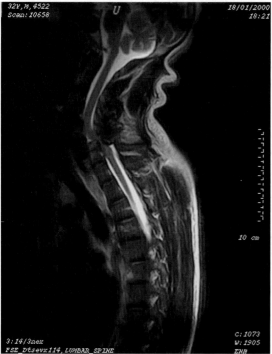

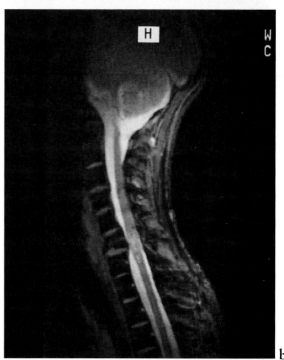

Fig. 5.16 - Acute cervical spine flexion trauma. The MRI examination shows anterior dislocation of C6-C7 associated with marked stenosis of the central spinal canal. The spinal cord is severely compressed at this level, revealing oedema and swelling of the cord above and below the compression. [**a**) sagittal T1-weighted MRI; **b**) sagittal T2-weighted MRI].

Fig. 5.17 - Acute cervical spine trauma. The MRI images reveal straightening of the physiologic cervical lordotic sagittal spinal curvature. In addition, there is a compression fracture of the C6 vertebral body. The spinal cord is swollen and is hyperintense on T2*-weighted MRI due to oedema associated with cord contusion, but no evidence of acute haemorrhage can be identified. [**a**) sagittal T1-weighted MRI; **b**) Sagittal T2*-weighted MRI].

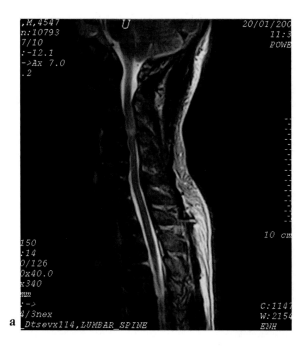

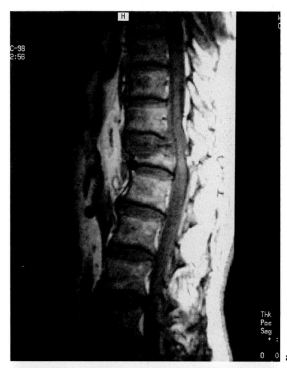

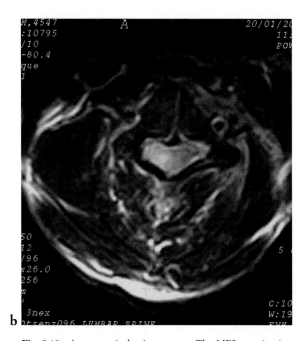

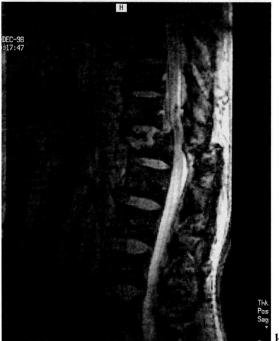

Fig. 5.18 - Acute cervical spine trauma. The MRI examination shows a loss of the physiologic cervical lordotic sagittal spinal curvature and pre-existent central spinal canal stenosis. A focal area of spinal cord contusion (i.e., oedema and swelling) can be seen on the right side at the C4 level as well as a presumed traumatic posterior disk herniation associated with underlying spinal cord compression. [**a**, sagittal T2-weighted MRI; **b**) axial T2-weighted MRI].

Fig. 5.19 - Acute thoracic spine trauma. The MRI acquisitions reveal a compression fracture of the body of T12 associated with T12-L1 anterior subluxation and central spinal canal narrowing. In addition, there is a small anterior epidural haematoma at T11. MRI signal hypointensity is present within the spinal cord on the T2* acquisition due to acute haemorrhagic contusion (deoxyhaemoglobin). **a**) [sagittal T1-weighted MRI; **b**) sagittal T2*-weighted MRI].

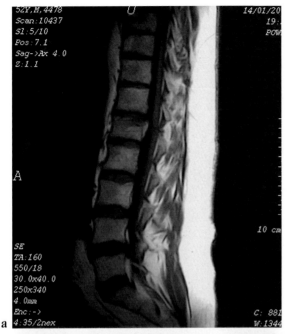

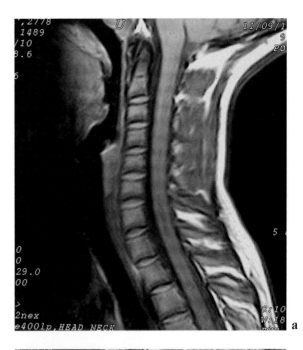

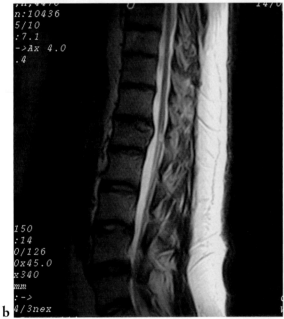

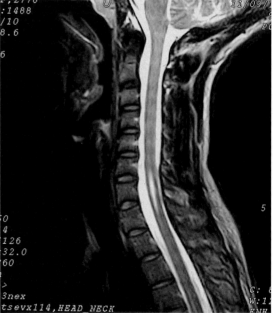

Fig. 5.20 - Chronic spinal cord trauma. MRI images in a case of late follow up of a burst fracture of L1 revealing diffuse spinal cord atrophy and a focal area of myelomalacia within the conus medullaris. [**a**) sagittal T1-weighted MRI; **b**) sagittal T2-weighted MRI].

Fig. 5.21 - Chronic spinal cord trauma. MRI in the chronic phase following spinal cord trauma reveals a posttraumatic syringomyelia cavity extending from C6-T1. [**a**) sagittal T1-weighted MRI; **b**) sagittal T2-weighted MRI, **c**) axial T2-weighted MRI].

the brain due to the reduced oxygen tension in the spinal cord (16). In the chronic phase, the presence of haemosiderin in the macrophages causes a marked signal hypointensity on T2-/T2*-weighted sequences.

The spinal cord is often more easily assessed in the sagittal plane due to the simplicity of determining an alteration in the continuity and uniformity of the medullary MR signal along the longitudinal axis of the cord. Axial and

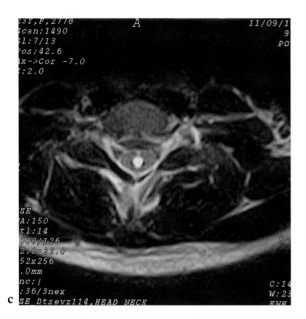

Fig. 5.21 (cont).

coronal images will help to clarify the complex traumatic changes. Multiplanar imaging is also often helpful in cases of spinal cord lacerations.

Sequelae of spinal cord trauma include cord atrophy, localized non-cystic and cystic myelo-malacia and frank syringomyelia formation, the latter of which may be progressive. Spinal cord atrophy appears as a reduction in the calibre of the cord both at the level of trauma as well as caudally. Non-cystic/cystic myelomalacia appears as an area that is hyperintense on T2-weighted images in the chronic phase following trauma. This alteration is often poorly visualized if at all on T1-weighted sequences, and is associated with cord atrophy (Fig. 5.20). Syringomyelia is easily demonstrated on both T1- and T2-weighted sequences, may be well de-

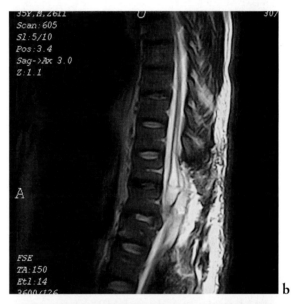

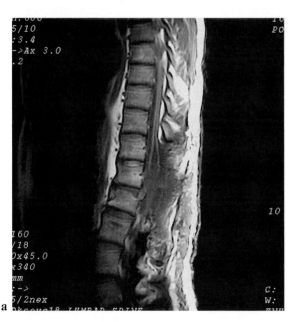

a

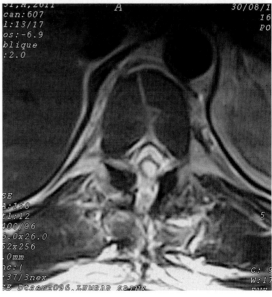

b

c

Fig. 5.22 - Chronic spinal cord trauma. MRI examination several years following flexion injury and spinal cord contusion shows postsurgical changes and a multisegmental syringohydromyelia cavity of the lower thoracic spinal cord. [a) sagittal T1-weighted MRI; b sagittal T2-weighted MRI, c) axial T2-weighted MRI].

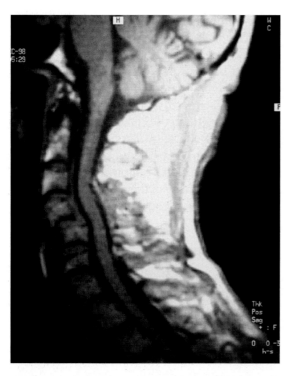

Fig. 5.23 - Acute spinal trauma. Sagittal T1-weighted MRI reveals anterior C4-C5 subluxation associated with a multilevel anterior epidural haematoma deflecting the spinal cord posteriorly.

marcated and is associated with expansion of the spinal cord (Figs. 5.21, 5.22).

It is important to point out that in some patients with posttraumatic neurological deficits related to the spinal cord MRI of the spinal cord can be completely negative in the acute phase. These are usually transitory clinical deficits usually encountered in adult subjects, which regress completely in the first few hours after the injury. This syndrome, sometimes known as SCIWORA (spinal cord injuries without radiological abnormalities) originated during the conventional radiographic era; currently, with the advent of MRI the acronym has become known by some as SCIWMRA (spinal cord injuries without magnetic resonance abnormalities) (2, 7, 30). The transient syndrome can be explained by the mechanisms of stretching or temporary compression of the spinal cord during the traumatic event, resulting in a type of spinal cord "concussion", analogous to cerebral concussion. An association between

this clinical syndrome and severe degrees of preexisting cervical spondylosis and therefore central spinal canal stenosis has been established (30).

In cases of posttraumatic epidural haematoma, as mentioed above, the MR signal varies according to the oxidation state of the haemoglobin molecules and the strength of the magnetic field of the MR unit (Figs. 5.15, 5.23). In the acute phase, extradural collections are isointense as compared to the spinal cord on T1-weighted images and isointense with regard to CSF on T2-weighted sequences. The IV administration of gadolinium can be useful in some cases for better demarcating the enhancing peripheral rim of the haematoma (26).

Root avulsions are traditionally diagnosed using myelography and CT myelography. At the levels of the avulsion, the associated pseudo-meningocele is filled by the intrathecal contrast medium used for the myelogram. However MRI is also able to identify the pseudo-meningocele, demonstrating hyperintensity of the intra- perispinal cavity on T2-weighted sequences. In some cases MRI with gadolinium can also document the interrupted nerve roots, in particular at the point where the root is partially-completely avulsed, an expression of blood-nerve barrier disruption (18). Although not universally approved, the most recent myelographic MR techniques are potentially capable of replacing conventional invasive myelography in many or all of its applications (8).

REFERENCES

1. Beers GJ, Raque GH, Wagner GG et al: MRI imaging in acute cervical spine trauma. J CAT 12(5):755-761, 1988.
2. Beltramello A, Piovan E, Alessandrini F et al: Diagnosi neuroradiologica dei traumi spinali. In Dal Pozzo G, Syllabus XV congresso nazionale AINR. Centauro, Bologna: 11-18, 1998.
3. Carella A, D'Aprile P, Farchi G: Reperti RM nei traumi vertebro-midollari. Studio con tecniche di acquisizione con eco di gradiente. Rivista di Neuroradiologia 3:45-55, 1990.
4. Chakeres DW, Flickinger F, Bresnahan JC et al: MRI Imaging of acute spinal cord trauma. AJNR 8(1):5-10, 1987
5. Curati WL, Kingsley DPE, Kendall BE et al: MRI in chronic spinal cord trauma. Neuroradiology 35:30-35, 1992.

6. Daffner RH, Deeb ZL, Goldeberg AL et al: The radiological assessment of post-traumatic vertebral stability. Skeletal Radiology 19:103-108, 1990.

7. Davis SJ, Teresi LM, Bradley WG et al: Cervical spine hyperextension injuries: MRI findings. Radiology 180(1):245-251, 1991.

8. Demaerel P, Van Hover P, Broeders A et al: Rapid lumbar spine MR mielography: imaging findings using a single-shot technique. Rivista di Neuroradiologia 10:181-187, 1997.

9. Denis F: The three column spine and its significance in the classification of acute thoraco-lumbar spinal injuries. Spine 8:817-831, 1983.

10. Denis F: Spinal instability as defined by the three-column spine concept in acute spinal trauma. Clin Orthop 189:65-76, 1984.

11. Faccioli F: La biomeccanica del trauma vertebro-midollare. In: Dal Pozzo G, Syllabus XV congresso nazionale AINR. Centauro, Bologna: 7-10, 1998.

12. Falcone S, Quencer RM, Green BA et al.: Progressive post-traumatic myelomalacic myelopathy. AJNR 15:747-754, 1994.

13. Flanders AE, Croul SE: Spinal trauma. In: Atlas SW: Magnetic resonance imaging of the brain and spine. 2° edition. Lippincott-Raven: 1161-1206, 1996.

14. Flanders AE, Tartaglino LM, Friedman DP et al: Application of fast spin-echo MRI imaging in acute cervical spine injury. Radiology 185(P):220,1992.

15. Goldberg AL, Rothfus WE, Deeb ZL et al: The impact of magnetic resonance on the diagnostic evaluation of acute cervico-thoracic spinal trauma. Skeletal Radiol 17(2):89-95, 1988.

16. Hackney DB, Asato LR, Joseph P et al: Hemorrhage and edema in acute spinal cord compression: demonstration by MRI imaging. Radiology 161:387-390, 1986.

17. Hall ED, Braughler JM: Central nervous system trauma and stroke. II. Physiological and pharmacological evidence for involvement of oxygen radicals and lipid peroxidation. Free Radical Biol Med 6:303-313, 1989.

18. Hayashi N, Yamamoto S, Okubo T et al: Avulsion injury of cervical nerve roots: enhanced intradural nerve roots at MR Imaging. Radiology 206:817-822, 1998.

19. Janssen L, Hansebout RR: Pathogenesis of spinal cord injury and newer treatments. A review Spine 14:23-32, 1989.

20. Jones KM, Mulkern RV, Schwartz RB et al: Fast spin-echo MR Imaging of the brain and spine: current concepts. AJR 158:1313-1320, 1992.

21. Kakulas BA: Pathology of spinal injuries. CNS Trauma 1:117-129, 1984.

22. Kalfas I, Wilberger J, Goldberg A et al: Magnetic resonance imaging in acute spinal cord trauma. Neurosurgery 23(3):295-299, 1988.

23. Kwo S, Young W, De Crescito V: Spinal cord sodium, potassium, calcium and water concentration changes in rats after graded contusion injury. J Neurotrauma 6:13-24, 1989.

24. Levitt MA, Flanders AE: Diagnostic capabilities of magnetic resonance and computed tomography in acute cervical spinal column injury. Am J Emerg Med 9(2):131-135, 1991.

25. Meldrum B: Possible therapeutic applications of anthagonists of excitatory aminoacid neurotransmitters. Clin Sci 68:113-122, 1985.

26. Pellicanò G, Cellerini M, Del Seppia I: Spinal trauma. Rivista di Neuroradiologia 11:329-335, 1998.

27. Posse S, Aue WP: Susceptibility artifacts in spin-echo and gradient-echo imaging. J Magn Reson 88:473-492, 1990

28. Quencer RM, Sheldon JJ, MJD et al: MRI of the chronically injured cervical spinal cord. AJR 147:125-132, 1986.

29. Ramon S, Dominguez R, Ramirez L et al: Clinical and magnetic resonance imaging correlation in acute spinal cord injury. Spinal Cord 35:664-673, 1997.

30. Rogenbogen VS, Rogers LF, Atlas SW et al: Cervical spinal cord injuries in patients with cervical spondylosis. Am J Radiol 146:277-284, 1986.

31. Scarabino T, Polonara G, Perfetto F et al: Studio RM Fast Spin-Echo dei traumi vertebro-midollari acuti. Rivista di Neuroradiologia 9:565-571, 1996.

32. Tarr RW, Drolshagen LF, Kerner TC et al: MRI Imaging of recent spinal trauma. J CAT 11(3):412-417, 1987.

33. Tartaglino LM, Flanders AE, Vinitski S et al: Metallic artifacts on MRI images of the postoperative spine: reduction with fast spin echo techniques. Radiology 190:565-569, 1994.

34. Tator CH, Fehlindgs MJ: Review of the secondary injury theory of acute spinal cord trauma with emphasis on vascular mechanisms. J Neurosurg 75:15-26, 1991.

35. Tien RD: Fat suppression MR imaging in neuroradiology: techniques and clinical application. Am J Roentgenol 158:369-379, 1992.

36. Weirich SD, Cotler HB, Narayana PA et al: Histopathologic correlation of magnetic resonance signal patterns in a spinal cord injury model. Spine 15(7):630-638, 1990.

37. White AA, Panjabi MM: Clinical biomechanics of the spine. PA JB Lippincott, Philadelphia: 169-275, 1990.

5.4

EMERGENCY IMAGING OF THE SPINE IN THE NON-TRAUMA PATIENT

G. Polonara, M.G. Bonetti, T. Scarabino, U. Salvolini

INTRODUCTION

Non-traumatic spinal emergencies include all those clinical situations that present with acute and/or rapidly progressive signs and symptoms of spinal cord-spinal nerve/root compromise. These can be a result of extrinsic spinal radiculomedullary compression or of intrinsic pathology.

All of these conditions require rapid diagnostic analysis: the recognition of a compressive or expanding spinal cord-canal lesion makes it possible to determine a surgical solution, whereas its exclusion guides diagnosis and treatment in other directions. The main causes of non-traumatic acute and subacute myelopathic and/or radiculopathic syndromes are given in Table 1.

IMAGING TECHNIQUES

Worsening acute and/or subacute radiculomedullary compression constitutes the most frequent cause of non-traumatic spinal emergency. In the case of rapid onset of a severe neurological syndrome (e.g., sudden paraplegia), diagnostic imaging must be conducted as rapidly as possible in order to proceed swiftly with surgical decompression if deemed appropriate.

Conventional radiography makes it possible to analyse the entire spine in a very short inter-

---

EXTRADURAL PATHOLOGY

Vertebrodiscal pathology:	– vertebral metastases
	– disk herniation
	– severe spondylosis and arthrosis
	– haemolymphopathies
	– benign tumours
	– primitive malignant tumours
	– spondylodiskitis
Epidural pathology:	– lymphoma
	– metastasis
	– haematoma
	– arachnoid cyst

INTRADURAL PATHOLOGY
Extramedullary intradural tumours
Spinal cord tumours
Multiple sclerosis
Spinal cord infarcts
Spinal cord arteriovenous malformations
Spinal arteriovenous fistulae
Dural arteriovenous fistulae
Cavernous angioma
Myelitis and spinal cord abscesses
Acute disseminated encephalomyelitis
Radiation myelopathy

Tab. 5.1 - Causative factors of emergency non-traumatic clinical spinal syndromes.

val of time, highlighting abnormalities in the physiological curvature, bony spinal canal stenoses, vertebral collapse and other structural alterations. A negative x-ray examination, however, does not exclude the presence of bony, intervertebral disk or ligamentous pathology and in any case it does not provide information, except very rarely, on the presence of the pathology affecting the contents of the central spinal canal.

Today, almost all patients with acute syndromes of neurological radiculomedullary impairment can be rapidly sent to a diagnostic centre where MRI equipment is available even without the delay entailed in an initial conventional x-ray examination. MRI is currently the most sensitive and specific technique available for studying the spine. This methodology makes it possible to acquire images in various spatial planes without having to move the patient. It clearly enables the visualization of the spinal column (vertebrae, disks, ligaments and paravertebral soft tissues) and its contents (epidural space, thecal sac, spinal cord and roots/nerves) in a direct, thorough and panoramic way. In addition to establishing the focus of the lesion and the extent of the process, the nature of the condition can often be surmised.

Although the cortical bone is best studied using x-rays and computed tomography, MRI is the method of choice in studying vertebral bone marrow. In selected cases, a CT examination focused on a precise location identified using MRI can be a useful complement in non-traumatic radiculomedullary syndromes due to the greater contrast resolution of bone achieved with CT.

Myelography is rarely used in those cases where the usual exclusions of MRI exist (e.g., pacemakers, MRI-incompatible metal surgical cerebral aneurysm clips). In such cases it is used to search for indirect signs of non-osseous causes of compression of the thecal sac and underlying spinal cord/cauda equina. *Bone scintigraphy* can be useful for a non-specific analysis of possible active lesions in the skeleton as a whole. In selected cases it can also be useful in studying pathology limited to the spinal column.

CAUSES

In this section, the most frequent causes of non-traumatic spinal emergencies will be considered, making a distinction between extradural (pathology affecting the vertebrae, intervertebral disks, spinal ligaments and epidural space) and thecal sac, intradural-extramedullary and neural pathology (disease of the meninges, subarachnoid space, spinal cord and/or spinal nerves/roots).

EXTRADURAL PATHOLOGY

Back pain is the most frequent symptom of epidural pathology. Signs and symptoms of spinal cord and/or radicular involvement are precipitated by pathological conditions that primarily affect the bony structures of the spinal column, with or without the collapse of the vertebrae at the site of the pathology. This is in turn followed by extraosseous involvement of the central spinal canal and neural foramina and the subsequent onset of myelopathic and radiculopathic compression syndromes.

The pathogenesis of vertebral collapse can be benign (e.g., osteoporosis, vertebral haemangiomas, spondylodiskitis) or malignant (e.g., primary or metastatic neoplastic disease). Symptomatic vertebral collapse is most often caused by neoplastic metastases, haematological/lymphatic neoplastic conditions (i.e., haemolymphopathies) and spondylodiskitis. All of these can be responsible for radiculomedullary compression even without vertebral collapse due to extraosseous neoplastic or inflammatory mass-forming collections.

In some instances MRI makes it possible to distinguish between benign and malignant spinal column collapse, and it is also the most sensitive method of identifying the overlying spinal cord involvement in cases of extradural pathology.

Spinal neoplasia and haemolymphopathies

Spinal neoplasia can be primary (benign 10%, malignant 10%), or secondary (metastases 80%).

Up to 5% of patients with known neoplastic conditions have symptomatic spinal metastases.

The most common type of primary "tumour" of a vascular nature affecting the spine is vertebral *haemangioma* (Fig. 5.24), benign lesions that are usually discovered incidentally. They can affect any part of the spine, however the thoracolumbar spine is the most frequent site. Haemangiomas usually only affect the vertebral body, but can also involve the posterior bony arch and spread into the perivertebral soft tissues, thereby potentially causing neural compression syndromes (Fig. 5.25).

CT typically reveals a diminution in number but thickening of the individual trabeculae within the affected vertebral marrow space. However, in certain cases it can be difficult to differentiate these benign vascular lesions from true neoplasia on the basis on CT alone.

On MR examinations using T1-weighted sequences, haemangiomas have an irregular appearance due to the simultaneous presence of hyperintense areas (adipose tissue) and hypointense areas (thickened bony trabeculae). On T2-weighted images they appear generally hyperintense due to their high cellularity and perhaps the collection of blood within the haemangioma itself.

Some *rarer forms of benign tumour* include osteochondromas, osteoid osteomas, osteoblas-

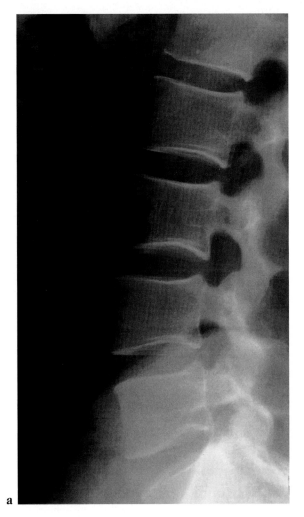
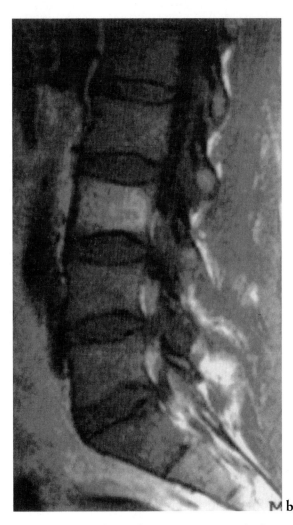

a   b

Fig. 5.24 - Vertebral haemangioma. The lateral radiographic examination shows the typical vertical striations consistent with a bone marrow haemangioma at the L3 level. The T1-weighted MRI reveals bone marrow hyperintensity typical of vertebral haemangioma. [**a**) Lateral radiograph of lumbar spine; **b**) sagittal T-1 weighted MRI].

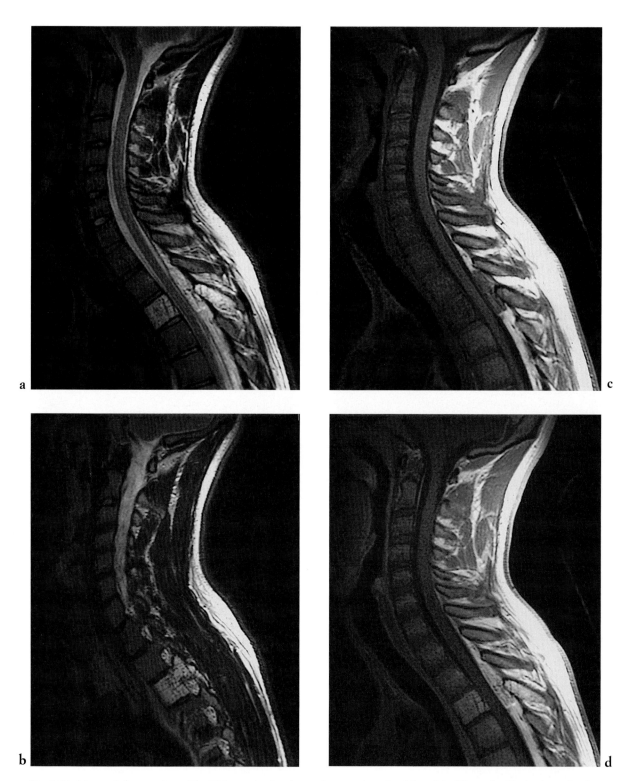

Fig. 5.25 - Metameric haemangioma. The MRI examination shows a haemangioma involving of the T3 vertebral body, the peduncles, the articular processes, the posterior arch and the posterior epidural space with minor compression of the thecal sack and spinal cord. The internal vascular component of the haemangioma is observed to enhance following IV gadolinium (Gd) administration. [**a**), **b**) sagittal T2-weighted MRI; **c**) unenhanced sagittal T2-weighted MRI; **d**) sagittal T1-weighted MRI following IV Gd; **e**) axial T1-weighted MRI following IV Gd].

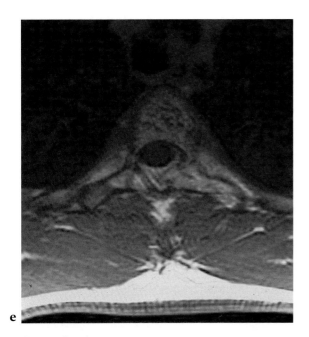

e

Fig. 5.25 (*cont.*).

tomas (Fig. 5.26) and aneurysmal bone cysts, all of which are clearly visualized on both radiographs and CT (7).

Rare malignant primary tumours include osteosarcomas (including those presenting as a malignant degeneration of Paget's disease of the spine), chondrosarcomas, Ewing's sarcomas, and fibrosarcomas. Chordomas, having an intermediate histological status between benign and malignant, originate from elements of the notochord and are particularly common in the sphenoid bone, the clivus and the sacrum. In these cases MR is the best imaging technique for defining the extent of the tumour within the spine as well as determining the involvement of the perispinal soft tissues.

Undoubtedly the most frequent type of neoplastic spinal involvement is haematogenously borne *metastatic disease*, which replaces the bone marrow tissue and destroys the bony cortex of the vertebrae. Statistically, 10% of cases of metastatic neoplastic disease affect the cervical spine, 77% the thoracic and upper lumbar levels and 13% involve the lumbar and sacral segments. The vertebral body is more frequently involved than are the posterior bony elements, with the exception of the vertebral pedi-

cles which are often affected. Epidural metastatic disease is often present, either secondary to primary disease, or in some cases as the sole spinal location.

In most cases bony spinal metastatic disease has an osteolytic appearance on x-ray and CT imaging, however depending upon the histological type, it may be sclerotic or mixed lytic-sclerotic.

Metastatic replacement of the bone marrow is clearly visible on MRI. Destructive lesions demonstrate areas of relative hypointensity on T1-weighted imaging and comparative hyperintensity on T2* STIR/chemical saturation fat-suppressed and T2-weighted sequences (Fig. 5.27). The presence and extent of the tumour in the spinal canal and the perivertebral tissues is well documented after the administration of IV gadolinium contrast medium on T1-weighted images, especially when combined with fat-suppression techniques.

On MRI, an appearance similar to that described for metastases can be observed in cases of vertebral lymphoma, multiple myeloma and plasmocytoma affecting the spine (Fig. 5.28). Lymphomas, like metastatic neoplastic disease, can also have a solely epidural localization.

Infectious processes involving the spine

The early diagnosis of vertebral osteomyelitis, diskitis or epidural abscess formation by means of medical imaging (Fig. 5.29) facilitates suitable treatment to be instituted rapidly, even though the clinical signs, symptoms and laboratory tests are frequently not specific (10). In cases of spondylodiskitis, 2-8 weeks can elapse from the onset of clinical symptoms until visible signs are present on conventional radiographic studies. These findings can include a reduction in the height of the intervertebral disk space, alterations in the vertebral end plates (e.g., erosion, blurring of margins, reactive bony sclerosis) and the presence of an extraosseous paravertebral soft tissue mass. The vertebral bodies can variably be destroyed, however the pedicles are rarely involved in cases of infection, with the exception of spinal tuberculosis.

CT, preferably performed after the IV administration of iodinated contrast medium, typically reveals the existence of a mass in the perivertebral soft tissues and epidural space, and the fragmentation and destruction of vertebrae.

On MRI, spondylodiskitis has a characteristic appearance that includes the involvement of the two contiguous vertebrae (hypointense marrow signal on T1-weighted images; hyperintense marrow signal on T2-weighted sequences) and the intervening intervertebral disk (reduction of height of disk space; hyperintense signal on T2-weighted images) (Fig. 5.30). In addition, MRI demonstrates bony erosions of the vertebral end plates, inflammatory epidural and perivertebral soft tissue masses and semifluid abscess collections (Fig. 5.31). Postcontrast images acquired with fat suppression are most sensitive in defining the extent of the complex inflammatory processes.

It should be noted that while spinal metastatic neoplasia reveals signal alteration of the vertebrae similar to those described for spondylodiskitis, involvement of the adjacent intervertebral disk and adjacent vertebral end plates is not present.

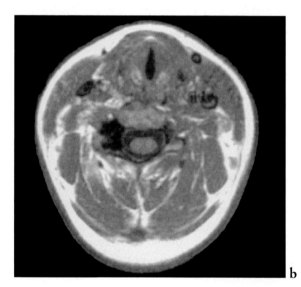

b

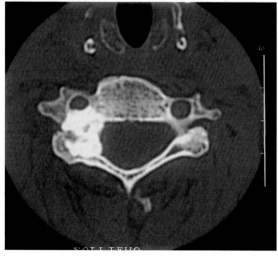

c

a

Fig. 5.26 - Osteoblastoma of the posterior arch of C5. The MRI examination reveals a hypointense lesion within the posterior arch of C5 on the right. The CT study shows a sclerotic mass lesion of the posterior arch of C5. [**a**) oblique-sagittal T1-weighted MRI; **b**) axial T1-weighted MRI; **c**) axial CT].

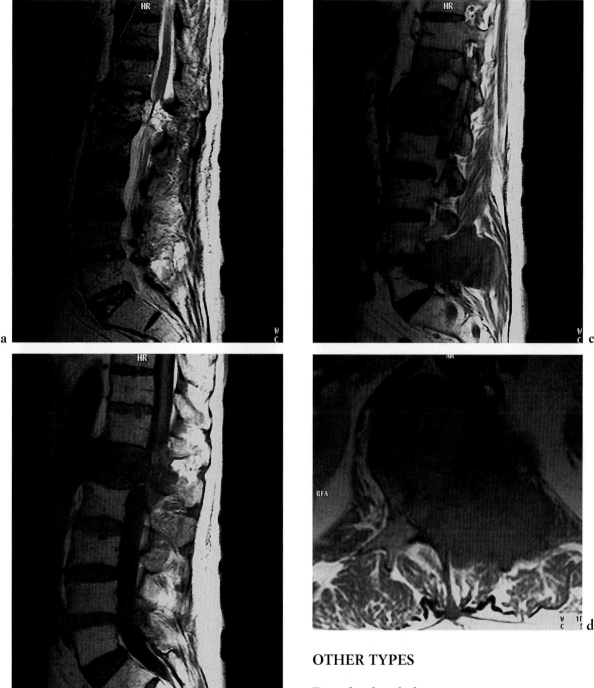

Fig. 5.27 - Multiple vertebral neoplastic metastases from primary colon cancer. The MRI examination shows partial collapse and expansion of the L1 vertebral body and the presence of an epidural soft tissue mass that compresses the thecal sac, the conus medullaris and the roots of the cauda equina. In addition, there is neoplastic involvement of T11, L5 and the adjacent perispinal soft tissues. [**a**) sagittal T2-weighted MRI; **b**), **c**) sagittal T1-weighted MRI; **d**), **e**) axial T1-weighted MRI; **f**) coronal T2-weighted MRI].

OTHER TYPES

Extradural pathology

The differential diagnosis of acute clinical radiculomedullary syndromes must also take into consideration other types of pathology (10, 12), including: *posterior spinal facet joint and interspinous spondylosis* (Fig. 5.32); *disk herniations-protrusions; osteopenic-osteoporotic verte-*

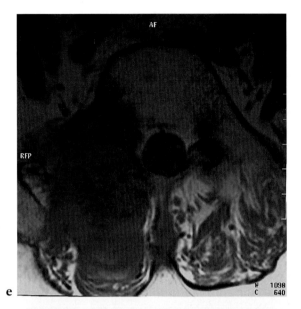

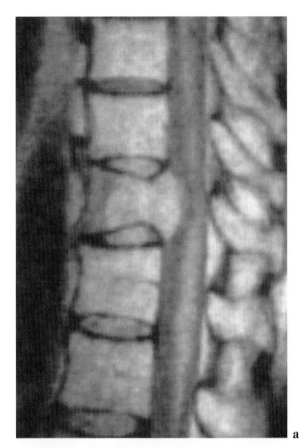

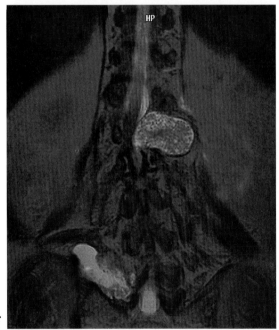

Fig. 5.27 (*cont.*).

bral collapse; osteonecrosis; and developmental spinal malformations especially at the cervico-occipital junction (Fig. 5.33).

The high contrast resolution of MRI regarding soft tissues enables a straightforward evaluation of degenerative/protrusive intervertebral disk pathology. T2-weighted images acquired in the sagittal plane characterize such degenerative

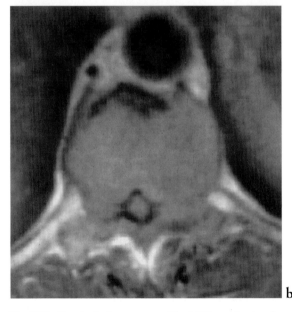

Fig. 5.28 - Vertebral plasmocytoma. The MRI examination the sagittal picture clearly shows the expansion and partial collapse of the T9 vertebral body with associated invasion of the paravertebral and epidural soft tissues. [**a**) sagittal T1-weighted MRI; **b**) axial T1-weighted].

alterations thanks partly to the "myelographic effect" of the high CSF signal. Spinal cord compression, with or without parenchymal oedema, is also well visualised on sagittal T2-weighted sequences; these alterations are generally less easily visible on axial T2-weighted images. T1-

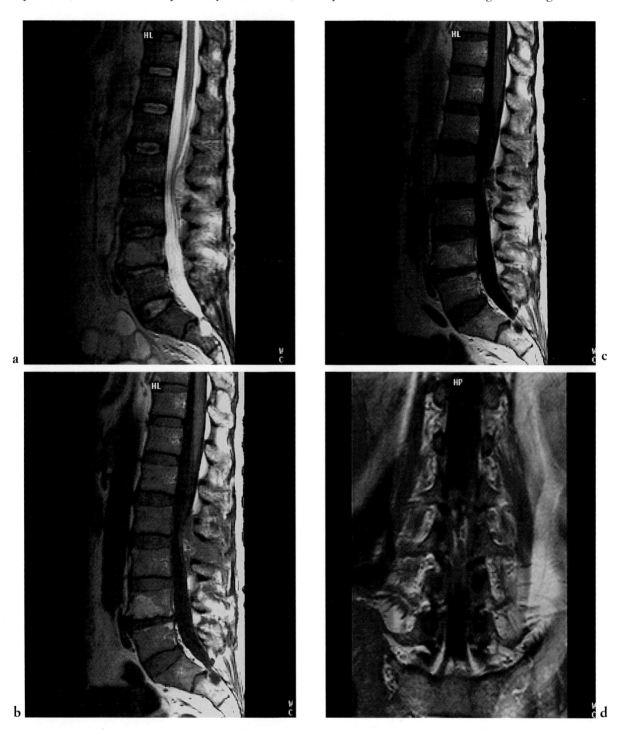

Fig. 5.29 - Iatrogenic epidural abscess. The MRI study shows a mass forming posterior epidural lesion that displaces the nerve roots of the cauda equina forwards. There is inhomogeneous enhancement of this process following IV Gd administration. [**a**) sagittal T2-weighted MRI; **b**) unenhanced sagittal T1-weighted MRI; **c**) sagittal T1-weighted MRI following IV Gd; **d**) coronal T1-weighted MRI following IV Gd].

weighted acquisitions, that provide greater visibility of epidural and neural foramen fat, further assist in the diagnostic evaluation in the thoracic and lumbar regions. Finally, MR myelography utilizing T2-wieghted sequences can facilitate evaluating the presence or absence of a radicular compression.

Of the causes of compression emanating directly from the epidural space, *spontaneous haematomas* (Fig. 5.34), *and extradural arachnoid cysts* should be considered. Epidural haematomas will typically demonstrate no other related findings on imaging studies; the MRI characteristics will be the same as those previously described for acute-subacute spinal haematomas. CT and MR examinations in cases of arachnoid cyst reveal smooth bony erosion, including: widening of the central spinal canal, pedicle erosion, widening of the affected neural foramen and erosion of the adjacent surfaces of the vertebral body. MRI shows an expanding lesion having signal similar or identical to that of CSF. Signs indicating an extradural nature of the cyst are cranial and caudal displacement of the adjacent epidural fat, anterior displacement of the subarachnoid space and the spinal cord and extension into the neural foramen (8, 10) (Fig. 5.35).

Intradural pathology

In cases of extramedullary masses, radicular symptoms usually precede medullary ones, they are segmental and can be sensory and/or motor. Intramedullary masses most often present with non-specific, gradual, progressive signs and symptoms; pain may be the first symptom. Sensory deficits vary according to the location of the lesion. Bladder and bowel dysfunction and impotence are rare and appear late in the clinical course (1).

Fig. 5.30 - Spondylodiskitis. The MRI examination demonstrates a pathologic process effecting simultaneous involvement of multiple thoracic vertebrae together with the intervening intervertebral disks. In addition, there is associated disk and vertebral collapse, perivertebral and epidural soft tissue mass formation and spinal cord compression. These findings are consistent with nonspecific spondylodiskitis. [**a**] coronal T1-weighted MRI; coronal T2-weighted MRI; unenhanced sagittal T1-weighted MRI; sagittal T1-weighted MRI following IV Gd].

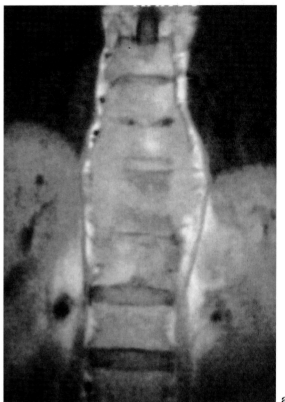

a

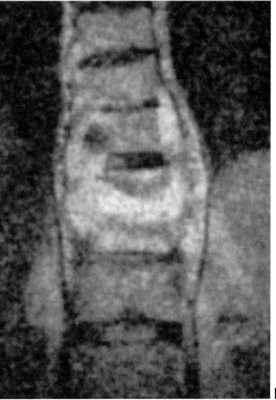

b

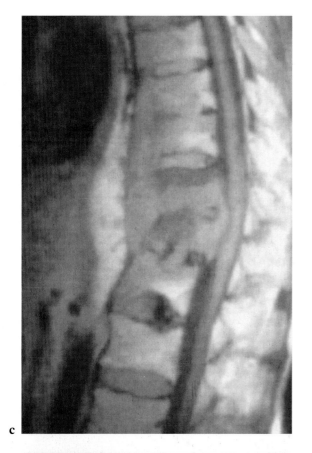

c

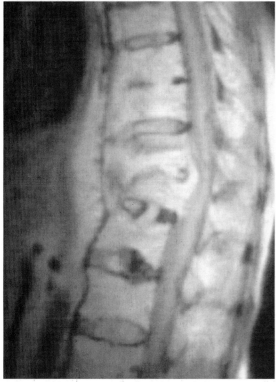

d

In the cases of intradural masses, x-rays may show a straightening of the physiological curvature of the spine or even progressive scoliosis. Especially in children with congenital intramedullary tumours, widening of the central spinal canal and thinning of the pedicles may be observed.

Myelography is rarely indicated, except in subjects where MRI is contraindicated or unavailable, or when MRI is not diagnostic, as when small neurinomas, vascular malformations and arachnoid lesions are suspected.

CT is not particularly helpful in these situations and should principally be reserved for osteoarticular pathology of the spinal column and following myelography.

Spinal angiography is indicated in the examination of vascular malformations and neoplasia as a preliminary stage for interventional radiology procedures and in preoperative evaluation.

MR is the examination technique of choice for imaging the subarachnoid space and the spinal cord, and should be the first study to be performed where available. The examination should include T1- and T2-weighted images, and T1-weighted images after the IV administration of gadolinium. The entire spine can be examined using dedicated phased-array surface coils. The images must be acquired in at least two different scan planes in order to clearly define the lesion in three planes and to assist in the differentiation between intra- and extramedullary masses.

Neoplasia and non-neoplastic mass forming processes

The most frequent types of intradural extramedullary neoplasia are meningiomas and neurinomas (1). *Meningiomas* are benign tumours that originate in the arachnoid mater, occur more frequently in females in the fifth decade of life and exert effects via mass effect. They are most often encountered in the tho-

Fig. 5.30 (*cont.*).

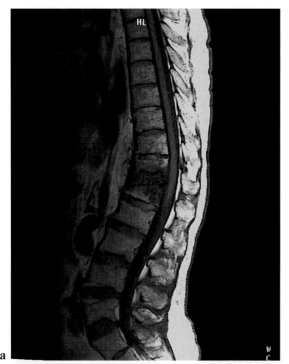

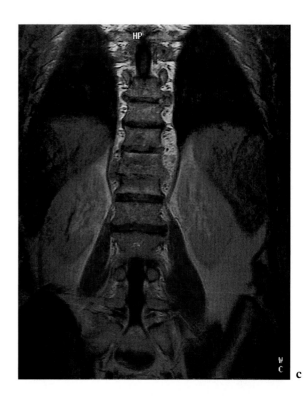

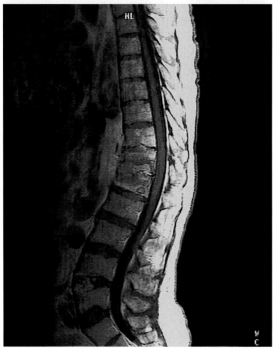

Fig. 5.31 - Subacute spondylodiskitis caused by brucella species. The MRI study shows a simultaneous pathologic involvement of two adjacent vertebrae and the intervening intervertebral disk. There is irregular contrast enhancement in all involved structures following IV Gd administration. The perivertebral soft tissues demonstrate limited involvement. [**a**) unenhanced sagittal T1-weighted MRI; **b**) sagittal T1-weighted MRI following IV Gd; **c**) coronal T1-weighted MRI following IV Gd].

racic spine. Only rarely are they multiple in the spine, and very seldom have large extradural components.

From a diagnostic imaging point of view, on x-rays it is only rarely possible to observe calcifications or signs of vertebral remodelling. Myelographic signs are indirect, typically appearing as an obstruction of flow of the subarachnoid contrast medium, typical of extramedullary intradural lesions, with associated displacement and compression of the spinal cord. On CT, meningiomas can be distinguished from the surrounding anatomical structures by their intrinsic hyperdensity relative to the spinal cord, calcifications when present and dense enhancement following the IV administration of iodinated contrast medium.

On MRI, meningiomas may have a similar intensity to spinal cord. Their identification is facilitated by the use of heavily T2-weighted sequences, and the administration of IV gadolinium contrast medium. Meningiomas typically reveal an intense, homogeneous pattern of enhancement after the gadolinium injection (Fig. 5.36).

Neurinomas originate from Schwann cells and favour the posterior spinal nerve roots as sites of origin. They are more frequently observed at cervical and thoracic spinal locations, but can involve the roots of the cauda equina. These neoplasms can be multiple in Recklinghausen's disease (Fig. 5.37). Neurinomas present in an intradural-extramedullary location, can extend into the neural foramen and even grow outside the spinal canal (i.e., hourglass-shaped mass). In such cases on x-rays it is possible to observe widening of the neural foramen and, if sufficiently large, the presence of a paravertebral mass. If voluminous, neurinomas can al-so cause scalloping of the posterior wall of the vertebral body(ies).

Concerning the intradural component of the neurinoma, myelography provides typical findings of spinal cord displacement and compression, and cup-shaped blockage of the contrast medium by the neoplasm; myelography provides no information on the extradural component of the lesion. CT following the myelogram, however, reveals the entire extent of the tumour together with the bony remodelling when present. Neurinomas generally show heterogeneous enhancement on CT after IV iodinated contrast medium administration.

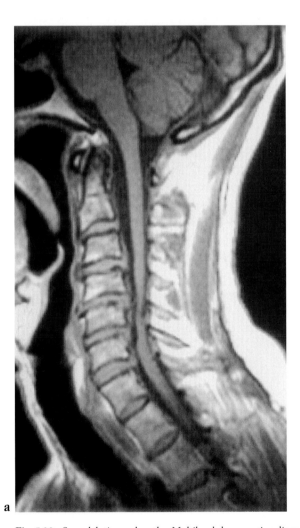

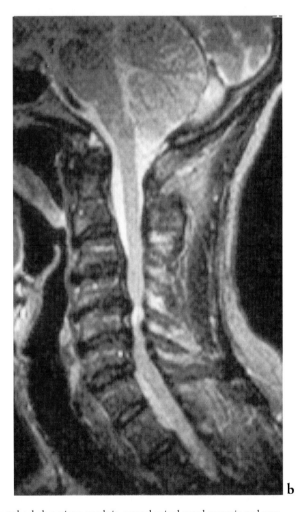

a   b

Fig. 5.32 - Spondylotic myelopathy. Multilevel degenerative discovertebral alterations result in central spinal canal stenosis and associated cervical spinal cord compression. In addition, a focal area of hyperintense MRI signal is observed on the T2-weighted image at the C5 level consistent with myelomalacia. [**a**) sagittal T1-weighted MRI; (**b**) sagittal T2-weighted MRI].

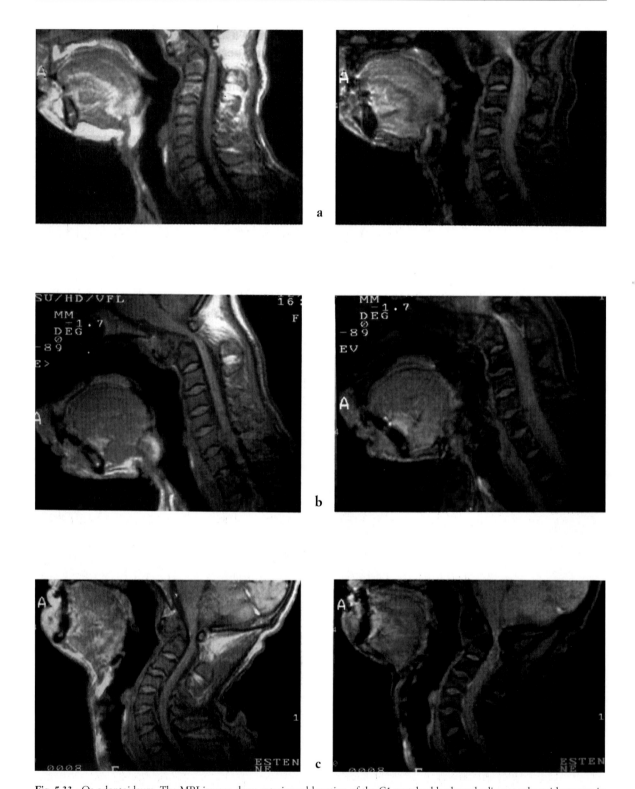

Fig. 5.33 - Os odontoideum. The MRI images show anterior subluxation of the C1 vertebral body and adjacent odontoid process in relationship to the vertebral body of C2. In addition, the spinal cord is compressed between the posterior bony arch of C1 and the vertebral body of C2, and the intervening spinal cord is hyperintense indicating underlying myelomalacia. Note the partial reduction of the dislocation in extension. [**a**): neutral T1- and T2-weighted sagittal MRI; **b**): flexion T1- and T2-weighted sagittal MRI; **c**): extension T1- and T2-weighted sagittal MRI].

Unenhanced MRI provides all the diagnostic information outlined above.

The *rarer mass-forming lesions* of the subarachnoid space include (in decreasing order of frequency) lipomas (most often associated with congenital dysraphic conditions), teratomas, and subarachnoid metastases (Fig. 5.38) that are typically multiple and widespread, fre-

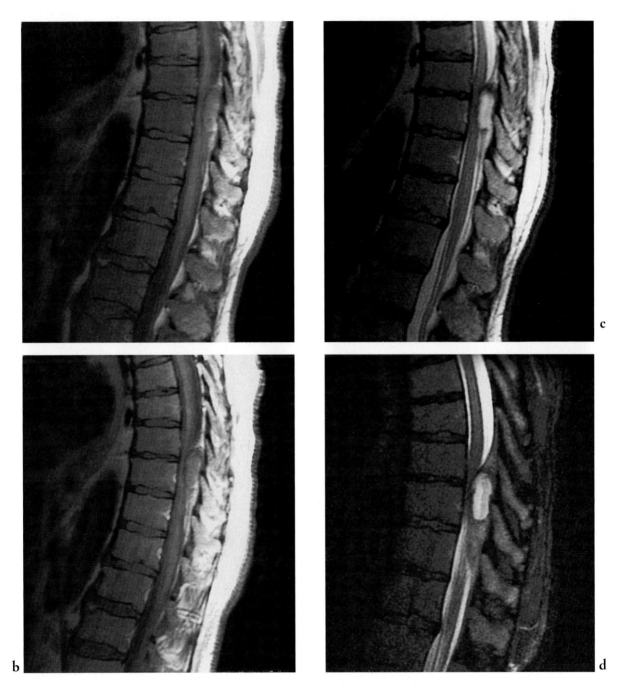

Fig. 5.34 - Spontaneous subacute epidural haemorrhage in patient with plasmacytopenia. The MRI examination shows mass forming posterior epidural haematoma. IV Gd enhanced MRI shows minor peripheral enhancement around the haematoma. The remaining MRI study reveals hypointensity of the margins of the haematoma consistent with early haemosiderin evolution and anterior spinal cord deflection-compression. [a) unenhanced sagittal T1-weighted MRI; **b**) T1-weighted MRI following IV Gd; **c**) T2-weighted MRI; **d**) sagittal T2-weighted MRI with fat suppression; **e**) axial T1-weighted MRI; **f**) axial T2-weighted MRI].

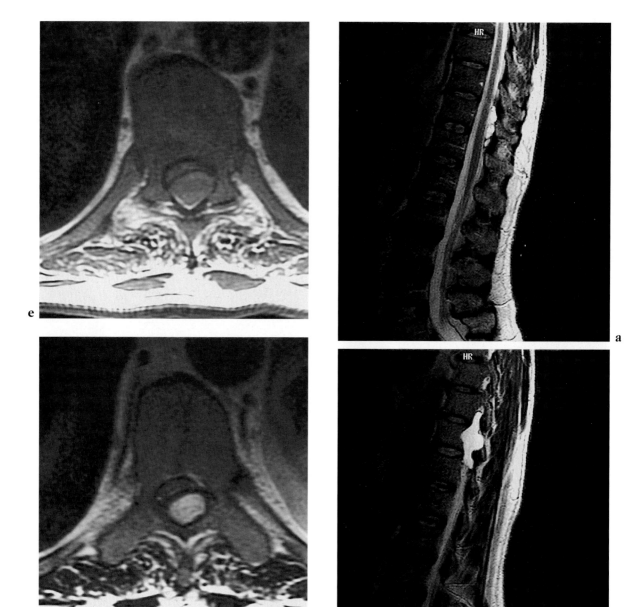

Fig. 5.34 (cont.).

quently covering the leptomeningeal surfaces of the spinal subarachnoid space (Fig. 5.39). All these pathological conditions are well documented using MRI. CT is excellent in documenting adipose tissue and, unlike MRI, is able to demonstrate tumour calcifications present in some neoplasms (e.g., teratomas).

MRI is also the best non-invasive technique for documenting *non-neoplastic expanding processes,*

Fig. 5.35 - Extradural arachnoid cysts. The MRI images show a posterolateral intraspinal mass lesion that has an MRI signal that is slightly higher than that of CSF. There is associated cranial and caudal displacement of the supra- and subjacent epidural fat surrounding the mass indicating its epidural location. There is also minor mass effect upon the thecal sac and extension of the cyst into the contiguous, expanded spinal neural foramen. [**a**) midline sagittal T2-weighted MRI; **b**) parasagittal T2-weighted MRI; **c**) midline T1-weighted MRI; **d**) coronal T1-weighted MRI; **e**) midlesion axial T2-weighted MRI; **f**) subjacent axial T2-weighted MRI].

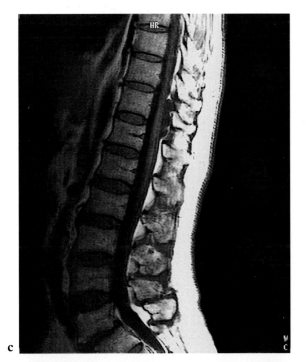

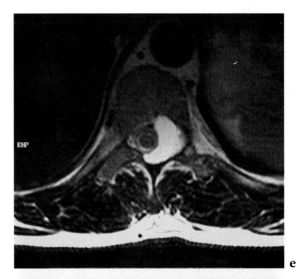

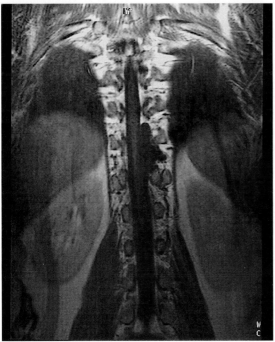

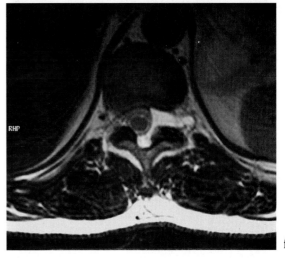

c

d

Fig. 5.35 (*cont.*).

e

f

including intradural arachnoid cysts and lateral spinal meningoceles (associated with von Recklinghausen's disease).

The most frequently encountered intramedullary neoplasms are astrocytomas, ependymomas and haemangioblastomas. Astrocytomas represent 25-30% of all intramedullary tumours presenting in adults and more than 90% of all spinal cord tumours in children. Typical astrocytomas cause a fusiform expansion of the spinal cord. If a cystic component is present, it is typically intratumoral, although satellite cysts and secondary syringomyelia are observed. Astrocytomas reveal moderate, irregular enhancement after IV contrast medium administration. The boundaries of the astrocytoma are usually poorly defined. The evolution of such lesions into glioblastoma multiforme is occasionally seen (Fig. 5.40).

Ependymomas are typically located in the cervical region and are often associated with

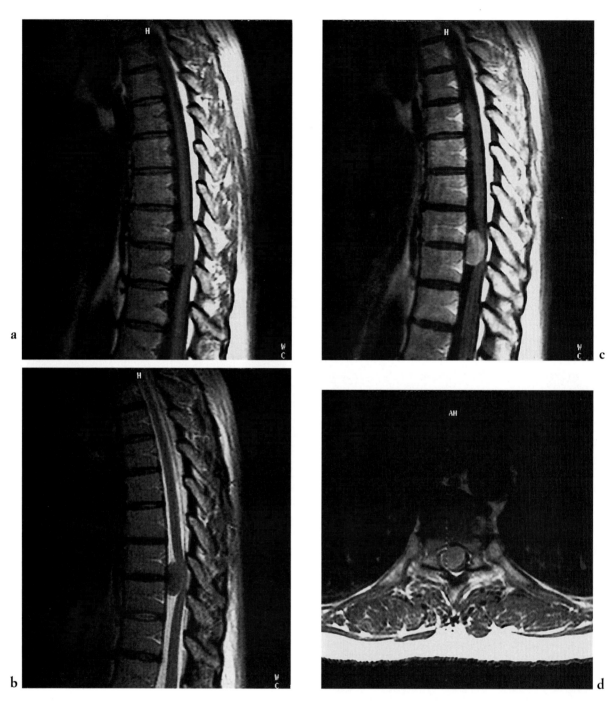

Fig. 5.36 - Spinal meningioma. The MRI images reveal a spinal canal mass having MRI signal that is very similar to that of the spinal cord. The heavily T2-weighted images demonstrate the intradural-extramedullary location of the tumour. The lesion shows intense, homogeneous contrast enhancement following IV Gd administration. [**a**) sagittal T1-weighted MRI; **b**) sagittal T2-weighted MRI; **c**), **d**), **e**) sagittal, axial and coronal T1-weighted MRI following IV Gd].

a large satellite cyst(s). Although not always seen, a low signal intensity area on T2-weighted MR typically surrounds the cranial and caudal boundaries of the lesion, representing repeated intralesional microhaemorrhages (Fig. 5.41). Ependymomas generally reveal well-defined boundaries and, with the exception of the often associated cystic component,

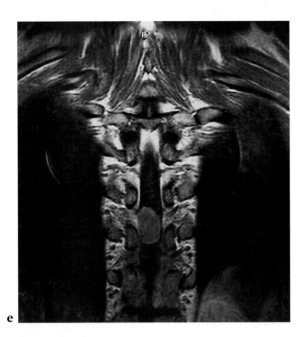

e

Fig. 5.36 (*cont.*).

demonstrate intense, rather homogeneous enhancement after IV gadolinium contrast medium administration. Originating from ependymal cells, they occupy a less eccentric location that astrocytomas. They are most commonly encountered in adolescents and young adults. Not uncommonly they may be located in the cauda equina because of embryonic rests of ependymal cells in the filum terminale (Fig. 5.42).

Haemangioblastomas represent 5% of all spinal cord neoplasia. This kind of tumour can be isolated or multicentric. In the latter case, they are associated with von Hippel-Lindau's disease. Tumour nodes are typically small, richly vascularized, generally located eccentrically in the cord and often associated with extensive syringomyelia formation and/or marked spinal cord oedema.

Rare tumours of the spinal cord include lymphomas (usually a spinal cord deposit of a systemic lymphoma), congenital lipomas, neoplastic metastases, gangliogliomas and oligodendrogliomas.

MRI is the examination of choice for studying spinal cord tumours, especially as it is able to identify the extent of the neoplasia and visualize various components of the

mass. The solid components of the tumour may or may not have well-defined boundaries. Generally speaking, low grade tumours such as ependymomas or haemangioblastomas have well-defined margins whereas infiltrating or more aggressive tumours have poorly limited confines. After IV contrast medium administration ependymomas typically reveal an intense, homogeneous enhancement pattern; astrocytomas on the other hand show a modest, inhomogeneous pattern of enhancement.

Intratumoral haemorrhages, often observed in spinal cord neoplasia, show increased signal on T1-weighted MRI images in the subacute phase (i.e., methaemoglobin) and reduced signal on T2-weighted sequences. In the late phases, if gradient-echo sequences are used, haemosiderin deposits will demonstrate marked areas of hypointensity.

Parenchymal oedema can be seem in up to 60% of cases of ependymoma, 23% of astrocytoma and almost always in haemangioblastomas, in which case it is usually extensive.

Intratumoral cystic components are usually located within the boundaries of the neoplastic lesion itself. The MR signal of this type of cyst is generally higher on T2-weighted images than that of the CSF due to the high protein content of the fluid; the walls of these intrinsic tumour cysts show enhancement after IV contrast medium administration. On the contrary, satellite cysts, which resolve spontaneously after surgical resection of the neoplasm, are found cranially and caudally in relationship to the solid tumour mass. They demonstrate MR signal characteristics similar to those of the CSF and the walls do not enhance after IV gadolinium administration.

Syringohydromyelia, which can be associated with spinal cord neoplasia, also disappears spontaneously after the total surgical removal of the neoplasm.

Spinal angiography may occasionally be useful in order to complete the diagnostic imaging examination in the presence of clinical clues or MR findings that suggest the presence of haemangioblastoma.

Non-mass forming spinal cord pathology

MRI is also useful for the diagnosis of acute spinal cord involvement in multiple sclerosis and sudden onset ischaemic medullary disease. *Multiple sclerosis* (MS) (6, 9) is a demyelinating disease that most frequently affects females, and which presents with variable neurological

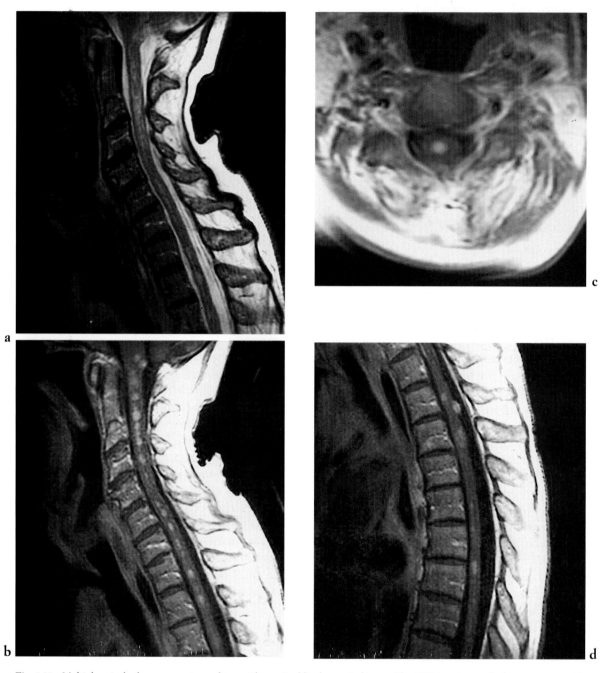

Fig. 5.37 - Multiple spinal schwannomas in a subject with von Recklinghausen's disease. The MRI imaging study demonstrates multiple intramedullary and intradural-extramedullary masses in the cervicothoracic region, which appear hyperintense on T2-weighted MRI, and show contrast enhancement following IV Gd administration. Also note the multiple perimedullary masses and the numerous masses within the nerve roots of the cauda equina. [**a**) sagittal cervicothoracic T2-weighted MRI; **b**) sagittal cervicothoracic T1-weighted MRI following IV Gd; **c**) axial cervical T1-weighted MRI following IV Gd; **d**) sagittal midthoracic T1-weighted MRI following IV Gd; **e**) axial upper thoracic T1-weighted MRI following IV Gd; **f**): sagittal lumbosacral T1-weighted MRI following IV Gd].

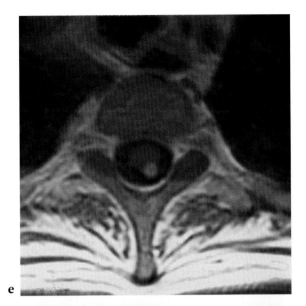

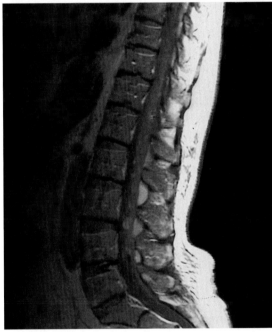

Fig. 5.37 (*cont.*).

signs and symptoms often in a relapsing-remitting pattern. Spinal cord involvement typically affects the dorsolateral regions of the cervical cord. Although isolated medullary involvement (i.e., in the absence of cerebral disease) can be observed in up to 10% of cases, nevertheless, when a spinal cord lesion of a probable demyelinating nature is identified using MRI, a supplemental brain scan is required to complete the investigation. MRI generally underestimates the number and presence of spinal cord demyelinative lesions, especially at a thoracic level, where fine detail can be reduced by artefacts caused by CSF pulsation, chest wall movement and motion of the cardiovascular system.

On T2-weighted MRI, MS lesions appear as single or more frequently multiple hyperintense areas of the spinal cord that generally extend for less than two spinal segments, located in the axial plane in the white matter of the lateral and posterior columns. Areas of acute demyelination can cause swelling of the spinal cord and enhancement after IV contrast medium administration (Fig. 5.43).

The combination of retrobulbar optic neuritis and a spinal cord lesion is termed Devic's disease. The question of whether this pathology is a variant of multiple sclerosis or a separate entity is still controversial. In Devic's disease, MRI shows widespread spinal cord lesions with cord swelling and inhomogeneous enhancement after IV contrast medium injection.

Spinal cord infarcts (3, 5, 11) are rarely isolated events, but instead are more often associated with spinal column trauma, inadvertent ligation of the afferent radiculomedullary arteries, spinal arteriovenous malformations, hypotension, vasculitis and neoplasia. The majority of spinal cord infarcts take place in the territory of the anterior spinal artery and have a propensity for the thoracolumbar region, where the normal blood supply to the spinal cord is most sparse. MRI using axial T2-weighted sequences demonstrates the ischaemic area as hyperintensity affecting the entire volume of the spinal cord over multiple segments associated with moderate swelling (Fig. 5.44). Spinal cord infarcts in the subacute phase (i.e., 2-6th day) may demonstrate contrast enhancement after IV gadolinium administration; chronic phase infarcts evolve to spinal cord atrophy.

Spinal cord arteriovenous malformations are congenital vascular abnormalities. They typically present in the young and are most frequently encountered in the thoracic or cervical region. The lesion is generally principally supplied by the anterior spinal artery. Patients present with

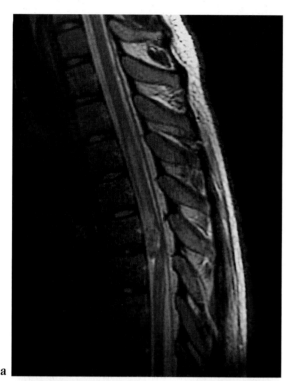

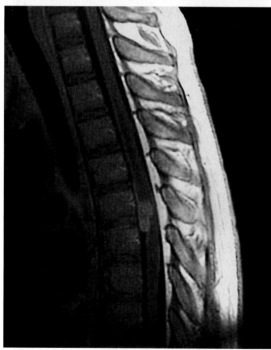

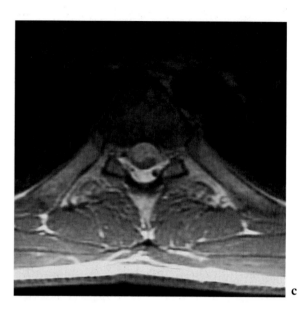

Fig. 5.38 - Intradural spinal metastasis in a patient with primary intracranial pinealoblastoma. The MRI examination shows that the spinal cord is compressed posterolaterally by an enhancing intradural-extramedullary mass consistent with subarachnoid dissemination of the pinealoblastoma. [**a**) sagittal T2-weighted MRI; **b**) sagittal T1-weighted MRI; **c**) axial T1-weighted MRI following IV Gd].

signs and symptoms of progressive myelopathy (venous congestion or arterial steal) or with the onset of an acute neurological deficit secondary to spontaneous intramedullary and/or subarachnoid haemorrhage. In such cases MRI demonstrates serpentine flow voids within abnormal coiled vessels, focal spinal cord swelling, haemorrhage in various stages, and hyperintensity on T2-weighted images adjacent to the nidus of the malformation, representing oedema, ischaemia and/or gliosis. After IV contrast medium administration, depending upon flow velocity and intravascular turbulence, enhancement is seen in some of the vascular component and occasionally within the surrounding parenchymal component if the latter has undergone insult from spontaneous adjacent parenchymal haemorrhage of the vascular malformation or if related cord infarction has occurred.

Spinal dural arteriovenous fistulae are acquired lesions, most frequently encountered in elderly subjects in the thoracic spinal region. In most cases the fistula is supplied by the posterior spinal artery and represents a direct communication between a dural branch of a radiculomedullary artery and a perimedullary intradural vein.

Dural arteriovenous fistulae represent approximately 80% of all spinal vascular malfor-

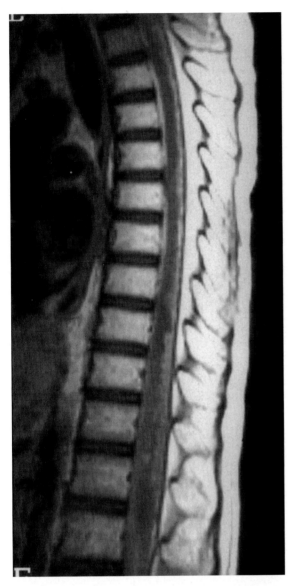

Fig. 5.39 - Metastatic neoplastic leptomeningeal spread in a case primary pineal region neoplasm. Sagittal T1-weighted MRI following IV Gd administration shows diffuse leptomeningeal contrast enhancement consistent with subarachnoid dissemination of the primary intracranial neoplasm.

Fig. 5.40 - Primary thoracic spine intramedullary glioblastoma with subarachnoid dissemination. The MRI imaging study shows diffuse spinal cord swelling associated with inhomogeneous MRI signal. Irregular contrast enhancement is present following IV Gd administration. Extramedullary masses are also present on the surface of the spinal cord as well as associated with the roots of the cauda equina and the posterior fossa due to leptomeningeal spread of the primary spinal cord neoplasm. [**a**) sagittal T2-weighted MRI; **b**) sagittal T1-weighted MRI; **c**), **d**) midline sagittal and parasagittal T1-weighted MRI following IV Gd].

mations. They do not typically cause haemorrhage, but instead patients present with either chronic signs and symptoms of progressive myelopathy secondary to spinal cord ischaemia that is generated by venous congestion, or acute clinical findings consistent with sudden

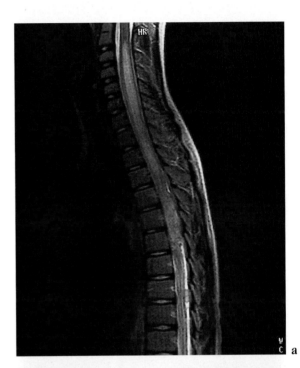

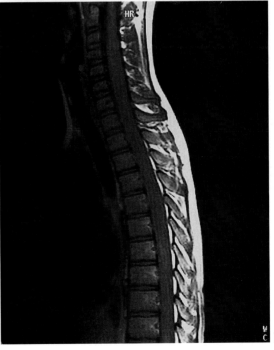

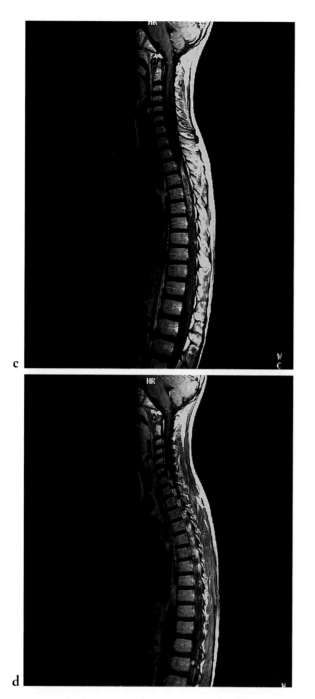

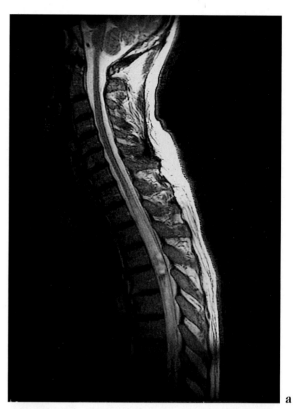

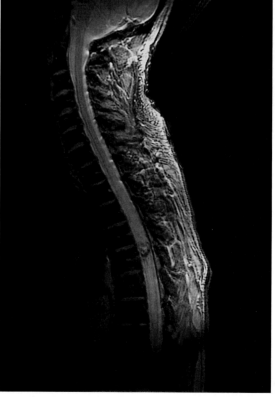

Fig. 5.40 (*cont.*).

Fig. 5.41 - Thoracic spine intramedullary ependymoma. The images reveal a thoracic intramedullary mass having peripheral low signal intensity on T2-weighted images at the cranial and caudal margins of the lesion, indicating repeated intratumoural microhaemorrhages. Note the extensive peritumoural hyperintense oedema on the T2-weighted images. [**a**) sagittal T2-weighted MRI **b**) sagittal T2*-weighted MRI; **c**), **d**) axial T2-weighted MRI].

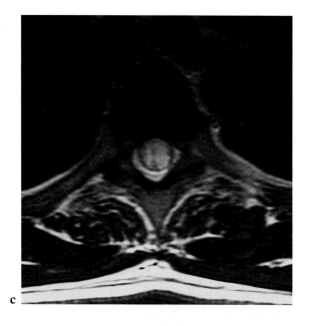

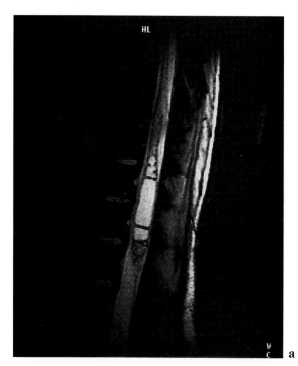

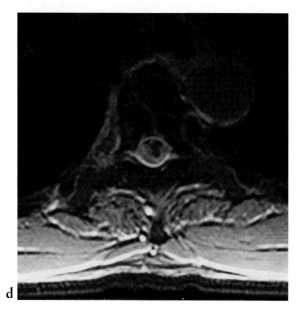

Fig. 5.41 (*cont.*).

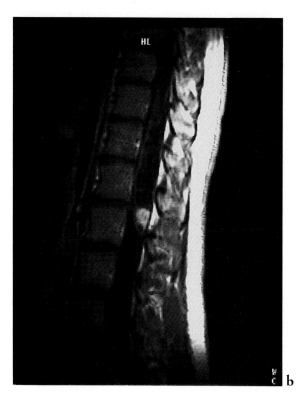

spinal cord infarction. T2-weighted MRI shows an indentation of the posterior surface of the spinal cord by dilated intradural-perimedullary veins (Fig. 5.45), a finding that can often be more clearly visible after IV gadolinium administration; multilevel intramedullary spinal cord hyperintensity is also observed in acutely presenting cases as a result of the evolving infarct

Fig. 5.42 - Ependymoma of the conus medullaris. The MRI study shows a septated partially cystic mass with a mural nodular area of contrast enhancement. [**a**) sagittal T2-weighted MRI, **b**) sagittal T1-weighted MRI following IV Gd].

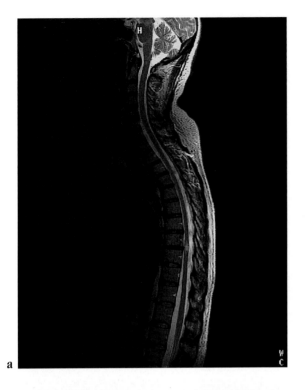

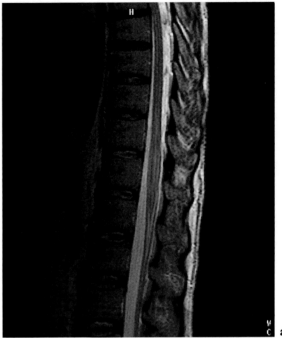

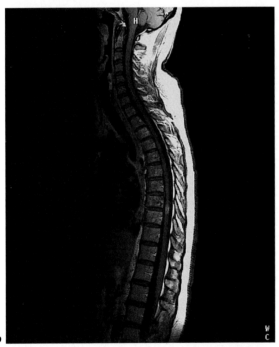

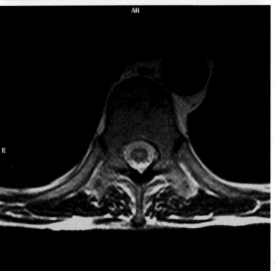

Fig. 5.44 - Ischaemia of the thoracic spinal cord associated with spinal dural arteriovenous fistula. T-2 weighted MRI demonstrates high signal intensity within the central region of the conus medullaris associated with central medullary hyperintensity and vascular flow voids over the posterior surface of the thoracic spinal cord. [**a**) sagittal T1-weighted MRI; **b**) axial T2-weighted MRI; **c**) axial T-weighted MRI].

Fig. 5.43 - Thoracic intramedullary multiple sclerosis. T2 weighted MRI shows an area of intramedullary high signal intensity at the T8-9 level associated with minor focal swelling of the spinal cord. Contrast enhancement is seen within the area of MRI signal abnormality following IV Gd administration. [**a**) sagittal T2-weighted MRI; **a**) sagittal T-1 weighted MRI following IV Gd].

which may also show homogenous multisegmental contrast enhancement (2). It has been shown that on occasion MRI can be equivocal or even falsely negative in instances that subsequently were proven to have spinal dural fistu-

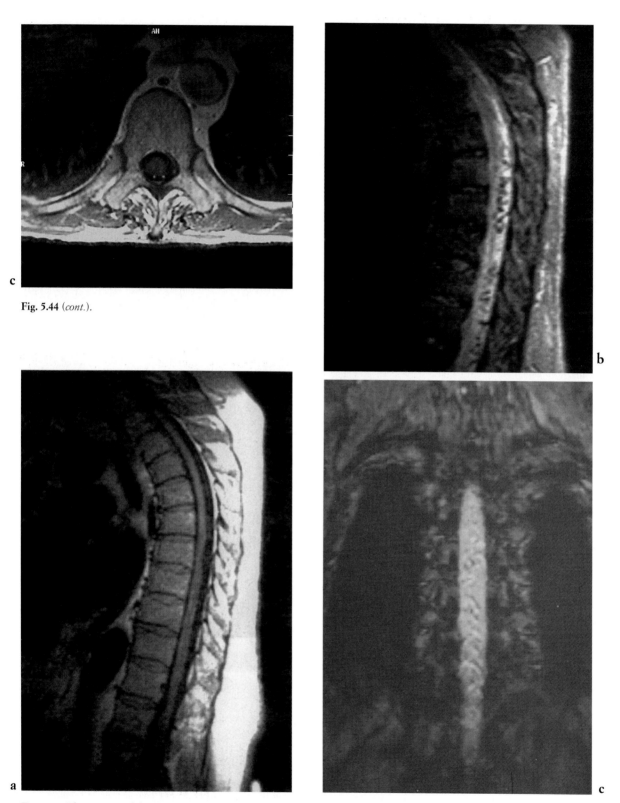

Fig. 5.44 (*cont.*).

Fig. 5.45 - Thoracic spinal dural arteriovenous fistula. The MRI study reveals subarachnoid space MRI signal irregularity posterior to the spinal cord, which becomes much more evident on the T2-weighted images due to the presence of serpentine vascular flow voids. [**a**) sagittal T1-weighted MRI; **b**) sagittal T2-weighted MRI, **c**) coronal T2-weighted MRI].

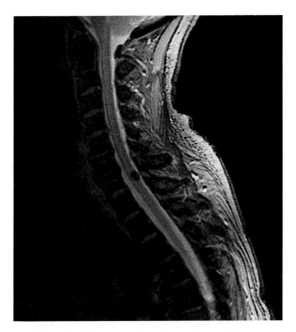

Fig. 5.46 - Chronic haemorrhage within thoracic intramedullary cavernous angioma. T2*-weighted sagittal MRI reveals hypointensity within the upper thoracic spinal cord as a consequence of deposition of haemosiderin associated with thrombosis-haemorrhage within an intramedullary cavernous angioma.

lae. In such clinically suspected but MRI-negative cases, myelography and spinal angiography may be indicated, and when positive will definitively reveal the site of the dural fistula, the feeding arteries and the dilated draining veins. In any case, angiography is a prerequisite for therapeutic dural fistula embolization, the treatment of choice in these patents.

Cavernous angiomas are usually indolent vascular malformations that are nevertheless prone to haemorrhage and intrinsic thrombosis. T1- and T2-weighted MRI typically shows a central hyperintense core with a peripheral margin or margins of hyper- and hypointensity due to the presence of mixed subacute and chronic haemoglobin metabolites (Fig. 5.46). Some cases demonstrate central enhancement after IV contrast medium administration, representing the residual patent vascular component of the angioma. Cavernous angiomas can present acutely with signs and symptoms related to intramedullary haemorrhage (Fig. 5.47).

Acute spinal cord syndromes can also be caused by viral or granulomatous infections. In

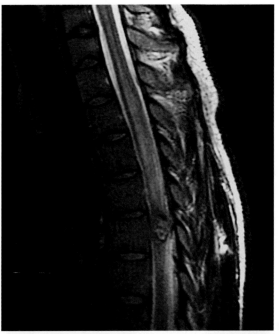

a

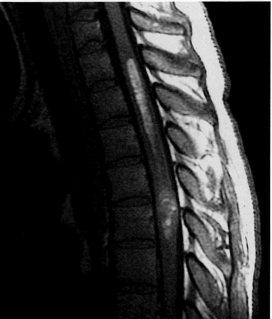

b

Fig. 5.47 - Acute haemorrhage within intramedullary cavernous angioma. The spinal T1-weighted spinal MRI images demonstrate an extensive acute-subacute (deoxyhaemoglobin and methaemoglobin) thoracic intramedullary haemorrhage associated with an intramedullary cavernous angioma showing intrinsic hypointensity on T2-weighted acquisitions consistent chronic peripheral microhaemorrhages (haemosiderin). The MRI of the brain showed several cavernous angiomas demonstrating the multicentric potential of this pathologic process. [**a**) sagittal T2-weighted spinal MRI **b**) sagittal T1-weighted weighted spinal MRI; **c**) sagittal T2*-weighted spinal MRI; **d**) axial T1-weighted spinal MRI; **e**) axial T2*-weighted cranial MRI].

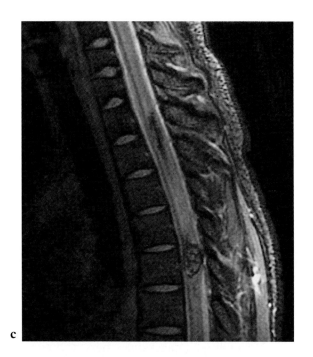

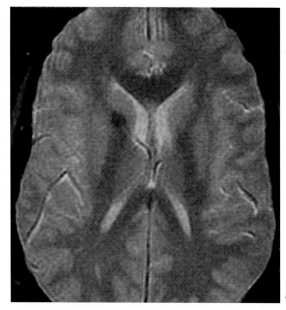

e

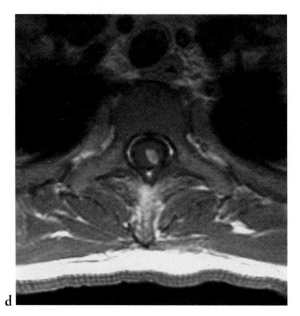

d

Fig. 5.47 (*cont.*).

cases of *infectious myelitis*, MRI demonstrates multisegmental non-specific intramedullary hyperintensity on T2-weighted sequences, with a variable enhancement after contrast medium administration.

Spinal cord abscess formation is rare and is usually caused by the direct extension of in-

fections from adjacent perispinal tissues or from penetrating trauma. T2-weighted MRI demonstrates an intramedullary mass that is hyperintense on T2-weighted sequences and reveals rim enhancement after IV gadolinium administration. Distinguishing this pattern from other spinal cord lesions such as neoplasia is not always possible on the basis of the images alone.

Acute transverse myelitis is an acute inflammatory process with a poor prognosis. The aetiology is unknown, however it is probably autoimmune in nature. Acute transverse myelitis can be associated with various conditions such as multiple sclerosis, paraneoplastic syndromes, prior vaccinations, vasculitis or known autoimmune disorders. Clinically there is an acute onset of a profound spinal cord neurological deficit in the absence of other findings. It is for this reason that transverse myelitis is always a diagnosis of exclusion. On MRI, acute transverse myelitis demonstrates areas of hyperintensity on T2-weighted imaging associated with spinal cord swelling and irregular contrast enhancement following gadolinium administration due to an associated breakdown in the blood-cord barrier. In the chronic phase, the spinal cord

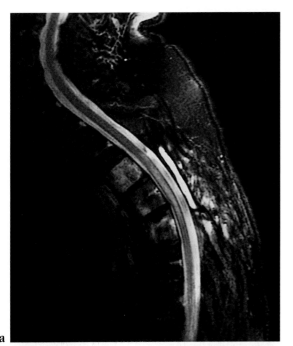

a

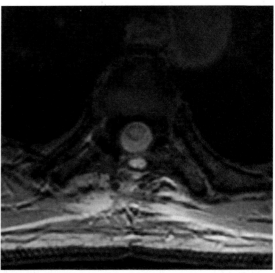

c

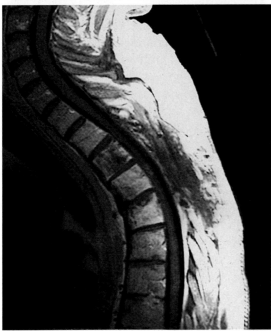

b

Fig. 5.48 - Radiation induced thoracic myelitis/spondylitis three years following radiotherapy. T2-weighted MRI with fat suppression shows hyperintense MRI signal within the thoracic spinal cord and within the bone marrow of several contiguous vertebral bodies, both of which are caused in this case by the preceding radiation therapy. Axial T2*-weighted images demonstrate again the intramedullary location of the pathologic process. No contrast enhancement of the intramedullary process can be identified. Note the postsurgical alterations. [a) sagittal T2-weighted MRI; b) sagittal T1-weighted MRI following IV Gd; c) axial T2*-weighted MRI].

can appear atrophic, and areas of high signal on T2-weighted images may persist due to gliosis.

Acute disseminated encephalomyelitis is a monophasic autoimmune disease that follows within days or weeks of an antiviral vaccination or viral infection. As the name indicates, it involves the brain but also concomitantly affects the spinal cord. Pathologically the lesions are similar to those of MS. The prognosis is typically good and the majority of patients respond rapidly to steroid treatment. MRI shows hyperintense areas on T2-weighted sequences within the parenchyma of the brain and spinal cord that enhance after IV gadolinium; the spinal cord may be swollen.

The development of *radiation myelopathy* in part depends on the dose of radiation and the time period over which it was administered. In the acute milder forms, typically presenting approximately three months after radiation is applied to the spinal cord, the patient experiences sensations similar to electric shocks in the lower limbs; MRI may show no abnormality. However in severe cases the patient reveals a severe, rapidly progressive myelopathy; in such cases, the spinal cord is swollen, hyperintense on T2-weighted images and enhances following IV contrast injection. Evolution of spinal cord atrophy will occur over time (Fig. 5.48).

REFERENCES

1. Baleriaux DL: Spinal cord tumours. Eur Radiol 9 (7):1252-1258, 1999.
2. Chen CJ, Chen CM, Lin TK: Enhanced cervical MRI in identifying intracranial dural arteriovenous fistulae with spinal perimedullary venous drainage. Neuroradiology 40: 393-407, 1998.
3. Fortuna A, Ferrante L, Acqui M et al: Spinal cord ischemia diagnosed by MRI. J Neuroradiol 22:115-122, 1995.
4. Karampekios S: Inflammatory, vascular and demyelinating diseases of the spine and spinal cord. Eur Radiol (S1)10:36, 2000.
5. Liou RJ, Chen CY, Chou TY et al: Hypoxic - ischaemic injury of the spinal cord in systemic shock: MRI. Neuroradiology 38:S 181-183, 1996
6. Lyclama à Nijeholt GJ, Uitdehaag BMJ et al: Spinal cord magnetic resonance imaging in suspected multiple sclerosis. Eur Radiol 10:368-376, 2000.
7. Obenberg J, Seidi Z, Plas J: Osteoblastoma in lumbar vertebral body. Neuroradiology 41:279-282, 1999.
8. Rimmelin A, Clouet PL, Salatino S et al: Imaging of thoracic and lumbar spinal extradural arachnoid cysts: report of two cases. Neuroradiology 39:203-206, 1997.
9. Rocca MA, Mastronardo G, Horsfield MA et al: Comparison of three MR sequences for detection of cervical cord lesions in patients with multiple sclerosis. AJNR 20:1710-1716, 1999.
10. Silbergleit R Brunberg JA, Patel SC et al: Imaging of spinal intradural arachnoid cysts: MRI, myelography and CT. Neuroradiology 40:664-668, 1998.
11. Suzuki K, Meguro K, Wada M et al: Anterior spinal artery syndrome associated with severe stenosis of the vertebral artery. AJNR 19:1353-1355, 1998.
12. Wilmink JT: MR imaging of the spine: trauma and degenerative disease. Eur Radiol 9 (7):1259-1266, 1999.
13. Yamada K, Shrier DA, Tanaka H et al: A case of subacute combined degeneration: MRI finding. Neuroradiology 40: 398-400, 1998.

VI

NEUROPAEDIATRIC EMERGENCIES

6

NEUROPAEDIATRIC EMERGENCIES

N. Zamponi, B. Rossi, G. Polonara, U. Salvolini

INTRODUCTION

This chapter covers the most common emergency situations encountered in neuropaediatrics, including cerebrovascular disease, head injuries, infections of the central nervous system (CNS) and intracranial hypertension.

CEREBROVASCULAR DISEASE

Cerebrovascular disease (15, 32) is rare in infants and newborns and when encountered does not have the same aetiological factors as in adults: the most common causes in the young age group are congenital vascular abnormalities and those secondary to systemic illnesses. Various areas of the brain show significant differences in their susceptibility to cerebral vasculopathy. In addition, there are also important physiological differences in the blood vessels of different areas of the brain. The pathological conditions of cerebrovascular disease are haemorrhage and ischaemia.

Haemorrhage

Newborns at term and young infants

In newborns at term, a large number of possible pathological events may result in intracranial haemorrhage: a) trauma: subdural haematoma, epidural haematoma. subarachnoid haemorrhage, intracerebral haemorrhage, intracerebellar haemorrhage, b) clotting disorders: clotting defects, thrombocytopenia, c) vascular disorders: aneurysms, arteriovenous malformations, d) metabolic disorders, and e) idiopathic intraparenchymal haemorrhage.

The clinical signs of an intracranial haemorrhage lesion in a newborn are often modest and non-specific: apathy or irritability/hyperexcitability without focal neurological signs, seizure, tremors, breathing disorders. Frequently acidosis, hypoglycaemia and hypotension are associated with such haemorrhages.

a) *Labour trauma* is the most frequent cause of bleeding in newborns.

Subdural haematomas and *subarachnoid haemorrhage* are the most common types of haemorrhagic lesion. The most frequent site of subdural bleeding is over the cerebral convexity and within the temporal fossa, however haemorrhages can also be encountered adjacent to the falx cerebri, tentorium cerebelli and in the posterior cranial fossa.

Intraparenchymal haemorrhages are less frequent and can be associated with subarachnoid and subdural haemorrhage, should the bleeding extend into the ventricles. The prognosis of small lesions is good, however serious sequelae are typically observed following larger haemorrhages.

Diagnostic imaging should first include CT, which demonstrates the presence, site and extent of the cerebral bleed at an early stage; on the other hand, haemorrhages associated with cerebral infarcts will only become evident some days after the ischaemic event.

Ultrasound may not show epidural or subdural haemorrhages localized to the cranial convexity or in the posterior fossa, whereas larger haemorrhages are clearly visible on ultrasound images as hyperechoic areas, and later hypo- anechoic regions.

Both ultrasound and CT are capable of documenting and sequentially monitoring the most important sequelae: porencephalic cysts and hydrocephalus.

Porencephalic cysts usually form off of the bodies of the lateral ventricles. They typically develop from a haemorrhage that ruptures into the lateral ventricle or the subarachnoid space. Associated posthaemorrhagic hydrocephalus develops in 10-15% of patients with intraventricular haemorrhage. The hydrocephalus halts or improves in most cases; more rarely it progresses and can require surgical ventricular-peritoneal shunt placement.

b) Various *clotting and platelet disorders* can result in intracranial haemorrhage in newborns. The most frequent causes of thrombocytopenia are the use of medicines during pregnancy, maternal infections, immunological disorders and disseminated intravascular coagulation.

c) *Vascular malformations* and *intracranial aneurysms* may present with intracranial haemorrhages in newborns in rare occasions.

Ultrasound may prove useful in diagnosis, especially in infants with aneurysmal dilatation of the vein of Galen. This is a rare congenital disorder wherein abnormal arteriovenous formations drain into the deep, dilated vessels of the galenic system. These direct connections with the vein of Galen can be by large fistulae or by multiple smaller arteriovenous connections. The pathogenesis would seem to involve intrauterine vascular thrombosis or absence of formation of the superior sagittal venous sinus.

In 90% of cases, signs and symptoms of vasculopathy arise in early infancy: intracranial haemorrhage (intraparenchymal or subarachnoid) and rapidly progressive hydrocephalus are the most frequent presentations. In newborns these complications are frequently associated with cardiac insufficiency, the final pathophysiological result of a preexistent congenital haemodynamic anomaly (e.g., increase in blood flow across an arteriovenous fistula, increase in blood return to the right atrium, right-to-left blood flow through cardiac defects). In addition, the large blood flow through the fistula can create a secondary state of cerebral ischaemia.

In newborns, the aneurysmal dilatation of the vein of Galen can be simply diagnosed using ultrasound. On colour Doppler images, turbulent flow can usually be seen.

On CT without IV contrast medium, the vein of Galen appears as a rounded mass in the region of the tentorial incisura and straight venous sinus; aqueduct compression may cause obstructive hydrocephalus. After IV contrast medium administration, intense enhancement is typically seen within the aneurysmally dilated vessel which is smooth and well defined. In the presence of thrombosis of this structure, variable degrees of non-enhancement will be observed.

On MRI the vascular malformation appears hypointense on both T1- and T2-weighted sequences due to the rapid blood flow within the abnormal vessels. The arteries that supply the malformation can be reasonably well shown with MRA. Conventional selective angiography will still better define the arterial feeding vessels and the draining venous structures and may assist in presurgical planning (27, 32, 37).

PREMATURE NEWBORNS

Subependymal and *intraventricular haemorrhages* are more frequently encountered in premature newborns than in those born at term (3, 5, 11). Babies with a gestational age of less than 35 weeks or a birth weight of less than 1.5 kg have a higher risk of such haemorrhages, which commonly present during the second or third day of life. The haemorrhage originates from the germinal matrix that surrounds the lateral cerebral ventricles. Small haemorrhages remain confined to the subependymal regions, however, when the bleeding is larger it can extensively involve the cerebral parenchyma or rupture into the ventricular system. Certain factors make haemorrhage in this area more likely. The vessels of the germinal matrix are fragile and contain little connective tissue. This germinal matrix begins to involute at approximately the 35th week of gestation. Until that time it has a high arterial perfusion with consonantly elevated venous and capillary pressure.

Two clinical syndromes have been described in association with subependymal and intraventricular haemorrhage. The *catastrophic syndrome* has an acute onset and a rapid evolution towards coma; the mortality rate is high. The *salt losing syndrome* is a disorder of consciousness, accompanied with a reduction in spontaneous movements, hypotonia and oculomotor abnormalities; these signs evolve slowly and are often followed by a period of stabilization followed by a second phase of deterioration. The mortality rate is lower for this syndrome than for the catastrophic syndrome.

From the standpoint of medical imaging, germinal matrix haemorrhages can be broken down into 4 stages: stage I is characterized by a small germinal matrix haemorrhages together with a small intraventricular haemorrhage; stage II is characterized by germinal matrix haemorrhage accompanied by a large intraventricular haemorrhage; stage III is characterized by a subependymal haemorrhage, intraventricular haemorrhage, and hydrocephalus; and, stage IV indicates the spread of the parenchymal haemorrhage into one or both cerebral hemispheres.

The use of ultrasound, which can be performed safely at the bedside, has lead to an increase in the identification and characterization of neonatal subependymal and intraventricular haemorrhages. On ultrasound, stage I germinal matrix subependymal haemorrhage appears as a hyperechoic mass lesion, which is either uni- or bilateral and is primarily located in the head of the caudate nucleus. Generally speaking, in order to be visualized, it must measure 4-5 mm in diameter. A Stage II haemorrhage appears as hyperechoic material within the lateral ventricle(s). A stage III haemorrhage is represented by a dilatation of the ventricular system and the presence of intraventricular hyperechoic blood. The intraparenchymal component of a stage IV haemorrhage appears on ultrasound as an intensely hyperechoic lesion located in the deep white matter of the centrum semiovale.

Subsequent ultrasound scans will show progressive stages of resolution of the subependymal-intraventricular haemorrhage. An extensive haemorrhage can evolve over 2-3 months towards the formation of porencephalic cysts or the development of cystic encephalomalacia.

On CT, acute germinal matrix haemorrhages appear as hyperdense foci, usually adjacent to the lateral ventricle near the head of the caudate nucleus. MRI is also fairly sensitive and specific in demonstrating acute germinal matrix haemorrhage.

In premature neonates with the hypoxic-ischaemic syndrome white matter alterations are also frequently detected: periventricular leukomalacia appears on ultrasound as widespread, poorly defined hyperechoic periventricular regions. These are especially prominent in the ventricular trigone regions and adjacent to the foramina of Monroe. The hyperecho findings are due to oedema and petechial haemorrhage. The abnormality is generally bilateral, but is often asymmetric. After 2-3 weeks, small cysts form within the hyperechoic region that coalesce to form a multicystic lesion, before collapsing, fusing and being replaced by glial scars. In this late phase of glial scarring the ultrasound findings are usually unremarkable.

During the acute phase of ischemia, CT can be normal or can show a minor attenuation in the parenchyma of the periventricular regions; during the subacute phase it is only possible to identify medium-sized cysts, whereas chronic glial scarring is not usually visible on CT (Fig. 6.1).

MRI is rarely used in the acute phase, however it is the best technique for highlighting chronic periventricular leukomalacia. On T2-weighted scans the residual glial scars localized to the periventricular areas appear hyperintense. These areas generally border the ventricles and typically spread into the adjacent white matter in a flame-shaped configuration. A thin-

ning of the posterior body and splenium of the corpus callosum are seen in the chronic phase as a result of degeneration of the transcallosal fibres, ventricular dilatation and atrophy of the hemispheric white matter (Fig. 6.2).

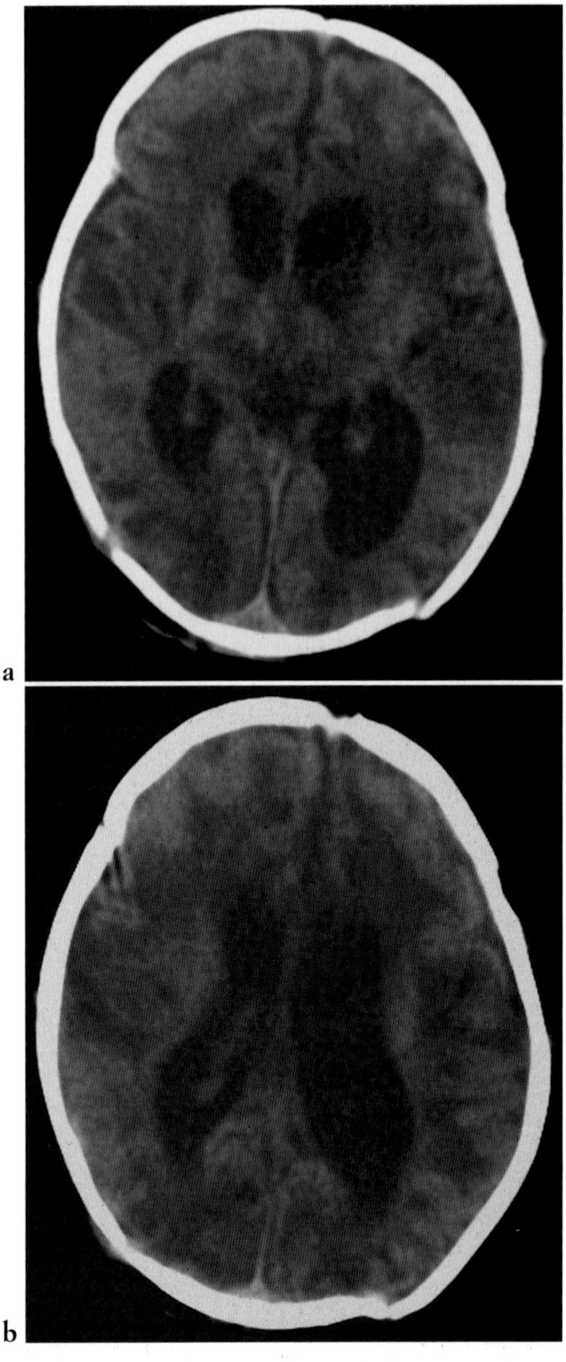

INFANTS

Vascular malformations are the most common cause of haemorrhage in infants (15, 32) and can be broken down into four main types: arteriovenous malformations, venous angiomas, capillary telangiectasias and cavernous angiomas. The most common clinical manifestations are headache and seizures rather than haemorrhage; however, if the latter do occur, they may be subarachnoid, intraparenchymal or combined.

Arteriovenous malformations (AVM's) consist of an aggregate of abnormal vessels with thin walls (i.e., nidus) in which there is direct continuity between dilated arteries and veins without the interposition of capillaries. Approximately 90% are superficial and are located within the cerebral hemispheres. AVM's are responsible for up to 40% of spontaneous intracranial haemorrhages in infants. The mortality rate associated with the rupture of an AVM is approximately 10%.

On unenhanced CT, a typical AVM appears as a heterogeneous area with slightly increased density compared to the normal surrounding parenchyma. After IV contrast medium administration, intense enhancement of the malformation and its afferent and efferent vessels is observed.

On MRI the fast blood flow within AVM's creates flow voids on spin echo sequences. The nidus appears as a tangle of tubular shaped black vessels. However, in order to obtain an accurate anatomical map of the vascular malformation, an angiographic examination is required. Typically a tangle of small, irregular blood vessels supplied by dilated and twisted arteries and drained by dilated veins that fill rapidly.

In the case of haemorrhage, unenhanced CT details the haemorrhagic spread into the sub-

Fig. 6.1 - Hypoxic-ischaemic injury in newborn. **a, b**) Unenhanced CT shows widespread hypodensity of the subcortical and periventricular white matter and enlargement of the cerebral ventricular system.

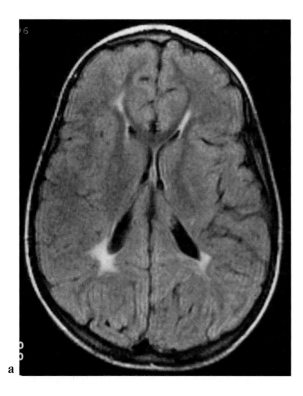

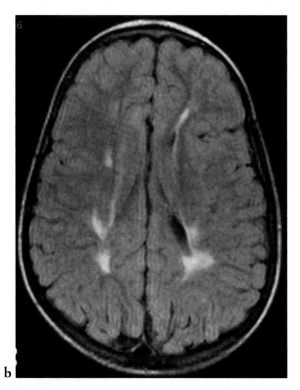

Fig.6.2 - Periventricular leukomalacia. **A, b**) Axial FLAIR MRI shows an increase in the subependymal and periventricular white matter MR signal with sickle shape of the cerebral ventricles.

arachnoid space, cerebral parenchyma and cerebral ventricles. In severe cases haemorrhage can obscure the underlying vascular malformation. In the acute phase the haematoma appears hyperdense and relatively homogeneous (Fig. 6.3); in the chronic phase, encephalomalacia, rarely accompanied by calcifications, may result.

Cavernous vascular malformations consist of a tangle of dilated vessels that do not possess the characteristics of normal arteries or of veins. With the exception that thrombi can be present, the draining veins and arteries usually have a normal calibre. The malformation may contain small intrinsic areas of neural tissue. Most of these lesions are located in the cerebral parenchyma, and although they are usually isolated they can also be multiple and have a familial pattern of expression. The clinical presentation is typically seizures, but more rarely it can be cerebral haemorrhage. In fact, subclinical haemorrhages often occur. The diagnosis is currently based on MRI due to the characteristic imaging findings, including a mixed signal core surrounded by a hypodense haemosiderin ring on T2-weighted sequences.

Venous malformations are often incidentally detected on MR or CT scans. The risk of bleeds is generally low. MRI, which is more sensitive than CT, shows a branching network of small draining veins that unite to form a single, large terminal vein. In the venous phase, conventional angiography shows a collection of abnormal veins (i.e., "Medusa head") that drain into a single large collecting vein before emptying into a superficial cortical vein or dural venous sinus.

Aneurysms are rare in children under the age of ten years; males are more frequently affected than are females. The clinical presentation is typically a subarachnoid haemorrhage, however, some patients present with seizures. Aneurysms in children under 2 years usually originate from the anterior cerebral or the internal carotid arteries. Such aneurysms are usually larger than 1 cm in diameter.

CT at presentation shows an acute subarachnoid haemorrhage. If the aneurysm is sufficiently large it will demonstrate intense en-

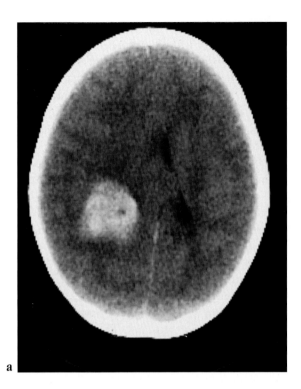

a

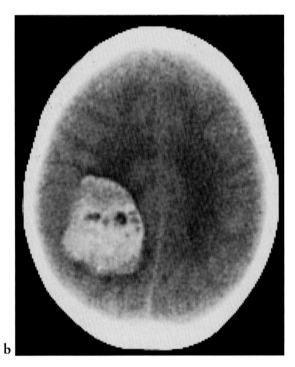

b

Fig.6.3 - Intraparenchymal haematoma caused by AVM haemorrhage. **a, b)** Unenhanced CT demonstrates inhomogeneous right frontoparietal intraparenchymal haemorrhage associated with compression of the right lateral ventricle and contralateral shift of the midline structures.

hancement with a smooth, round or oval configuration after IV contrast medium administration. Internal thrombosis may be observed. While MR and angio-MR better define the aneurysm, conventional angiography definitively visualizes the lumen and neck of the aneurysm, and its relationship to the vessel of origin.

ISCHAEMIA

Cerebrovascular occlusions may occur in arteries, veins or capillaries, as a single acute event, a recurrence or a progressive phenomenon. They can be associated with a number of pathological conditions including inflammation, infection, cardiac disease, neoplasia, trauma, primary arterial dysplasia, vascular malformations and metabolic disease (26, 32).

The clinical symptoms vary according to the age of the infant and the vascular territory involved. The most common sign of internal carotid occlusion is acute hemiplegia. A vascular occlusion in the vertebrobasilar circulation can result in pyramidal and cerebellar signs, hemiparesis, paralysis of the cranial nerves, lateral conjugate deviation of the eyes, dizziness, nausea and vomiting.

Acute phase CT is typically normal. After 24-48 hours the infarction appears as a hypodense area with poorly defined margins and is accompanied by varying mass effect. After the second to third week, enhancement is usually observed after IV contrast medium administration. In the later stages encephalomalacia, porencephalic cyst formation and focal atrophy are typical terminal sequelae.

MRI is more sensitive in detecting acute/subacute postinfarction oedema, which appears hyperintense relative to the normal cerebral parenchyma on T2-weighted sequences. MRA (Fig. 6.4) may reveal vascular thrombosis of the cranial circulation (Fig. 6.5).

Despite the fact that it is the most sensitive technique for examining the cranial vascular system, in infants angiography is reserved for selected cases where it will clearly influence future therapy or when the diagnosis is in doubt (12).

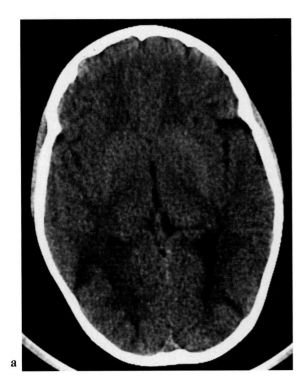

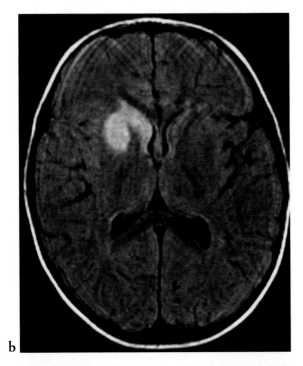

Fig.6.4 - Ischaemia of the basal ganglia. **a)** Unenhanced CT shows hypodensity in the head of the caudate nucleus and the frontal aspect of the putamen on the right side, with involvement of the anterior limb of the internal capsule. **b)** Corresponding MRI.

THE MOYA-MOYA PHENOMENON

The moya-moya phenomenon (6, 32) is a disorder that characteristically affects children and adolescents. Approximately 70% of cases are diagnosed within the first 20 years of life. The disorder consists of an idiopathic progressive stenosis of the supraclinoid internal carotid arteries. A prominent collateral circulation is formed by small branches of the rubrothalamic arteries and the lenticulostriate arteries, resulting in an MRA and conventional angiographic appearance similar to that of a puff or cloud of smoke (moya-moya means foggy in Japanese).

The aetiology and pathogenesis are unknown, although there are many pathological conditions that are sometimes associated with moya-moya type angiographic patterns (e.g., neurofibromatosis, tuberculosis, Down's syndrome, tuberous sclerosis, prior radiation therapy, etc.). Nevertheless, in certain cases the disease presents as an isolated phenomenon. In infants, moya-moya phenomenon clinically reveals transient-relapsing ischaemic episodes, with the appearance of neurological deficits and convulsions. In adolescents, headaches and cerebral haemorrhages are the most common clinical presentations.

Unenhanced CT typically reveals the presence of multiple cerebral infarcts in different stages of evolution. In certain cases, enhanced CT may demonstrate absence of visualization of the proximal internal carotid vessels and the vessels of the circle of Willis. These findings are more clearly visible on MRI and MRA. Sufficiently large collateral vessels are seen at the base of the brain in the region of the basal ganglia (Fig. 6.6). In time regional cerebral encephalomalacia and intracranial calcifications may develop.

The definitive diagnosis is angiographic: the supraclinoid sections of the internal arteries are stenotic or completely occluded as may be the proximal segments of the anterior and middle cerebral arteries. Distal to the occlusion the collateral vessels appear as a tangle of dilated, twisted vessels. The marked, dense blood flow within these small collateral vessels

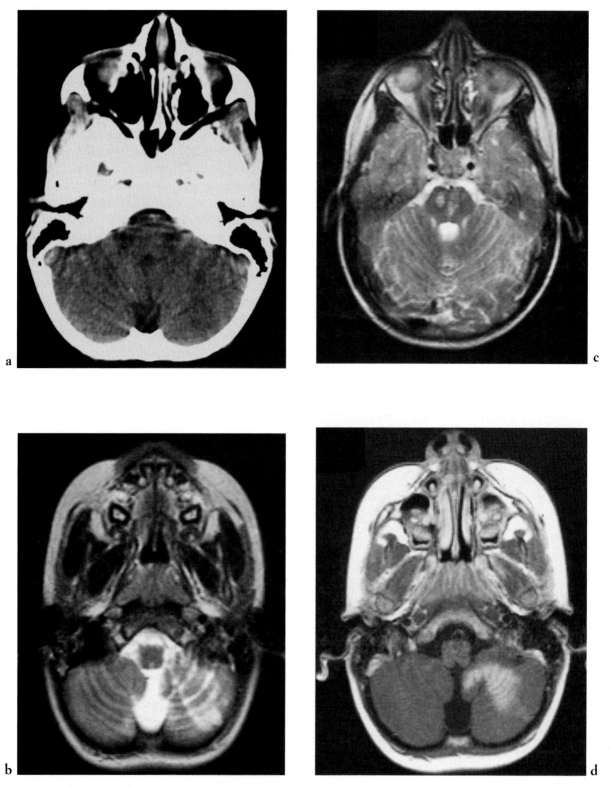

Fig.6.5 - Left cerebellar ischaemia. **a**) Unenhanced CT scan shows minor cortical-subcortical hypodensity. **b, c**) Unenhanced T2-weighted MRI demonstrates areas of increased signal in the left cerebellar hemisphere and midbrain-pontine junction. **d**) Enhanced T1-weighted MRI reveals breakdown in the blood-brain barrier following IV gadolinium administration.

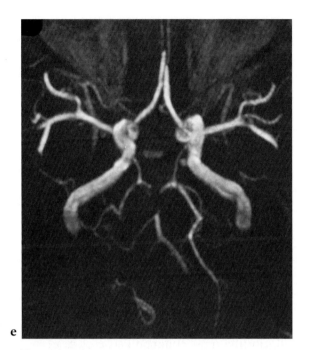

e

Fig. 6.5 (*cont.*).

can produce the typical cloud of smoke appearance.

FIBROMUSCULAR DYSPLASIA

This is a rare progressive idiopathic condition typically encountered in children and adolescents and adult women. The most common

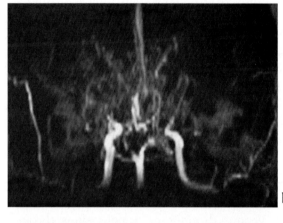

b

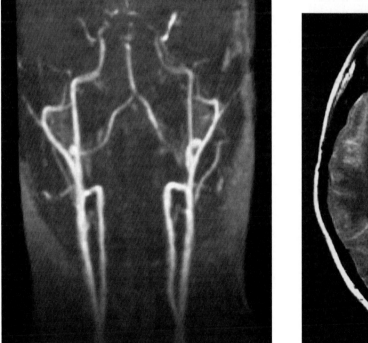

a

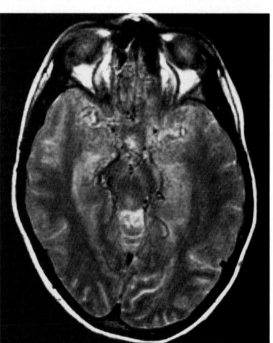

c

Fig.6.6 - Moya-Moya syndrome. **a**) coronal MR angiogram shows that the flow signal of the internal carotid arteries is not visible in an intracranial vessels above the supraclinoid segments of the internal carotid artery siphons. **b**) MR angiogram reveals absence of flow signal in the arterial vessels of the circle of Willis, which have been replaced by a number of small, irregular vessels at the base of the brain. **c**) T2-weighted MRI demonstrates poor visualisation of the anterior and middle cerebral arteries and the presence of numerous irregular vascular structures.

form consists of concentric rings of mural fibrous proliferation and smooth muscle hyperplasia resulting in thickening of the media associated with destruction of the elastic lamina. In addition to the cervical and intracranial arteries, this disease process can also affect the renal arteries. The findings are frequently bilateral although asymmetric. The diagnosis is an angiographic one, having the appearance of a typical string of beads pattern as a result of a series of multiple constrictions alternating with dilatations along the course of the artery involved. Signs and symptoms may result from either dissection of the diseased vessel and/or thrombosis as well as spontaneous intracranial haemorrhage. Intracranial aneurysms also may be associated with this condition, and may themselves lead to haemorrhage upon rupture.

CEREBROVASCULAR OCCLUSIONS SECONDARY TO SYSTEMIC ILLNESSES

Venous thromboses, venous sinus thromboses and arterial embolic disease are not infrequent consequences of cyanogenic congenital heart malformations, in particular tetralogy of Fallot and the transposition of the great vessels. The initial signs/symptoms are typified by the sudden onset of focal neurological deficits and/or intracranial hypertension. Venous thrombosis is the most commonly encountered complication, often related to the polycythaemia typically present in such patients.

Arterial embolism usually occurs as a consequence of right-to-left vascular/cardiac shunts or the presence of septic endocarditis. Falciform cell anaemia results in stroke in up to 8% of cases, especially in the 5-10 year age group. A condition of homozygous protein C deficit, one of the components of the antithrombotic system, may present in newborns with a purpura fulminans and cerebral venous/venous sinus thrombosis.

The MELAS syndrome (i.e., mitochondrial encephalomyopathy, lactic acidosis and stroke-like episodes) presents with repeated migraine-like events, with vomiting at onset and repeat-ed stroke-like episodes later in the evolution of the disease. Children may be short in stature, with multisystem involvement. MR shows multifocal hyperintense areas on T2-weighted sequences that involve the cerebral cortex and the subcortical white matter. MR spectroscopy may demonstrate characteristic patterns with a certain degree of specificity (25, 43, 45).

HEAD INJURIES

Head injuries (9, 18, 30, 33) are a not uncommon cause of disability and death in the infant population. Approximately one in ten children experiences posttraumatic loss of consciousness during childhood. However, most traumatic incidents are minor and do not require hospitalization or any specific treatment. Falls are the most common cause of head injuries in children under ten and road traffic accidents are the most frequent cause in adolescents.

Head injuries can be classified in various ways: according to the general type of trauma (e.g., closed or open), the location and extent of the traumatic lesion (e.g., skull fracture, focal intracranial lesion, widespread intracranial lesion) and the severity of the traumatic lesion (e.g., minor, moderate, severe). The severity of head injuries is clinically defined using the Glasgow Coma Scale (GCS) score, modified to suit children with the Paediatric Coma Scale. Severe head injuries are associated with a GCS score lower than or equal to 8, moderate head injuries with a GCS between 9 and 13 and minor head injuries with a GCS score between 13 and 15.

MINOR/MODERATE DEGREE HEAD INJURIES

Patients with minor or no external signs of trauma, who are awake and cooperative with a normal orthopaedic and neurological examination, and who have no symptoms with the exception of slight headache and/or nausea-vomiting, do not necessarily require emergency medical imaging examinations (e.g., skull x-ray,

CT), but they should be hospitalized for an observation period of 24 hours. Should they require general anaesthesia in order to operate on trauma to other body parts, cranial CT should be performed prior to the surgery.

Brief immediate posttraumatic loss of consciousness and/or confusion and disorientation are not necessarily indicators of cerebral structural damage, however, CT should be considered in such cases.

In general, the indications for CT in cases of minor/moderate head trauma include: the onset/progression of neurological signs; progressive reduction of the level of consciousness; and patients whose mental status is difficult to evaluate.

Currently, certain practitioners recommend abandonment of the use of standing-order skull radiography in favour of CT. However, certain cases of minor/moderate head injury, and specific situations such as x-ray evidence of fractures (e.g., depressed fracture, skull base fracture, etc.), can mandate the need for hospitalization for clinical observation as well as for emergency CT.

SEVERE DEGREE HEAD INJURIES

Children with severe head injuries have a GCS of less than 9 and are incapable of fulfilling simple commands due to their impaired state of consciousness. The disability and mortality associated to this type of trauma can be dramatically reduced by the rapid initiation of specific treatment (e.g., stabilization of the vital functions, respiratory control, reduction of intracranial hypertension) in order to curb the consequences of the primary traumatic lesion as well as the sequelae resulting from hypotension, hypoxia, hypercapnia, ischaemia and oedema.

The initial imaging examination of choice in cases of severe head trauma is unenhanced CT, using 5 mm thick slices for the base of the skull and posterior fossa, and 10 mm thick slices for the remainder of the brain. Cervical spine CT should also be included in the protocol. Diagram 6.1 illustrates a recommended diagnostic pathway (21).

Extracranial traumatic lesions

In newborns, the presence of a *cephalohaematoma* (i.e., subperiosteal scalp haematoma) is most frequently a consequence of the application of the forceps during delivery, but can also occur in 1% of unassisted vaginal births. Cephalohaematomas appear on ultrasound, CT and MRI as a crescent-shaped extracranial soft tissue mass directly adjacent to the outer table of

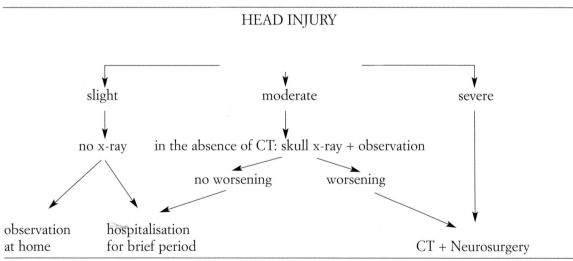

HEAD INJURY

slight — moderate — severe

slight → no x-ray

moderate → in the absence of CT: skull x-ray + observation

no worsening

worsening

no x-ray → observation at home / hospitalisation for brief period

severe → CT + Neurosurgery

Diagram 6.1

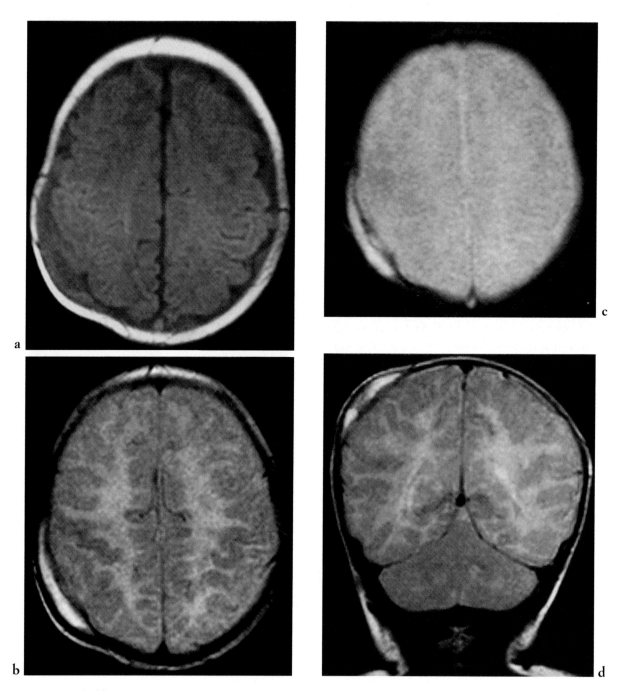

Fig.6.7 - Cerebral haematoma. **a)** T1-, **b)** T2-, **c)** T2*-, **d)** T1-weighted MRI shows a large extracranial haemorrhage in the right parietal region.

the skull, limited by the cranial sutures (Fig. 6.7). On CT in the acute phase, cephalohaematomas are hyperdense, becoming progressively hypodense in the chronic phase. Calcification may occur late in the evolutionary process.

Another common post-partum posttraumatic lesion is so-called *caput succedaneum* characterized by haemorrhagic oedema of the scalp secondary to a trauma occurring in the vagina at the time of labour and delivery. They can be distinguished from cephalohaematomas by their superficial site and the fact that they traverse the cranial suture lines.

The third type of extracranial posttraumatic lesion encountered in newborns is the *subgaleal haematoma*, which consists of a haematoma delineated externally by the calvarial aponeurosis that covers the scalp beneath the frontal and occipital scalp muscles.

Traumatic bony lesions

Fractures of the vertex and the base of the skull can be linear or stellate, depressed or non-depressed. Subgaleal haematomas are often associated with skull fractures of the calvaria. Therefore the detection of such haematomas in a child would indicate the performance of a skull x-ray.

A "ping-pong ball" type depressed fracture in newborns may be a consequence of the use of the forceps during labour or due to falls from a height. In most cases, cerebral pulsation re-establishes the normal bone contour within weeks of the initial injury.

The so-called "growing fracture" or *leptomeningeal cyst* on the other hand occurs when the leptomeninges are entrapped between the edges of a skull fracture. Vascular and CSF pulsations result in the progressive enlargement of the fracture site.

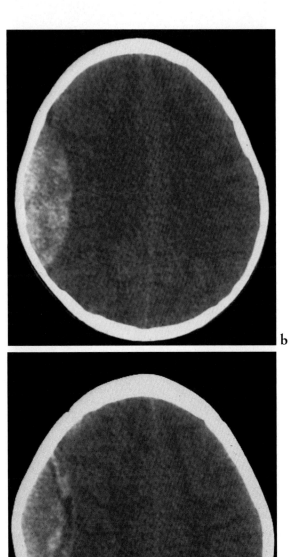

a

b

c

Fig.6.8 - Acute extradural haematoma. CT shows a biconvex extradural haemorrhage in the right frontoparietal region. Marked mass effect upon the underlying cerebral structures is present.

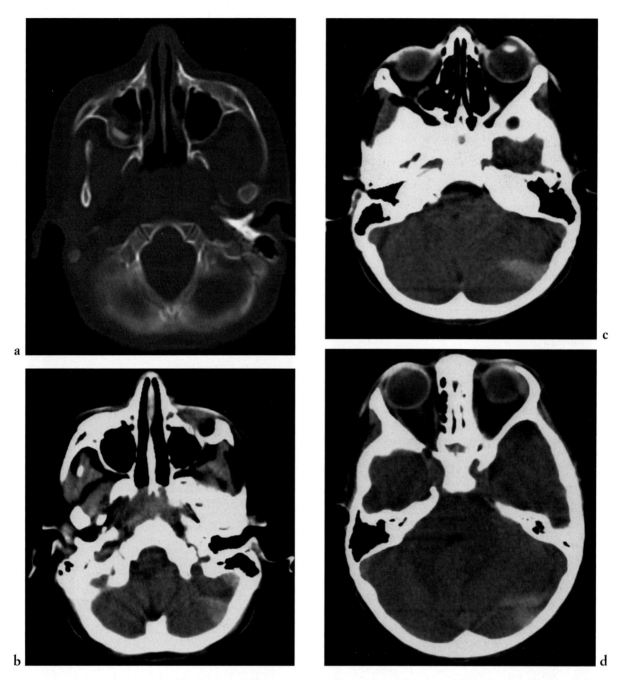

Fig. 6.9 - Posterior fossa extradural haematoma. **a**) CT shows a fracture of the base of the skull involving the occipital bone on the left with anterior extension into the left petrous bone. **b, c** and **d**) CT reveals a posterior fossa extradural haemorrhage with signs of compression on the left cerebellar hemisphere and the 4th ventricle.

Depressed skull fractures are a consequence of major traumatic impact and are often associated with serious underlying cerebral injury. Therefore, CT must always be performed even when there are no clinical neurological signs or symptoms. This being said, most depressed fractures smaller than 1 cm in diameter do not require surgical elevation. Fractures of the skull base must be suspected in cases of periorbital or retroauricular ecchymoses. They can sometimes be associated with oto- or rhinorrhea and mandate the performance of a CT scan.

Meningeal lesions

Epi- or extradural haematomas usually occur following arterial laceration in the space between the inner and outer layers of the cranial

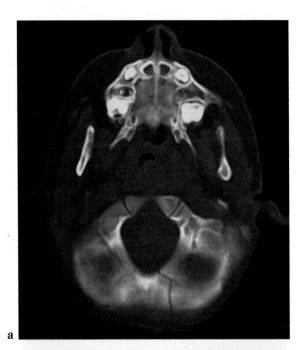

a

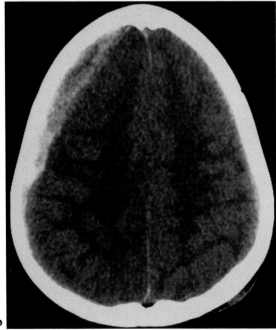

b

Fig.6.10 - Acute subdural haematoma. Unenhanced CT shows **a)** a left occipital skull fracture and **b)** an acute right frontal subdural haematoma.

dura mater. The haematoma can potentially extend to the margins of the dura mater, only being delimited by the cranial sutures. These haematomas appear as a sickle-shaped or biconvex/lens-shaped lesion in cross section on CT (Figs 6.8, 6.9). Approximately 75% of these haematomas are associated with overlying skull fractures. If there are no other cranial lesions, the patient may remain conscious and devoid of neurological deficits until the intracranial structures are significantly compromised (i.e., the clinically lucid interval); if the haematoma continues to enlarge, this early phase if followed by a rapid deterioration in consciousness and the onset of focal neurological symptoms. At this point, surgical drainage becomes imperative, and if performed swiftly typically results in a good outcome. In infants, the lucid interval may be longer and the clinical signs less rapidly progressive. This is due, at least in part, to the open state of the sutures in infancy which allows for a limited expansion of the cranial case in the presence of a growing haematoma. About half of infants do not lose consciousness. Another complication, anaemia and hypovolemic shock, may be observed in smaller babies.

Subdural haematomas are usually a consequence of the rupture of the bridging veins between the brain and the dura mater. On CT acute subdural haematomas appear as a crescent-shaped extraaxial hyperdense collection (Fig. 6.10). There may be associated lesions of the underlying cerebral parenchyma. In patients under one year of age, peripheral subdural haematomas, parenchymal haematomas and/or parafalcian haematomas are typical of the battered child syndrome. These findings are in turn frequently associated with extracranial soft tissue ecchymoses and cranial fractures which are often star-shaped or depressed. Other bony structures may also be fractured in battered children, especially the ribs and limbs (Fig. 6.11).

Shaking trauma is a common cause of intracranial traumatic lesions. When babies are grasped by the chest and shaken violently the head is subject to intense whiplash and rotation forces due in part to the relative weakness of

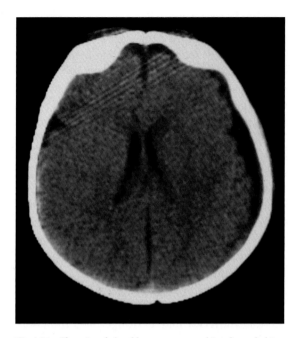

Fig.6.11 - Chronic subdural haematoma resulting from shaking injury in child. Unenhanced CT demonstrates a chronic left hemisphere subdural haematoma with a fluid-fluid level due to the sedimentation of the haemorrhagic content. Also note the signs of compression of the left lateral ventricle and shift of the midline cerebral structures.

the muscles of the neck and to the disproportionate size of the head as compared to the body at this age. This type of movement can cause the rupture of the bridging veins. Interhemispheric or convexity haematomas can evolve into the chronic stage. In such cases CT reveals low density blood collections, whereas MRI shows low signal on T1-weighted scans and high signal on T2-weighted sequences.

Neuroradiological investigations may reveal the simultaneous presence of acute and chronic haematomas, the consequences of repeated traumatic abuse. Subarachnoid haemorrhage and extradural haematomas are less frequently encountered, being more typically an expression of direct, nonshaking trauma. Physically abused children may also show a variety of parenchymal lesions, including: oedema, nonhaemorrhagic contusions, and intraparenchymal haematomas.

In subjects who have suffered severe rotational forces, there may be a sudden rapid compression of the cervical spinal cord with a consequent contusion with or without haemorrhage, typically observed first at the grey-white matter junction (10, 16, 24, 29).

Subarachnoid haemorrhage. In the more severe cranial injuries, there may be a widespread haemorrhage into the subarachnoid space, which exposes the patient to the risk of subsequent development hydrocephalus due to abnormalities in CSF reabsorption. CT reveals hyperdensity within the basal subarachnoid cisterns, the parietal subarachnoid spaces or the interhemispheric fissure.

Posttraumatic parenchymal lesions

On CT *oedema* appears as a focal hypodense lesion that is sometimes on the opposite side of that of the traumatic impact. Alternatively, widespread swelling associated with small ventricles and flattening of the cerebral sulci against the overlying inner table of the skull. Oedema can also typically be detected on the periphery of acute/subacute haemorrhagic lesions after the first few hours following the event.

The *malignant cerebral oedema syndrome* is encountered exclusively in children, with an average age at presentation of 6 years. The pathogenesis is not clear, however it is probably related in part to a loss of cerebrovascular autoregulation with resultant uncontrolled hyperaemia. CT shows collapsed cerebral ventricles and an obliteration of the cranial subarachnoid spaces. Frank oedema is more clearly visible in the peripheral regions of the cerebral hemispheres; it is usual to observe relative sparing of the basal ganglia, thalami and structures of the posterior cranial fossa.

Cerebral contusion. Parenchymal contusion is the manifestation of direct trauma to the brain tissue. Its macroscopic appearance derives from oedema, haemorrhage and necrosis. On CT, the appearance of brain contusion depends upon the components of the haemorrhage: in most cases haemorrhage appears as a heterogeneous hyper- hypodense, mixed signal lesion with indistinct margins. Multiple contusions are the sign of widespread cerebral damage. These extensive injuries are particularly well shown on MRI.

Diffuse axonal injury (DAI) is caused by acceleration-deceleration phenomena that affect different areas of the brain as the diffusion of the forces are applied on impact. The appearance of DAI on CT can vary from minor degrees having a reduction in the differentiation between white and grey matter, small cerebral ventricles and small quantities of intraventricular blood, to more severe situations with multiple brain contusions, diffuse brain swelling, disappearance of the basilar subarachnoid cisterns and involvement of the brainstem. The initial CT appearance may lead to an underestimation of the severity of the lesion, however the patient's clinical condition rapidly worsens. DAI may progress over the first 48-76 hours of the traumatic incident, making serial CT re-evaluations necessary. A system for classifying the severity of DAI has recently been proposed, based on the obliteration of the basal subarachnoid cisterns and on the degree of midline shift when present (Tab. 6.1) (28, 42).

MRI is presently assuming a more important role in the evaluation of paediatric patients with acute head injuries. The advantages of the technique include safety, multiplanar imaging capability, excellent anatomical definition, major blood vessel identification without using contrast agents and critical posterior fossa analysis absent of artefacts typically present on CT. The technique's main disadvantages are the relatively long acquisition times and the unsuitability of the method in critical patients requiring continuous extracorporeal monitoring and life support devices.

Therefore, with the exception of certain situations (e.g., very small extraaxial haematomas over the cranial convexity or the posterior cranial fossa, small contusions, DAI), the technique of choice in the acute phase of cranial trauma remains CT. MRI is of greater diagnostic utility in the subacute phase (e.g., subacute/chronic haematomas that may be isodense on CT, posttraumatic white matter lesions such as DAI) and in the evaluation of late sequelae (e.g., hydrocephalus, atrophy, monofocal/multifocal encephalomalacia) (46).

CNS INFECTIONS

CNS infections are a rather varied group of disorders. Acute *meningitis* is an inflammation of the meninges and the CSF spaces. *Encephalitis* is an inflammation of the cerebral parenchyma. Encephalitis may result as an extension of a meningitic process or as a *de novo* isolated event.

The associated clinical symptoms vary in part with age: in children the onset is abrupt, with fever, headache, vomiting, neck stiffness and gait abnormality that may or may not be associated with disorders of consciousness. In newborns and infants the clinical signs and symptoms are dominated by alterations of behaviour and the sleep-wake pattern, digestive disorders, hypotonia and tension/protrusion of the cranial fontanels.

Meningitis

In the absence of complications, neuroradiological investigations may not be useful in *viral meningitis* (4, 35, 40). If performed, CT and MRI may be entirely normal or may show evi-

DEGREE OF DIFFUSE LESION	CT APPEARANCE	DEATH RATE
I	Normal	9.6%
II	Cisterns present/Shift < 5mm	13.5%
III	Cisterns compressed/Shift < 5mm	34%
IV	Shift > 5mm	56.2%

Tab. 6.1.

dence of minor extraaxial fluid accumulation surrounding the cerebral hemispheres (2). In *bacterial meningitis* CT and MRI can be normal, show an increase in the density of the CSF or variable, diffuse enhancement of the meninges after IV contrast medium administration.

During the course of the illness, the persistence of fever and the appearance of seizures, focal neurological signs and/or signs of intracranial hypertension suggest the presence of complications and indicate the need for the execution of diagnostic imaging examinations. In young infants with purulent meningitis (esp. *Haemophilus influenzae*) it is possible to observe the formation of extraaxial subdural fluid collections that may be either uni- or bilateral. The pathophysiologic mechanism that leads to the formation of such collections has not been clarified. The fluid is serous-haematic, rich in polymorphonucleocytes, and is usually sterile. On CT, such collections show increased density as compared to the normal CSF and following IV contrast medium injection, enhancement of the overlying meninges is typically observed (Fig. 6.12). In most cases spontaneous resolution of the extraaxial collections occurs; more rarely, these collections become chronic, may progressively increase and can undergo fibrinous organization.

Approximately 90% of newborns with bacterial meningitis present with concomitant ventriculitis, an occurrence that is more rarely encountered in older children. On CT or MRI dilatation of the cerebral ventricles is observed, often associated with intense contrast enhancement of the ventricular ependyma. Cerebral parenchymal alterations can also be seen in cases of purulent meningitis. Typically these alterations are small superficial infarctions due to septic microemboli. On CT these infarcts appear as hypodense, oedematous areas near the grey-white matter junction. On occasion there may be enhancement after IV contrast medium administration. More widespread cerebral infarctions caused by septic thrombosis or spasm of the major cerebral arteries are rare.

Thromboses of the cranial venous sinuses, especially the sagittal sinus, are only rarely encountered. Early in the process, CT demonstrates hyperdensity of the venous sinus involved. Subsequently, the thrombus becomes isodense in relation to the cerebral parenchyma; at this point the IV administration of contrast media shows an absence of enhancement

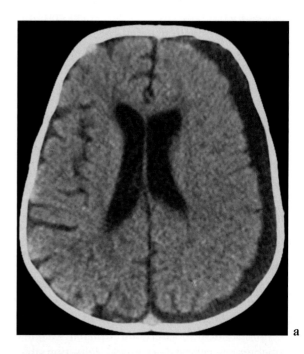

a

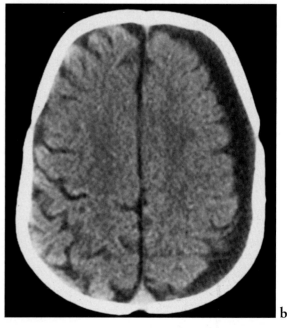

b

Fig. 6.12 - Subdural hygroma associated with haemophilus meningitis. CT shows a left hemispheric subdural hygroma with signs of mass effect upon the midline structures.

of the intraluminal thrombus (i.e., delta sign) and marked enhancement of the collateral dural venous draining structures. On MRI, thrombosis of a venous sinus appears as a hyperintense signal on T1-weighted scans associated with partial/complete loss of the normal flow void within the sinus itself.

A possible complication of bacterial meningitis and septic embolization is the formation of a *cerebral abscess*. A parenchymal abscess appears as a heterogeneous mass resulting in the displacement of adjacent structures. On CT following IV contrast medium administration there is typically peripheral enhancement in the form of a thin, regular thickness ring surrounding a hypodense round-oval center. In more advanced stages, the abscess may be multilocular, and adjacent secondary satellite abscesses may be identified. The abscesses are typically located at the grey-white matter junction.

On MRI, during the initial phases of abscess formation, the wall of the lesion appears hyperintense on both T1- and T2-weighted sequences, whereas the centre appears hypointense on T1- and hyperintense on T2-weighted images. In mature abscesses, the wall is isointense on T1-weighted scans and markedly hypointense in T2-eighted acquisitions; the necrotic central portion is slightly hypointense on T1-weighted and hyperintense on T2-weighted scans. The enhancement pattern after IV contrast medium injection is the same as that described for CT.

Tuberculous (TB) meningitis is today a relatively rarely encountered disease process in industrialized countries, although with the AIDS epidemic, the infection is once again on the rise in incidence. TB meningitis has a bimodal distribution, affecting young infants and the elderly. The involvement of the central nervous system results from haematogenous dissemination of the bacilli, usually from a site in the lung; TB meningitis in infants almost always coincides with primary pulmonary TB. The clinical presentation in this young age group often differs from that of classic bacterial meningitis (e.g., inconsistent fever, stiff neck, headache, non-specific prodromal signs, greater incidence of focal neurological deficit, involvement of the cranial nerves, disorders of consciousness including coma). The involvement of the meninges can be secondary to the rupture of a small tuberculoma of the adjacent cerebral cortex or spinal cord, or to direct haematogenous dissemination to the meninges. A gelatinous exudate fills the basal subarachnoid cisterns; vasculitis and thrombosis of the lenticulostriate and thalamoperforating arteries frequently result from this exudate and communicating hydrocephalus is common (i.e., 50-75% of cases).

The typical CT finding in TB meningitis is homogeneous hypodensity within the basal subarachnoid cisterns, with marked enhancement after IV contrast medium administration. MRI shows a hyperintensity of the basal cisterns on T1-weighted sequences. Septic emboli leading to the formation of tuberculomas localized at the grey-white matter junction may be isolated or multiple and supra- and/or infratentorial. On CT tuberculomas appear hypodense with indistinct margins with mass effect and intense enhancement after IV contrast medium injection.

The differential diagnosis in such cases includes other forms of granulomatous/neoplastic meningitis, such as cryptococcosis, coccidioidomycosis, sarcoidosis and diffuse carcinomatosis.

Encephalitis

Viral *encephalitis* (23, 34, 36, 44) caused by HSV1 (herpes virus 1) is one of the most common forms of cytotoxic encephalitis encountered in infancy and childhood. The clinical syndrome in infants is characterized by the presence of fever, seizures that are often unilateral, disorders of consciousness including coma and focal neurological signs. In newborns, patients may be asymptomatic, but the ultimate mortality is higher than in the older age groups. The diagnosis is based on CSF data (e.g., the presence of specific IgM antibodies, the demonstration of viral replication through PCR), EEG recordings (e.g., temporal, periodic, slow wave abnormalities) and medical imaging findings.

CT is the first diagnostic imaging examination performed in emergency situations in these cases. The initial findings may be negative, in

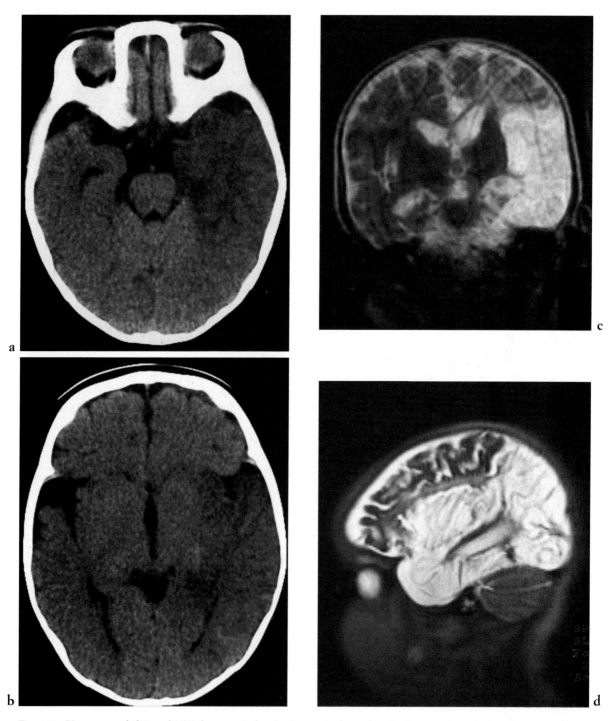

Fig. 6.13 - Herpes encephalitis. **a, b**) CT shows cortical and subcortical temporal-insular hypodensity with signs of associated cerebral swelling. Corresponding **c**) coronal T2-weighted and **d**) sagittal T2-weighted MRI in the subacute phase.

part due to the relatively poor resolution of the temporal fossae as a result of bone-related artefacts. A negative CT examination must not exclude immediate, specific antiviral treatment.

Some days later, CT may show hypo- hyperdensity of one or both temporal lobes, oedema/mass effect and sometimes contrast enhancement.

MRI is far more sensitive in detecting these parenchymal alterations, even within the first 24-48 hours from onset of the event. In the acute phase after contrast medium administration selective enhancement of the hippocampus may be observed, demonstrating the affinity of the virus for the hippocampal, parahippocampal and insular cortex. In the case of widespread infection, MRI may reveal lesions in the central/anterior temporal cortex, the insula and the grey matter nuclei of the cerebral hemispheres (Fig. 6.13). At a later stage, MRI shows atrophy in one or both of the two amygdaloid nuclei (70-80% of cases) associated with hippocampal atrophy. Overall, CT shows a sensitivity of 73% and a specificity of 89% during the first 5 days of the illness and 90% and 92% respectively from the 6th day onwards. However, there are many other pathological conditions that can simulate herpesvirus encephalitis including cerebritis, early abscess formation, TB meningoencephalitis, cryptococcosis and even some brain tumours.

In newborns, the most frequently encountered form of herpesvirus encephalitis is HSV type 2. This viral particle is transmitted to the infant during delivery via an infected birth canal. The risk of such infection is greater during delivery, whereas intrauterine infection is rare. The typical clinical manifestation is represented by a mucocutaneous vesicular eruption; without treatment, 75% of cases evolve into encephalitis. The disease usually presents during the second week of life. Common clinical signs and symptoms include poor appetite, lethargy, seizures, fever and signs of sepsis.

On CT and MRI the most frequent finding of herpes encephalomyelitis is focal oedema localized in most cases in the temporal lobes. However, these patients may also present with involvement of the frontal or parietal lobes or even the entirety of one or both hemispheres. In the later phases, widespread cortical atrophy with areas of porencephalic cyst formation is the most common finding; calcifications both in the cortex and the white matter are also frequently observed. There is cerebellar involvement in 50% of cases.

Acute Disseminated Encephalomyelitis

Acute disseminated encephalomyelitis (ADEM) is a demyelinating disorder associated with a previous viral infection or antiviral immunization that acts through an autoimmune mechanism (17, 31). Many viral infections can precede ADEM, including measles, mumps, chickenpox, influenza, viral hepatitis and also infections from *Campylobacter*, mycoplasm, and rarely streptococci.

The clinical onset is characterized by the sudden appearance of signs and symptoms involving scattered areas of the CNS associated to headache and dizziness and, more uncommonly, minor fever. MRI shows multifocal demyelinating lesions, sometimes of considerable size, which can pose problems of differential diagnosis with MS (Fig. 6.14). However, the clinical pattern is monophasic; there is a tendency towards slow resolution over time. Typically there are residual chronic areas of gliosis on imaging studies.

INTRACRANIAL HYPERTENSION

Normal intracranial pressure is the result of the pressures exerted by the cerebral parenchyma, blood vessels and CSF; on average, the cerebral tissue and the support structures occupy 70% of the intracranial volume, whereas the vascular component, CSF and interstitial water portion account for 10% each of the remainder. Intracranial hypertension in children is defined as a condition in which intracerebral pressure is higher than 15 torr in babies or more than 7 torr in newborns (1, 20, 39).

As in adults, regarding pathophysiology there are three different potential sources of intracranial hypertension: abnormalities of the cerebral parenchyma, the CSF compartment and the vascular tissue. The previous chapter should be consulted for parenchymal and vascular causes; attention will be paid here to the CSF compartment, and in particular, hydrocephalus.

The clinical characteristics with which intracranial hypertension presents are variable, depending on the compensating mechanisms and the age of the patient.

Compensated intracranial hypertension

The signs and symptoms of intracranial hypertension include headache, vomiting and visual problems as well as other less specific conditions such as tinnitus, dizziness, behavioural alterations, irritability, mood swings, and systemic vasomotor abnormalities that are manifested by paleness or intense flush.

The headache may present in a frontoorbital or occipital location, often has an intermittent character, and it tends to worsen with the evo-

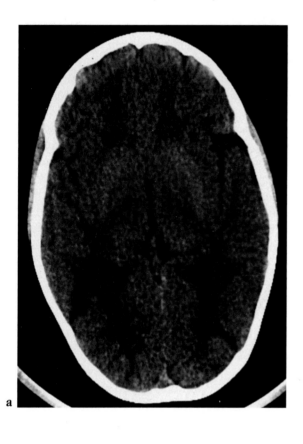

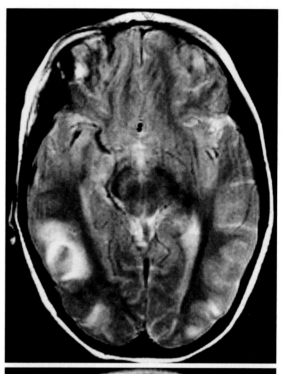

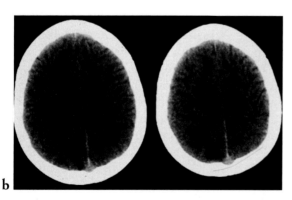

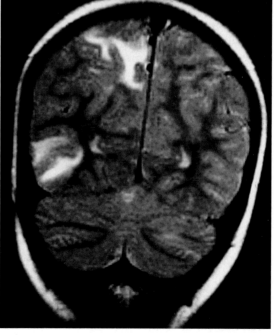

Fig. 6.14 - Acute disseminated encephalomyelitis (ADEM). **a, b)** CT demonstrates areas of hypodensity of the subcortical white matter. **c-e)** axial T2-weighted and **d)** coronal T2-weighted MRI reveals regions of signal alteration in the subcortical white matter with associated mass effect.

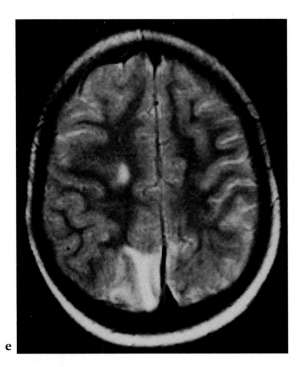

e

Fig. 6.14 (*cont.*).

lution of the illness. In cases where there is a mobile intraventricular mass lesion, the headache has a positional character whereby head movements can alter its intensity. These headaches are refractory to even the most powerful analgesics. The vomiting is sudden and "projectile" in character, and is not preceded by nausea; it is often the first sign of illness.

Visual involvement is represented by horizontal diplopia caused by a uni- or bilateral paralysis of the 4th cranial nerves; the 3rd cranial nerves are less frequently affected. On occasion there may be a frank reduction in vision, although this suggests an unfavourable course that can lead to ischaemia of the optic nerve and permanent loss of sight. Ophthalmoscopic examinations may detect papillary oedema when intracranial hypertension has been present for some days; whitish exudates along the course of the peripapillary vessels may be observed together with flame-shaped haemorrhages of a venous origin, both of which are negative prognostic factors relative to irreversible visual loss.

Patients with elevated intracranial pressure may present with anoxic-ischaemic attacks secondary to low cerebral perfusion pressure. These events have a limited duration and a complete remission; clinically an intense asthenia can be observed, together with problems of vigilance, changes in muscle tone and extremity tremors. If intracranial pressure is higher, internal herniation of the cerebral parenchyma may occur, which in turn can lead to serious clinical consequences. According to the anatomical site, these internal herniations include: lateral herniation of the cingulate gyrus beneath the free edge of the falx cerebri, lateral midline shifts, downward herniation of the structures of the medial temporal lobe through the tentorium cerebelli, downward herniation of the cerebellar tonsils through the foramen magnum, downward herniation of the diencephalon and the brainstem, and upward herniation of the posterior fossa contents through the tentorium cerebelli.

The clinical presentations can be subdivided into central, temporal or cerebellar involvement. In central involvement, the clinical signs include:
- diencephalic: disorders of consciousness, alteration of muscle tone, absence of photomotor reflex, myosis, Cheyne-Stokes respiration;
- mesencephalic: coma, decerebration, Cheyne-Stokes respiration or shallow hyperventilation, non-reactive pupils, altered ocular-vestibular reflex;
- pontine: rapid shallow breathing, non-reactive pupils in intermediate position, absence of oculovestibular reflex;
- medullary: slowed breathing alternating with phases of apnoea and gasping, dilated non-reactive pupils.

In temporal involvement, the clinical signs include:
- ipsilateral/bilateral pupil dilation caused by the compression of the 3rd cranial nerve(s);
- contralateral hemiplegia or hemiparesis due to the compression of the cerebral peduncles;
- cortical blindness due to haemorrhagic infarction of the mid-inferior portion of the occipital lobe secondary to the compression

of the ipsilateral posterior cerebral artery against the free edge of the tentorium cerebelli;
– bradycardia, disorders of consciousness, decerebrate posturing and hyperventilation in response to nociceptive stimuli secondary to compression of the brainstem.

In cerebellar involvement, the clinical signs include:
– opistotonus;
– nystagmus.

The clinical picture will vary yet more if the intracranial hypertension occurs before closure of the cranial sutures. Tab. 6.2 shows the clinical difference between an acute increase of the intracranial pressure in children over and under the age of two.

Clinical presentation in children under two years of age

Intracranial hypertension presents physically with a rapid increase in the skull circumference; repeated measurements are particularly important as the rapidity of growth provides an estimate of the degree of severity.

Clinically, macrocephalia (defined as skull circumference >98° percentile or >2 standard deviation than average for that age) is manifested by symmetric enlargement of the cranium. The anterior fontanel is tense or even outward-ly bulging and pulsating. The cranial sutures are widened and palpable, the scalp appears thin and the superficial veins are dilated.

Ocular examination may show a "setting sun" phenomenon, characterised by a conjoined deviation of the glance downwards so that the iris is covered by the lower eyelid, whereas the sclera is exposed at the top; nystagmus, proptosis and a reduction in the pupillary reflex to light complete the clinical picture.

Clinical presentation in children over two years of age

Intracranial hypertension that arises later in childhood presents with signs and symptoms that include: headache on awaking that improves when in an erect position, vomiting, papilloedema, strabismus, cerebellar signs and motor spasticity. Moreover, the chronic compression of the hypothalamic-pituitary axis caused by the dilatation of the inferior recesses of the 3rd ventricle can cause endocrine abnormalities.

Hydrocephalus

Making a diagnosis of the precipitating cause of hydrocephalus (1, 22, 39) is important as the prognosis is in part connected to the mechanism that caused the ventricular dilatation. Estimates in paediatric cases indicate that

Specific signs	Common signs	Specific signs
Child under 2		Child over 2
Papilloedema Macrocrania Tense fontanelle	Mental alterations Strabismus Signs of cerebral herniation «Setting sun» sign	Headache
Suture diastasis	Alteration of vital parameters	Papilloedema

Tab. 6.2.

38% of cases are caused by congenital cerebral malformations, 20% by neoplasia or other space-occupying lesions, 15% by haemorrhages, 7% by meningitis and the remainder by undetermined conditions.

From the standpoint of pathogenesis, there are two types of hydrocephalus: that due to an excessive production of CSF and that due to an obstruction of flow or insufficient absorption of CSF (Fig. 6.15).

Congenital cerebral malformations

Congenital hydrocephalus may result from a variety of cerebral malformations:
- Dandy-Walker malformation: enlargement of the 4th ventricle accompanied by partial or complete agenesis of the cerebellar vermis; in many cases hydrocephalus is not present at birth but develops during the first year of life;
- Neural tube closure defects;
- Cerebral aqueduct stenosis;
- Arnold-Chiari malformations: especially type II, in which in addition to the cerebral malformation myelomenigocele is also present;
- Malformation of the vein of Galen: compression of the aqueduct of Silvius resulting from aneurysmal dilation of the vein of Galen;
- Premature craniosynostosis.

Neoplasia and space-occupying lesions

The manner in which a space-occupying lesion within the cranium produces signs and symptoms is partially linked to the position of the mass and its rapidity of growth.

Neoplasia is a relatively common cause of hydrocephalus in infancy. The location of brain tumours during childhood is somewhat age-dependent: in the first six months of life neoplasia has a preferential supratentorial localization; between the 7th and 12th months tumours have a balanced incidence of supra-subtentorial localization; and after the first year of life, neoplasia is typically localised in the posterior fossa.

The most common primary neoplasia in this young age group includes medulloblastomas, ependymomas and those tumours recently defined as "scarcely differentiated embryonic tumours". Papillomas of the choroid plexuses, although only representing 2-5% of intracranial tumours in childhood, often result in hydrocephalus due to an excessive production of CSF. Typically they are located in the lateral ventricles and less frequently in the 3rd and 4th ventricles.

Haemorrhages

Haemorrhage can cause hydrocephalus for various reasons. In the acute phase blood clots may cause an intraventricular obstruction; in the chronic phase obstruction may be the result of meningeal adhesions or granular ependymitis. Spontaneous haemorrhages arise most frequently in preterm newborns.

Infectious processes

Acute or chronic meningeal infections may precipitate hydrocephalus if adhesions and subarachnoid pathway stenosis arise. The types of meningitis most frequently responsible for hydrocephalus include toxoplasmosis, cystercercosis and tubercular meningitis.

Neuroimaging techniques (e.g., ultrasound, CT and MR) are fundamental in determining the presence and aetiology of hydrocephalus. In complex abnormalities, the site of the obstruction can be documented using a CT utilizing intrathecal contrast medium, administered via lumbar puncture. A uterine diagnosis of hydrocephalus using prenatal ultrasound has potential therapeutic implications.

Dilated ventricles under normal pressure can be associated with passive cerebral atrophy (i.e., *ex vacuo* ventricular dilatation), cerebral malformations (e.g. developmental cerebral white matter hypoplasia such as lissencephaly

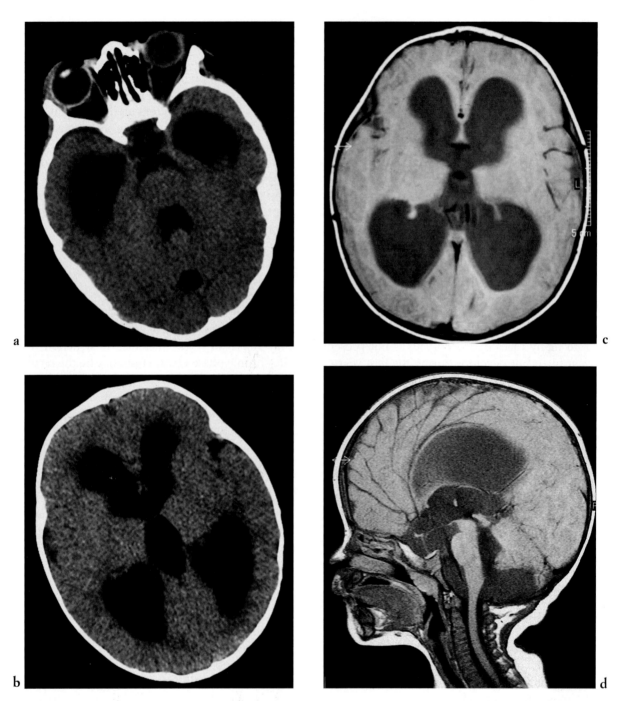

Fig. 6.15 - Communicating hydrocephalus. **a** and **b**) CT shows marked dilatation of the entire cerebral ventricular system. **c**) axial PD-weighted MRI again demonstrates the marked ventricular dilatation. **d**) Sagittal T1-weighted, and **d**, **e**) sagittal T2-weighted MRI reveals the patency of the aqueduct of Sylvius, ventricular dilatation, thinning and upward expansion of the corpus callosum, and expansion of an "empty" the sella turcica. In the posterior fossa, note the enlargement of the extraventricular cranial subarachnoid spaces and a prominent cisterna magna.

and culpocephaly) and arrested, non-progressive hydrocephalus. The radiological characteristics that suggest a high pressure hydro-cephalus include compressed superficial sulci and periventricular oedema (i.e., transependymal CSF absorbtion/penetration).

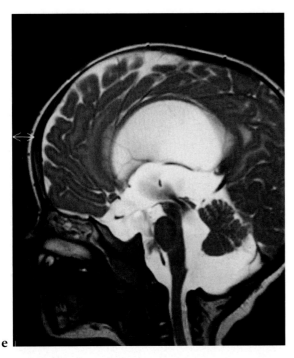

Fig. 6.15 (*cont.*)

Cerebral neoplasia in childhood

Generally speaking, intracranial neoplasia (7, 8, 13, 19, 22, 38, 41) in childhood represents the most frequent group of neoplasia after leukaemia. The diagnosis of neoplasia is confirmed by neuroimaging techniques. The clinical signs and symptoms vary with age, the child's neuropsychiatric condition and tumour location. The most common clinical manifestations are those that can be attributed to intracranial hypertension, although focal signs may be present and suggest the site of the primary lesion.

In most cases, MRI with or without IV contrast agent administration or CT after IV contrast medium injection can of course provide excellent definition of space-occupying lesions of the brain. MRI in particular is able to reveal lesions that are situated in regions that may be difficult to visualize using CT (e.g., posterior fossa, spinal canal). T1-weighted images provide an excellent definition of the anatomy and T2-weighted acquisitions clearly identify both the tumour and the surrounding oedema when present. Long image acquisition times and the

need for sedation represent limiting factors of MRI in smaller children.

Other diagnostic techniques tend to be less valuable: angiography provides information regarding the vascularization of the tumour and excludes the possibility of a vascular malformation; MRA replaces this examination in many cases of gross hypervascularization.

Analytical details concerning the various forms of cranial neoplasia are provided in other chapters; we will therefore presently discuss the neuroradiological characteristics of the tumours most frequently encountered in the paediatric population.

Medulloblastoma

This is the most frequent type of neoplasm encountered in the posterior fossa during infancy. Up to 40% of medulloblastomas are diagnosed in children five years of age or under. The main signs and symptoms include nausea, vomiting, headache, ataxia and macrocephaly. On CT, medulloblastomas are typically well-defined mass lesions originating from the cerebellar vermis with or without extension into the cerebellar hemispheres. On unenhanced CT, these tumours are hyperdense lesions surrounded by a perilesional hypodense oedema. Contrast enhancement of the neoplasm may be homogeneous or irregular. In up to 20% of cases, medulloblastomas contain cystic or necrotic areas and more rarely calcifications. In a high percentage of patients the compression or invasion of the 4th ventricle results in obstructive hydrocephalus. On MRI the mass is typically hypointense on T1-weighted images and slightly hyperintense on T2-weighted sequences in relation to the normal cerebellar parenchyma. Considerable enhancement of the tumour is usually observed after IV gadolinium injection (Fig. 6.16).

Cerebellar Astrocytomas

Astrocytomas can originate in any point of the cerebellum and spread to the cerebellar

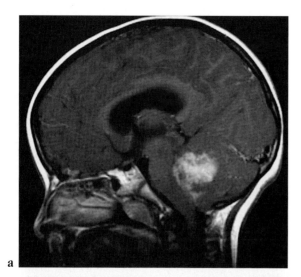

a

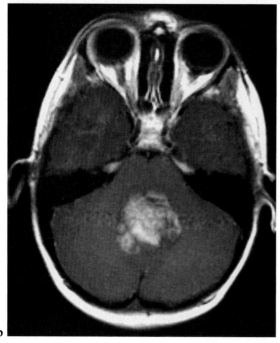

b

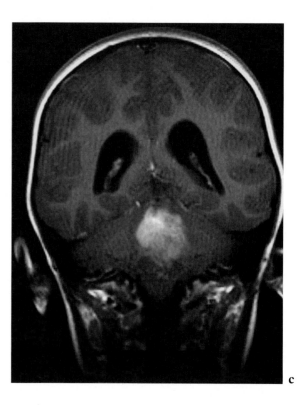

c

Fig.6.16 - Obstructive hydrocephalus associated with posterior fossa medulloblastoma. **a**) sagittal, **b**) axial and **c**) coronal T1-weighted MRI following IV gadolinium administration reveals inhomogeneous enhancement of a midline posterior fossa mass associated with poorly defined borders and with signs of compression of the 4th ventricle and brainstem. Note the early obstructive hydrocephalus.

hemispheres in 30% of cases. They are generally quite large, of a primarily cystic nature (e.g., pilocytic astrocytomas), but can also be solid with or without an intrinsic necrotic area.

On CT or MRI cerebellar astrocytomas in this age group typically present as a voluminous mass with a vermian or hemispheric location. They are frequently cystic and slightly hypodense on unenhanced imaging studies. After IV contrast medium administration, there is enhancement in up to 50% of cases. On MRI the solid components are typically hypointense on T1-weighted images and hyperintense on T2-weighted acquisitions. The signal characteristics of the cystic components depend on the content of the cavity. Uncomplicated, simple cysts yield an MR signal similar to that of CSF; intracystic necrotic material on the other hand produces a signal on T1-weighted images that is slightly hyperintense in comparison to CSF, which becomes yet more hyperintense on T2-weighted sequences.

Papillomas of the choroid plexus

These tumours represent 5% of supratentorial tumours and less that 1% of intracranial neoplasia in infants. This type of neoplasia originates from the epithelium of the choroid plexus and has papillary and/or carcinomatous characteristics. Signs and symptoms can be sec-

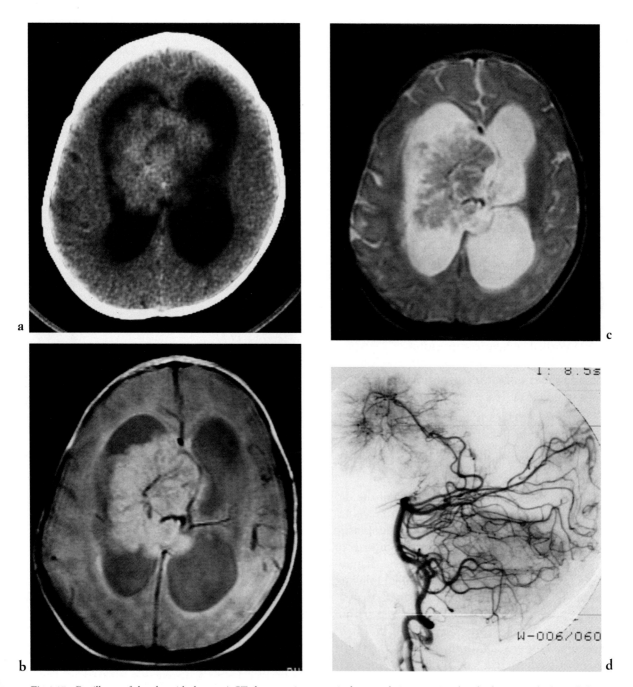

Fig.6.17 - Papilloma of the choroid plexus. **a**) CT shows an intraventricular mass lesion associated with obstructive hydrocephalus. **b**) PD-weighted and **c**) T2-weighted MRI shows an intraventricular mass lesion with inhomogeneous signal on long TR sequences, in part possibly due to intratumoural macroscopic neoplastic vasculature. Also noted is obstructive hydrocephalus and signs of transependymal resorption of CSF. **d**) digital angiogram confirms the neovascularisation of the intraventricular neoplasm.

ondary to hydrocephalus as well as local cerebral infiltration.

On CT choroid plexus papillomas appear as intraventricular masses with irregular boundaries and are generally isodense in rela-tion to the cerebral parenchyma; they are on occasion hyperdense and may show peritu-moural oedema. After IV contrast medium administration, one may observe a somewhat homogeneous enhancement of the lesion. Often, the papillomatous forms are associated with severe hydrocephalus. On MRI, these tumours appear homogeneous or non-homogeneous in intensity; the mass can be better visualized on T1-weighted scans; on both contrast enhanced studies and T2-weighted imaging the tumour and the CSF appear hyperintense and are therefore poorly differentiated (Fig. 6.17).

Pseudotumour cerebri (benign intracranial hypertension)

Pseudotumour cerebri (14) is a condition of intracranial hypertension whose salient clinical signs and symptoms are represented by headache, papilloedema, diplopia and progressive visual loss. The CSF reveals a high protein but a normal cellular composition.

Pseudotumour cerebri can be precipitated by a number of factors including obesity, various medicines (e.g., antibiotics, vitamin A and indometacin), and endocrinopathy, although most frequently it remains a pathological condition of unknown aetiology that is most commonly encountered in infants and adult female.

Neuroimaging techniques represent the definitive diagnostic method of patient evaluation by enabling the exclusion of neoplastic causes and cases resulting from thrombosis of the cranial dural venous sinuses. The diagnosis is made by showing normal cranial imaging findings; an ancillary imaging sign is distension of the optic subarachnoid space within the sheaths of the optic nerves, and in 1/3 of cases, an empty sella. In most cases, the treatment is medical (e.g., diuretics, steroids, and CSF drainage); patients usually recover, however permanent visual loss or even blindness may ensue in untreated cases.

REFERENCES

1. Aicardi J: Diseases of the Nervous System in Childhood. Mac Keith Press, London, 1992.
2. Archer BD: Computed Tomography before lumbar puncture in acute meningitis: a review of the risks and benefits. Can Med Ass, 148:961-965, 1996.
3. Bowerman RA, Donn SM, Di Pietro MA et al: Periventricular leukomalacia in the pretem newborn infant: sonographic and clinical features. Radiology 151:382-388, 1984.
4. Bruneel F, Wolff M: Méningites aigues. Encycl Méd Chir. Elsevier SAS, Paris. Neurologie 17-160-C-10, 2000.
5. Carson SC, Hertzberg Bs, Bowie JD et al: Value of sonography in the diagnosis of intracranial hemorrhage and periventricular leukomalacia: a postmortem study of 35 cases. AJNR 11:677-683, 1990.
6. Chabbert V, Ranjeva JP, Sevely A: Diffusion and magnetisation transfer-weighted MRI in childhood moya-moya. Neuroradiology 40(4):267-71, 1998.
7. Chanalet S, Chatel M, Grellier P et al.: Symptomatologique clinique et diagnostic radiologique des tumeurs intracraniennes. Editions Techiniques. Encycl. Méd. Chir. (Paris, France). Neurologie 17-210-A60-10, 1994.
8. Conway PD: Oechler HW, Kun LE et al.: Importance of histologic condition and treatment of pediatric cerebellar astrocytoma. Cancer 67:2772, 1991.
9. Crowe W: Aspects of Neuroradiology of head injury. Neurusurg Clin North Am 2:321, 1991.
10. Dias Ms, Backstrom J, Falk M, Li V: Serial radiography in the infant shaken impact syndrome. Pediatr Neurosurg 29 (2):77-85, 1998.
11. Flodmark O, Lupton B et al.: MR imaging of periventricular leukomalcia in childhood. AJNR 10:111-1118, 1989.
12. Ganesan V, Savv YL, Chong WK et al: Conventional cerebral angiography in children with ischemic stroke. Pediatr Neurol 20(1):38-42, 1999.
13. Garcia DM, Latifi AR, Simpson JR et al: Astocytomas of the cerebellum in children. J Neurosurg 71: 661-664, 1995.
14. Giusifelli V, Wall M, Siegel PZ: Symptoms and disease association in idiopathic intracra nial hypertension (pseudotumor cerebri) a case-control study. Neurology 41: 239-2444, 1991.
15. Golden GS: Cerebrovascular Diseases. In: Swaiman KF. Pediatric Neurology. Mosby eds. St. Louis, 1994.
16. Hadley MN, Sonntag VK, Rekate HC et al: The infant whiplash-shake injury syndrome: a clinical and pathological study. Neurosurgery 141: 536-540, 1989.
17. Hall MC, Barton LL, Johnson ML: Acute disseminated encephalomyelitis-like syndrome folllowing group A Beta hemolytic streptococcal infection. J Child Neurol 13, 7:354-355, 1998.
18. Harris BH: Management of multiple trauma. Pediatric Clin North-America 32:175, 1985.
19. Horowitz ME, Mulhern RK, Kun LE et al.: Brain tumors in the very young child. Cancer 61:428, 1988.
20. Irthum B, Lemaire JJ: Hypertension Intracranienne. Encycl. Méd. Chir. (Elsevier, Paris), Neurologie, 17-035-N-10, 8p, 1999.
21. Jan M, Aesch B: Traumatismes cranio-encéphaliques. Editions Techiniques-Encycl. Med. Chirurg Paris. Neurologie, 15785 A10, 15 p, 1991.
22. Jelink J, Smorniotopulos Db, Parisis JE: Lateral Ventricular Neoplasms of the Brain: differential Diagnosis Based on clinical CT and MR Findings. AJR 11:567-574, 1990.
23. Jonsson RT: Acute encephalitis. Clin Infect Dis 23:219-226, 1996.
24. Kalifa G, Cohen PA: The radiologic report in battered child syndrome. J Radiol 80(6):563, 1999.

25. Kimura M, Hasegawa Y, Yasuda K: Magnetic resonance imaging with fluid attenuated inversion recovery pulse sequences in MELAS syndrome Pediatr Radiol 27 (2):153-154, 1997.

26. Lanska MJ: Presentation, clinical course, and outcome of childhood stroke. Pediatr Neurol 7:333, 1991.

27. Lasjaunias P, Der Brugge K, Lopez-Ibor et al.: The role of dural anomalies in vein of Galen aneurysms: report of six cases and review of the literature. AJNR 8:185-192, 1988.

28. Marshall LF, Bowers-Marshall S, Klauber MR et al.: A new classification of head injury based on computerized tomography. J Neurosurgery 75 (Suppl):S14-20, 1991.

29. Merten DF, Osborne DR., Radkowski MA et al: Craniocerebral trauma in the child abuse syndrome: radiological observations. Pediatr Radiol 14:272-277, 1984.

30. Murgio A, Andrade FA, Sanchez Munoz MA: International Multicenter Study of Head Injury in Children. ISHIP Group. Childs Nerv Syst Jul 15 (6-7):318-21, 1999.

31. Pender MP: Acute disseminated encephalomyeilitis. In: Pender MP Mc Combe PM (eds): Autoimmune Neurological Diseases. Cambridge, Cambridge University Press pp. 155-165, 1995.

32. Roach ES, Riela AR: Pediatric cerebrovascular disorders. Futura Publishing Company Mount Kisco eds New York.

33. Rosman NP: Acute brain injury. In: Swaiman KF Mosby st Louis eds Pediatric Neurology: principles and practice.

34. Schmidbauer M, Podreka L, Wiimberger D et al.: SPECT and MR imaging in herpes simplex encephalitis. J Comput Assist Tomogr 15:811-815, 1991.

35. Schoemann J, Hewlett R: MR of childhood tubercolous meningitis. Neuroradiology 30:473-477, 1988.

36. Schroth G, Gawehn J, Thron A et al.: Early diagnosis of herpes simplex encephalitis by MRI. Neurology 37:179-183, 1987.

37. Seidnwurm D, Berenstein A et al.: Vein of Galen malformation: correlation of clinical presentation, arteriography and MR imaging. AJNR 12:347-354, 1991.

38. Starshak RJ, Wells RG, Sty JR et al: Testa collo e rachide. Diagnostica per immagini nel bambino. Momento medico, Salerno, 1996.

39. Swaiman K: Pediatric Neurology. Principles and practice. Mosby editor, St. Louis, 1994.

40. Syrogianopulos GA, Nelson JD. et al.: Subdural collection of fluid in acute bacterial meningitis in young children: a review of 136 cases. Pediatr Infect Dis 5:343-352, 1986.

41. Tores CF, Rebsamen S, Silber JH et al.: Survellaince scanning of children with medulloblastoma. N Engl J Med 330:892, 1994.

42. Toutant S, Klauber MR, Marshall L et al.: Absent or compressed basal cysterns of the first CT scan: ominous predictors of outcome in severe head injury. J Neurosurg 61: 691-694, 1984.

43. Volanne L, Ketonen L., Majander A et al.: Neuradiologic findings in children with mithocondrial disorders AJNR 19 (2):369-377, 1998.

44. Whitley RJ, Cobbs GC, Alford CA et al.: Diseases that mimic herpes simplex encephalitis. Diagnosis, presentation and outcome. JAMA 262:234-39, 1989.

45. Wilihowski E, Pouwels PJ, Frahm J: Quantitative proton magnetic resonance spectroscopy of cerebral metabolic disturbances in patients with MELAS. Neuropediatrics 30 (5):256-63, 1999.

46. Wison JT, Wiedman KD, Hadley DM et al: Early and late magnetic resonance imaging and neuropsycological outcome after head injury. J Neurol. Neurosurg Psychiatry 51: 391-6, 1988.

SUBJECT INDEX